Rapid Review
Laboratory Testing in
Clinical Medicine

Rapid Review Series

Series Editor
Edward F. Goljan, MD

Behavioral Science, Second Edition
Vivian M. Stevens, PhD; Susan K. Redwood, PhD; Jackie L. Neel, DO;
Richard H. Bost, PhD; Nancy W. Van Winkle, PhD; Michael H. Pollak, PhD

Biochemistry, Second Edition
John W. Pelley, PhD; Edward F. Goljan, MD

Gross and Developmental Anatomy, Second Edition
N. Anthony Moore, PhD; William A. Roy, PhD, PT

Histology and Cell Biology, Second Edition
E. Robert Burns, PhD; M. Donald Cave, PhD

Laboratory Testing in Clinical Medicine
Edward F. Goljan, MD; Karlis I. Sloka, DO

Microbiology and Immunology, Second Edition
Ken S. Rosenthal, PhD; James S. Tan, MD

Neuroscience
James A. Weyhenmeyer, PhD; Eve A. Gallman, PhD

Pathology, Second Edition
Edward F. Goljan, MD

Pharmacology, Second Edition
Thomas L. Pazdernik, PhD; Laszlo Kerecsen MD

Physiology
Thomas A. Brown, MD

USMLE Step 2
Michael W. Lawlor, MD

USMLE Step 3
David D. K. Rolston, MD; Craig Nielsen, MD

Rapid Review Laboratory Testing in Clinical Medicine

Edward F. Goljan, MD
Professor
Department of Pathology
Oklahoma State University Center for Health Sciences
College of Osteopathic Medicine
Tulsa, Oklahoma

Karlis I. Sloka, DO
Associate Professor and Chair
Department of Pathology
Oklahoma State University Center for Health Sciences
College of Osteopathic Medicine
Tulsa, Oklahoma

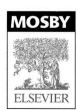

MOSBY

ELSEVIER

1600 John F. Kennedy Blvd.
Ste 1800
Philadelphia, PA 19103-2899

Library of Congress Cataloging-in-Publication Data

Goljan, Edward F.
  Rapid review laboratory testing in clinical medicine / Edward F.
Goljan, Karlis I. Sloka.
      p. ; cm.
  Includes bibliographical references and index.
  ISBN 978-0-323-03646-7
  1. Diagnosis, Laboratory–Outlines, syllabi, etc. I. Sloka, Karlis I. II. Title. III. Title: Laboratory testing in clinical medicine.
  [DNLM: 1. Laboratory Techniques and Procedures. 2. Clinical Medicine–methods. 3. Diagnostic Techniques and Procedures. QY 25 G626r 2007]
  RB37.G636 2008
  616.07′5—dc22

2007007544

Publishing Director: Linda Belfus
Acquisitions Editor: James Merritt
Developmental Editor: Katie DeFrancesco
Design Direction: Steven Stave

Printed in China

Last digit is the print number: 9   8   7   6   5   4   3   2   1

Working together to grow
libraries in developing countries

www.elsevier.com | www.bookaid.org | www.sabre.org

ELSEVIER   BOOK AID International   Sabre Foundation

To my Dad, who continues to be a source of inspiration for me to be all that I can be. And also to P.K., who is another welcome grandchild for me (Popie) to help make my life complete.

EFG

To my wife Vania, without whose help and inspiration this book would not have been possible.

KIS

Series Preface

The *Rapid Review Series* has received high critical acclaim from students studying for the United States Medical Licensing Examination (USMLE) Step 1 and high ratings in *First Aid for the USMLE Step 1*. We have created a learning system, including a print and electronic package, that is easier to use and more concise than other review products on the market.

SPECIAL FEATURES

Book

- **Outline format:** Concise, high-yield subject matter in a study-friendly format.
- **High-yield margin notes:** Key content that is most likely to appear on the exam is reinforced in the margin notes.
- **High-quality visual elements:** Abundant two-color schematics, full color images, and summary tables also enhance your study experience.
- **Practice questions:** USMLE Step 1–type multiple-choice questions appear at the end of each chapter; complete discussions (rationales) for all options are included.

New! Online Study and Testing Tool

- **Over 200 USMLE Step 1–type questions:** Multiple-choice and matching questions that mimic the current board format are presented. Complete rationales for all answer options are included. All the questions from the book are included so you can study them in the most effective mode for you!
- **Test mode:** Select from randomized 50-question blocks or by subject topics for an exam-like review session. This mode features a 60-minute timer to simulate the actual exam, a detailed assessment report that can be printed or saved to your hard drive, and direct links to all or only incorrect questions. The links include your answer, the correct answer, and full rationales for all answer options, so you can fully analyze your test session and learn from your mistakes.
- **Study mode:** Like the test mode, in the study mode you can select from randomized 50-question blocks or by subject topics to create a dynamic study session. This mode features unlimited attempts at each question, instant feedback (either on selection of the correct answer or using the "Show Answer" feature), complete rationales for all answer options, and a detailed progress report that can be printed or saved to your hard drive.
- **Online access:** This feature allows you to study from an Internet-enabled computer where and when it is convenient. This access can be activated through registration on www.studentconsult.com using the pincode printed inside the front cover.

Student Consult

- **Full online access:** You can access the complete text and illustrations of this book on www.studentconsult.com.
- **Save content to your PDA:** Through our unique Pocket Consult platform, you can clip selected text and illustrations and save them to your PDA for study on the fly!
- **Free content:** An interactive community center with a wealth of additional valuable resources is available.

Preface

It has been our observation that there are no concise review books covering the application and interpretation of commonly used laboratory tests in clinical medicine. Most of the existing texts provide long lists of diseases associated with a particular laboratory test result without explaining the mechanism for the abnormal test result in a particular disease. Furthermore, very few texts have discussions of laboratory tests along with high-quality photographs, figures, tables, and questions with discussions at the end of every chapter.

We feel that this book would be useful as a primary text in a laboratory medicine course; useful in performing well on USMLE and COMLEX exams parts 1, 2, and 3, residency exams, and specialty boards; and, most of all, useful in the day-to-day interpretation of laboratory test results in patients.

Special thanks to Katie DeFrancesco and Jim Merritt at Elsevier, who helped us through every stage of writing this book.

Edward F. Goljan, MD
Karlis I. Sloka, DO

Contents

CHAPTER 1

Laboratory Test Interpretation

I. Purpose of Laboratory Tests

A. Screen for disease

1. Mass screening
   - Example—phenylketonuria in newborns
2. Screening people without symptoms of a disease
   - Example—lipid profile
3. Screening people with symptoms of a disease
   - Example—serum antinuclear antibody test to rule autoimmune disease

B. Confirm disease

- Example—anti-Smith antibody to confirm systemic lupus erythematosus

C. Monitor disease status

- Example—serum glucose in a diabetic patient

D. Therapeutic drug monitoring

- Example—partial thromboplastin time in a patient taking heparin

II. Sensitivity and Specificity

A. Test results for people with a selected disease

1. True positive (TP)
   - Number of diseased people with a positive test result
2. False negative (FN)
   - Number of diseased people with a negative test result

B. Test results for nondiseased people

1. True negative (TN)
   - Number of nondiseased people with a negative test result
2. False positive (FP)
   - Number of nondiseased people with a positive test result

C. Sensitivity

1. Definition
   - Likelihood of having positive test results in people who have a selected disease
2. Formula for calculating sensitivity
   a. $TP/(TP + FN)$
   b. FN rate determines the test's sensitivity.

$Sensitivity = TP/(TP + FN)$; "positivity" in disease

3. Test with 100% sensitivity (no FNs)
   a. Normal test result excludes disease (must be a TN).
   b. Positive test result includes all people with disease.
      (1) Positive test result does *not* confirm disease.
      (2) Test result could be a TP or FP.
   c. Test is used most often as a screening test.

D. **Specificity**
   1. Definition
      • Likelihood of having negative test results in nondiseased people

Specificity = TN/
(TN + FP); "negativity" in
health

   2. Formula for calculating specificity
      a. TN/(TN + FP)
      b. FP rate determines the test's specificity.
   3. Tests with 100% specificity (no FPs)
      a. Positive test result confirms disease (must be a TP).
      b. Negative test result does *not* exclude disease.
         • Test result could be a TN or FN.

III. **Predictive Value**
   A. **Predictive value of a negative test result (PV−)**
      1. Likelihood that a negative test result excludes disease
      2. Formula for calculating PV−

Sensitivity 100% → PV−
100% → excludes
disease

         a. TN/(TN + FN)
         b. PV− best reflects the FN rate of a test.
      3. Tests with 100% sensitivity (no FNs) always have a PV− of 100%.
   B. **Predictive value of a positive test result (PV+)**
      1. Likelihood that a positive test result confirms disease
      2. Formula for calculating PV+

Specificity 100% → PV+
100% → confirms
disease

         a. TP/(TP + FP)
         b. PV+ best reflects the FP rate of a test.
      3. Tests with 100% specificity (no FPs) always have a PV+ of 100%.
   C. **Effect of prevalence on PV− and PV+**
      1. Definition of prevalence
         a. Total number of people with disease in the population under study
         b. Population includes disease and nondiseased people.
      2. Formula to calculate prevalence
         • (TP + FN)/(TP + FN + TN + FP)
      3. Low prevalence of disease (e.g., ambulatory population)
         a. PV− increases
            • More TNs than FNs
         b. PV+ decreases
            • More FPs than TPs
      4. High prevalence of disease (e.g., cardiac clinic)
         a. PV− decreases
            • More FNs than TNs
         b. PV+ increases
            • More TPs than FPs
   D. **Calculation of sensitivity, specificity, PV−, PV+, prevalence** (Fig. 1-1)

	Patients with SLE	Control group	Total
Positive test result	TP 100	FP 20	120
Negative test result	FN 0	TN 80	80
Total	100	100	200

Sensitivity = TP/TP + FN = 100/100 + 0 = 100%

Specificity = TN/TN + FP = 80/80 + 20 = 80%

PV– = TN/TN + FN = 80/80 + 0 = 100%

PV+ = TP/TP + FP = 100/100 + 20 = ~83%

Prevalence = TP + FN/TP + FN + TN + FP = 100/200 = 50%

1-1: *Serum antinuclear antibody (ANA) test results in patients with systemic lupus erythematosus (SLE) and a control population. In this study, the serum ANA has a sensitivity of 100% and a negative predictive value (PV–) of 100%, indicating that it is most useful as a screening test for SLE when the serum ANA is negative. Specificity is decreased (80%), because other autoimmune diseases also have a positive serum ANA (e.g., rheumatoid arthritis), which increases the false positive (FP) rate and decreases the positive predictive value (PV+ ~83%). Other tests that have high specificity for diagnosing SLE (e.g., anti-Smith antibody, specificity 100%, PV+ 100%) help to confirm the diagnosis of SLE. FN, false negative; TN, true negative; TP, true positive.*

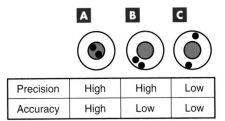

Precision	High	High	Low
Accuracy	High	Low	Low

1-2: *Precision and accuracy of a test. Using a target as an example, the bull's-eye is the true value of the test. Test A has both accuracy and precision. Test B has precision but is not accurate. Test C has neither precision nor accuracy.*

IV. **Precision and Accuracy**

A. **Precision**

1. Repetitive measurements on the same sample (Fig. 1-2)

a. High precision if the same test results are obtained

• Does *not* mean that the test is accurate (true value)

b. Low precision if different test results are obtained

2. Test result deviations usually have a random distribution

a. Standard deviation (SD) of a test

• Variation from the average mean value of a test performed in a normal population

b. Normal random (gaussian) distribution curve

(1) One SD encompasses 68% of the normal population.

SD reflects the precision of a test

        (2) Two SD encompasses 95% of the normal population.

        (3) Three SD encompasses 99.7% of the normal population.

    c. Tests with high precision have a low SD.

       • Example—serum electrolytes

    d. Tests with low precision have a high SD

       • Example—serum enzymes

B. **Accuracy**

  1. True value of the test (see Fig. 1-2)

  2. Evaluating accuracy of a test result

    • Laboratory measurement of control samples with known assay values

V. **Normal Range**

A. **Establishing normal range (reference interval)**

  1. Established by adding and subtracting 2 SD from the mean of the test

    a. Adding 2 SD to the mean establishes the upper cutoff point.

    b. Subtracting 2 SD from the mean establishes the lower cutoff point.

    c. Example

      • 2 SD = 10 mg/dL, mean = 100 mg/dL, normal range = 90–110 mg/dL

> Normal range: ±2 SD from the mean

  2. Out of normal range test results (outliers) occur in ~5% of normal people.

    a. Using ±2 SD, normal range encompasses 95% of normal population.

    b. Remaining 5% of the normal population are outliers.

  3. Likelihood of an outlier increases as the number of tests ordered increases.

    a. Likelihood of an outlier

      • $100 - (0.95^n \times 100)$, where n is the number of tests ordered

    b. Example—likelihood of an outlier if six tests are ordered:

$$100 - (0.95^6 \times 100) = {\sim}27\%$$

B. **Creating highly sensitive and specific tests**

  1. Ideal test (Fig. 1-3A)

    a. 100% sensitivity (PV− 100%)

    b. 100% specificity (PV+ 100%)

      • Note in the schematic that there are no FNs or FPs.

    c. Most normal ranges do *not* distinguish the normal from the disease population (see Fig. 1-3B and C)

      • Overlap between the normal and the disease population

  2. Establishing a test with 100% sensitivity and PV− (see Fig. 1-3B)

    a. Set the upper cutoff point at the beginning of the disease curve (A).

      (1) Creates a test with 100% sensitivity and 100% PV−

      (2) Excellent test to screen for disease

> ↑ Sensitivity: upper cutoff point at beginning of disease curve

    b. Increasing sensitivity always decreases specificity and PV+.

      • Due to a greater number of FPs

  3. Establishing a test with 100% specificity and PV+ (see Fig. 1-3C)

    a. Set the upper cutoff point at the end of the normal curve (B).

      (1) Creates a test with 100% specificity and 100% PV+

      (2) Excellent test for confirming disease

> ↑ Specificity: upper cutoff point at end of normal curve

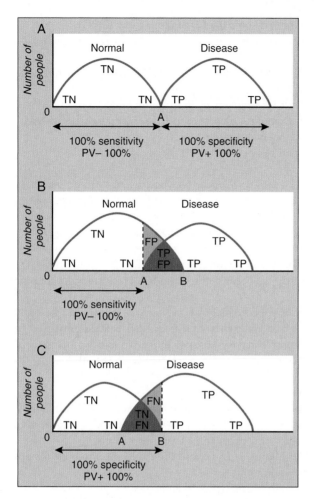

1-3: *Establishing tests with 100% sensitivity and specificity. Schematic A shows an ideal test with 100% sensitivity (100% PV–) and 100% specificity (100% PV+) when the normal range is 0 to A. Test results below the A cutoff point are all true negatives (TN), while those beyond the A cutoff point are all true positives (TP). Schematic B shows a test with 100% sensitivity (100% PV–) when the upper cutoff point is at A. Note that as sensitivity increases, the specificity and PV+ decrease owing to an increase in false positives (FP). Schematic C shows a test with 100% specificity (100% PV+) when the upper cutoff point is at B. Note that as specificity increases, the sensitivity and PV– decrease owing to an increase in false negatives (FN). PV–, predictive value of a negative test result, PV+, predictive value of a positive test result. (Adapted from Goljan EF: Pathology Review [Saunders Text and Review Series]. Philadelphia, WB Saunders, 1998, Fig. 1-2.)*

    b. Increasing specificity always decreases sensitivity and PV–.
       • Due to a greater number of FNs

VI. Variables Affecting Laboratory Test Results
  A. **Newborns**
    1. Increased hemoglobin (Hb) concentration compared to children and adults
      a. Due to increased concentration of HbF

b. HbF left-shifts the O_2-binding curve (OBC).
  (1) Less release of O_2 to tissue increases release of erythropoietin (EPO).
  (2) EPO stimulates an increase in RBC production and Hb synthesis.
2. Lack immunoglobulin (Ig) M
  a. Lack IgM isohemagglutinins in blood.
    • Example—blood group A newborns lack anti-B-IgM isohemagglutinin.
  b. Synthesis of IgM begins shortly after birth.

> *Clinical correlation:* Newborns who have an increase in cord blood IgM may have an underlying congenital infection (e.g., cytomegalovirus). Their blood should be screened for antibodies against the common congenital infections.

3. IgG antibodies are of maternal origin.
  • Newborns begin synthesizing IgG 2 to 3 months after birth.

Newborns synthesize IgM and IgG after birth

> *Clinical correlation:* A mother with a positive test for human immunodeficiency virus (e.g., IgG antibodies against gp120) transplacentally transfers IgG antibodies to the fetus. This does *not* mean that the child is infected by the virus.

B. **Children**
  1. Higher serum alkaline phosphatase (ALP) levels than adults
    • Due to increased bone growth and release of ALP from osteoblasts
  2. Higher serum phosphorus levels than adults
    • Phosphorus is required to drive calcium into bone for normal mineralization.
  3. Lower Hb concentration than adults
    a. Increased phosphorus increases synthesis of 2,3-bis**phospho**glycerate (BPG)
    b. Increased 2,3-BPG right-shifts the OBC, causing greater release of O_2 to tissue.

Children: ↑ serum ALP, phosphorus; ↓ Hb

C. **Adults**
  1. Serum iron, ferritin, and Hb levels are lower in women than in men.
    a. Women have menses.
    b. Women have less testosterone than men.
      • Testosterone stimulates erythropoiesis.
  2. Elderly
    a. Decreased glomerular filtration rate (GFR) and creatinine clearance (CCr)
      • Danger of drug toxicities if standard doses of drugs are used
    b. Increased serum ALP
      (1) Osteoarthritis (degenerative arthritis) invariably occurs in the elderly.
      (2) Articular cartilage wears down in weight-bearing joints.

Elderly: ↓ GFR, CCr; danger of drug toxicity

    (3) Reactive bone formation occurs at the joint margins (called osteophytes).
        • Reactive bone formation increases ALP.
  c. Males have a normal decrease in Hb concentration.
    (1) Hb is in the range of a normal adult woman.
    (2) Decrease in Hb parallels decrease in testosterone.
  d. May lose their blood group isohemagglutinins

> *Clinical correlation:* Elderly individuals may lose the isohemagglutinins associated with their blood group. For example, a blood group A individual may not have anti-B IgM antibodies or blood group B individuals may not have anti-A IgM antibodies. This explains why some elderly individuals transfused with the wrong unit of blood do not develop a hemolytic transfusion reaction. For example, a blood group A individual inadvertently transfused group B blood may not hemolyze the group B RBCs because they do not have anti-B IgM antibodies.

D. **Pregnancy**
  1. Greater increase in plasma volume (PV) than RBC mass
    a. RBC mass = total number of RBCs in mL/kg.
    b. Increased PV decreases Hb concentration.
      • Dilutional effect
    c. Increased PV increases GFR and CCr.
    d. Increased PV increases renal clearance of blood urea nitrogen, creatinine, and uric acid.
      • Causes a slight decrease in their serum concentration

Pregnancy: ↑ plasma volume; ↑ GFR, CCr

  2. Increased serum ALP
    • ALP is of placental origin.
  3. Increased serum human placental lactogen
    a. Inhibits the sensitivity of peripheral tissue to insulin
      • Produces the normal glucose intolerance in pregnancy
    b. Increased β-oxidation of fatty acids
      (1) Excess acetyl CoA is produced.
      (2) Increased liver synthesis of ketone bodies from acetyl CoA
        • Ketone bodies—acetone, acetoacetic acid, β-hydroxybutyric acid
  4. Mild respiratory alkalosis
    a. Estrogen/progesterone stimulate the respiratory center.
    b. Increased pulmonary clearance of CO_2
      (1) Decreased Pco_2 produces respiratory alkalosis.
      (2) Decreased Pco_2 causes corresponding increase in Po_2.
        • Arterial Po_2 is usually >100 mm Hg in pregnancy.
  5. Increased serum thyroxine (T_4) and cortisol
    a. Estrogen increases liver synthesis of their binding proteins.
      • Increased thyroid-binding globulin and transcortin
    b. Free hormone levels (metabolically active) are normal.
      (1) Serum thyroid-stimulating hormone (TSH) is normal.
      (2) Serum adrenocorticotropic hormone (ACTH) is normal.

E. **Hemolyzed blood specimen**
  1. Falsely increases serum potassium
     - Potassium is the major intracellular cation.
  2. Falsely increases lactate dehydrogenase (LDH)
     - LDH is present in RBCs.
  3. Must repeat the test using a different sample

F. **Effect of fasting on serum lipids**
  1. Does *not* significantly alter serum cholesterol (CH)
     a. Diet-derived CH is packaged in chylomicrons in the small intestine.
     b. CH accounts for <3% of the total lipid fraction in chylomicrons.
  2. Does *not* significantly alter high-density lipoprotein (HDL)-CH levels
  3. Significantly alters serum triglyceride (TG) levels
     a. Diet-derived TG is packaged in chylomicrons.
     b. TG accounts for 85% of the total lipid fraction in chylomicrons.
     c. Must be fasting to eliminate diet-derived TG.

G. **Drug/chemical effects on liver microsomal mixed function oxidase system**
  1. Located in the smooth endoplasmic reticulum (SER)
     a. Important in normal drug metabolism
     b. Key enzymes
        (1) NADPH-cytochrome P-450 reductase
        (2) Cytochrome P-450, which acts as a terminal oxidase
  2. Drug "induction" of the system
     a. Increased synthesis of the enzymes
        (1) Increased drug metabolism
        (2) May produce suboptimal drug levels
     b. Examples of inducing drugs and chemicals
        - Alcohol, barbiturates, phenytoin, polycyclic hydrocarbons (cigarette smoke)
     c. Increased synthesis of γ–glutamyltransferase (GGT)
        (1) GGT is normally located in the SER.
        (2) Excellent enzyme marker of induction
  3. Drug inhibition of the system
     a. Danger of drug toxicity
     b. Examples of inhibiting drugs
        - Imidazole drugs (cimetidine, ketoconazole), macrolides (erythromycin)

H. **Laboratory test alterations in ethanol abuse** (Fig. 1-4)
  1. Increased production of NADH in ethanol (alcohol) metabolism (step 1)
     a. Causes two-way reactions involving NADH to move in the direction of NADH
        (1) Pyruvate→ lactate
           (a) Produces lactic acidosis (step 2)
           (b) Produces fasting hypoglycemia (step 3)
              - Pyruvate is unavailable for gluconeogenesis.
        (2) Dihydroxyacetone phosphate (DHAP)→ glycerol 3-phosphate (G3-P)
           (a) Causes increased liver synthesis of TG (step 4)

Hemolyzed specimen:
↑ serum K⁺, LDH

Drug induction oxidase system: alcohol, phenytoin, barbiturates

Drug inhibition oxidase system: imidazole drugs, macrolides

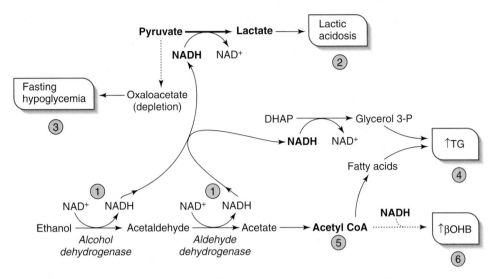

1-4: *Effect of ethanol on laboratory tests. See text for discussion. DHAP, dihydroxyacetone phosphate; β-OHB, β-hydroxybutyric acid; TG, triglyceride. (Adapted from Pelley JW, Goljan EF: Rapid Review Biochemistry, 2nd ed. St. Louis, Mosby, 2007, Fig. 9-6.)*

- G3-P is the substrate used by the liver to synthesize TG.
  - (b) Causes hypertriglyceridemia
    - Liver-synthesized TG is packaged in very low density lipoprotein.
2. Increased production of acetyl CoA in ethanol metabolism (step 5)
   a. Acetyl CoA is used to synthesize fatty acids and ketoacids.
   b. Fatty acids are used in TG synthesis (hypertriglyceridemia).
   c. Primary ketoacid produced is β-hydroxybutyric acid (β-OHB) (step 6).
      (1) Increased NADH causes acetoacetic acid to convert to β-OHB.
      (2) β-OHB is *not* detected in serum or urine with standard reagents.
3. Increased lactic acid and β-OHB interfere with renal excretion of uric acid.
   - Hyperuricemia may precipitate acute gouty arthritis.
4. Increased lactic acid and β-OHB produce an increased anion gap metabolic acidosis (Chapter 2).
5. Increased serum aspartate aminotransferase (AST)
   a. Ethanol damages mitochondria in the liver.
   b. AST is located in the mitochondria.
      - Alanine aminotransferase (ALT) is located in the cytosol.
   c. In ethanol abuse, AST is higher than ALT.
6. Increased serum GGT (see above)
7. Ethanol inhibits jejunal reabsorption of folate.
   - Produces folate deficiency with a macrocytic anemia (Chapter 5)
8. Ethanol damages mitochondria in RBC normoblasts in the bone marrow.
   a. Heme synthesis partly occurs in the mitochondria.
   b. Inhibition of heme synthesis cause sideroblastic anemia (Chapter 5).

Alcohol: ↑ lactate, β-OHB, TG, AST, GGT; ↓ glucose

I. **Laboratory test alterations in smokers**

1. Respiratory acidosis
   a. Retention of CO_2 occurs in smokers with chronic bronchitis.
   b. Respiratory acidosis produces hypoxemia (decreased arterial Po_2).
      (1) Increased alveolar Pco_2 causes a corresponding decrease in alveolar Po_2.
      (2) Decreased alveolar Po_2 causes a decrease in arterial Po_2.
   c. Decreased O_2 saturation (Sao_2)
      (1) Sao_2 is the percentage of heme groups in Hb occupied by O_2.
      (2) Decreased arterial Po_2 always causes a decrease in Sao_2.
         • Decreased Sao_2 produces cyanosis.
2. Increased carbon monoxide (CO) levels
   • CO is present in cigarette smoke.
3. Secondary polycythemia (increased RBC count)
   • Decreased arterial Po_2 and increased CO stimulate EPO release.
4. Absolute neutrophilic leukocytosis (Chapter 6)
   a. Metabolites in cigarette smoke decrease activation of adhesion molecules in neutrophils.
      (1) Adhesion molecules are required for neutrophils to adhere to endothelium.
      (2) Normally, 50% of the peripheral blood neutrophils adhere to endothelium.
         • Called the marginating pool
   b. In smokers, the marginating neutrophil pool becomes part of the circulating pool.
      • Causes an absolute increase in the neutrophil count

Smoking: ↓ arterial Po_2 causes ↑ RBC count, ↓ Sao_2

Questions

Each numbered item is followed by options arranged in alphabetical or logical order. Select the best answer to each question. Some options may be partially correct, but there is only *one best* answer.

1. A test for coronary artery disease is positive in 180 of 200 people with known coronary artery disease and negative in 140 of 200 people who do not have disease. If the test result returns positive, what is the likelihood that coronary artery disease is present?
   A. 50%
   B. 70%
   C. 75%
   D. 90%

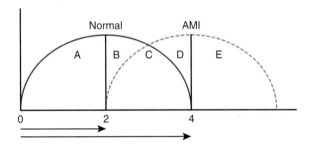

1-5: *Refer to question 2.*

2. The schematic in Figure 1-5 shows a normal control population (solid line) and a population of people with a 24-hour-old acute myocardial infarction (AMI; dotted line) who were evaluated with a new serum test to detect myocardial injury. Two normal ranges for the same test are noted, with the first extending from 0 to 2 and the second from 0 to 4. The areas under the two curves are subdivided into different populations of people, which are represented by the letters A through E. Depending upon the normal range selected, some of these areas contain people whose test results are true negatives (TN), false negatives (FN), true positives (TP), or false positives (FP). Which of the following correctly describes the test results in the lettered patient subpopulations for the two different normal ranges?

	Normal Range 0–2	**Normal Range 0–4**
A. Area A	TN	FN
B. Area B	FP	TN
C. Area C	TN + FN	TP + FP

D. Area D	FP		TP
E. Area E	FN		FN

3. A 65-year-old man with a history of coronary artery disease complains of severe substernal chest pain for the past 24 hours. He states that the pain also radiates down the left arm. A blood sample is drawn for electrolytes and serum creatine kinase (CK) isoenzyme MB. Owing to technical difficulties in collecting the blood, the sample is visibly hemolyzed. The serum potassium and CK isoenzyme MB are both increased. An electrocardiogram (ECG) shows a Q wave in the anterior leads; however, there are no T wave abnormalities present. Which of the following correctly describes the test results?

	Serum Potassium	**Serum CK-MB**
A.	False negative	True positive
B.	False positive	False positive
C.	False positive	True positive
D.	True positive	False positive
E.	True positive	True positive

4. A 55-year-old alcoholic, who also has chronic bronchitis secondary to cigarette smoking, is taking theophylline to improve breathing. His wife states that he is taking the medicine as prescribed and has not missed taking a single dose. A therapeutic drug level of serum theophylline is reported to be in a suboptimal range. Which of the following best explains this test result?
A. Decreased gastrointestinal reabsorption of the drug
B. Decreased renal excretion of the drug
C. Increased liver metabolism of the drug
D. Patient noncompliance

5. Study the data in Table 1-1 on a test performed on 100 patients who are known to have disease X and a control group containing 100 people who do not have disease X. Which of the following conclusions can be drawn from this study?

TABLE 1-1

	Disease X	Control Group
Positive test	100	20
Negative test	0	80

A. A negative test result excludes disease X.
B. A positive test result confirms disease X.
C. It is a poor screening test for disease X.
D. The predictive value of a positive test result is 100%.
E. The prevalence of disease is 60%.

6. Study the data in Table 1-2 on a test performed on 100 patients who are known to have disease Y and a control group containing 100 people who do not have disease Y. Which of the following conclusions can be drawn from this study?

TABLE 1-2

	Disease Y	Control Group
Positive test	70	0
Negative test	30	100

A. A negative test result excludes disease Y.
B. A positive test result confirms disease Y.
C. It is a poor test for confirming disease Y.
D. The predictive value of a negative test result is 100%.
E. The prevalence of disease is 60%.

7. A test is performed on 5 normal people who have the following test results: 48 mg/dL, 52 mg/dL, 50 mg/dL, 49 mg/dL, and 51 mg/dL. The standard deviation of the test is 4 mg/dL. What is the reference interval (normal range) for the test?
A. 40–60 mg/dL
B. 42–52 mg/dL
C. 42–58 mg/dL
D. 46–54 mg/dL

8. A medical student accidentally sticks his finger after drawing blood on a woman who is having elective surgery for removal of a benign breast mass. As part of the normal routine in handling accidental needle sticks, a baseline liver profile is ordered. The profile consists of a total bilirubin, serum aspartate aminotransferase (AST), serum alanine aminotransferase (ALT), serum alkaline phosphatase, and serum γ-glutamyltransferase. What is the approximate percent chance of one of these five tests having a value outside the normal reference interval for the test?
A. 10%
B. 13%
C. 23%
D. 35%
E. 47%

9. The upper limit of normal of the fasting blood glucose for diagnosing diabetes mellitus has been lowered from 140 mg/dL to 126 mg/dL. What effect does this change have on diagnosing diabetes mellitus?
A. Decreases the number of false positive diagnoses of diabetes
B. Decreases the sensitivity and increases the specificity of the test
C. Increases the number of false negative test results
D. Increases the predictive value of a negative test result
E. Increases the predictive value of a positive test result

10. In which one of the following clinical scenarios does the patient most likely have a false positive laboratory test result?
A. A 7-year-old child with a healing Colles' fracture has an increased serum alkaline phosphatase that is beyond the age-adjusted normal range.

B. A 35-year-old man has an increased serum cholesterol over previous baseline levels ~6 hours after eating bacon and eggs for breakfast.

C. A 45-year-old man who is an alcoholic has an increased anion gap metabolic acidosis. The physician suspects lactic acidosis and ketoacidosis. Lactic acid levels are increased; however, the serum and urine test for ketone bodies is negative.

D. A 70-year-old man with a normal serum blood urea nitrogen and creatinine level has a creatinine clearance of 65 mL/minute.

E. A 20-year-old woman with systemic lupus erythematosus, who is not sexually active, has a positive rapid plasma reagin (RPR) test. The physician orders a fluorescent treponemal antibody absorption (FTA-ABS) test, which returns negative.

11. A 22-year-old woman is in her third trimester of pregnancy. Physical examination, including examination of the thyroid gland, is normal. Laboratory studies show an increase in serum thyroxine and a normal serum thyroid-stimulating hormone (TSH). Which of the following best explains the increase in serum thyroxine?

A. Increase in the free thyroxine concentration

B. Increase in the synthesis of thyroid-binding globulin

C. Laboratory error in reporting the test

D. The patient is taking excess thyroid hormone

12. Which of the following groups of laboratory findings is commonly observed in smokers with chronic bronchitis?

A. Decreased arterial P_{CO_2}

B. Increased arterial pH

C. Increased serum aspartate aminotransferase (AST)

D. Increased serum erythropoietin

E. Normal oxygen saturation

13. A 25-year-old woman is in her third trimester. Which of the following laboratory test alterations is a normal finding in pregnancy?

A. Decreased arterial pH

B. Decreased creatinine clearance

C. Decreased plasma hemoglobin

D. Decreased serum cortisol

E. Increased serum blood urea nitrogen

14. A 45-year-old man with chronic bronchitis is taking theophylline for bronchodilation. He is also taking cimetidine for peptic ulcer disease to control gastric acidity. His drug level for theophylline is in the toxic range. Assuming that the patient is taking the appropriate dose of theophylline, what is the most likely cause for the toxic levels of the drug?

A. Decreased liver metabolism of the drug

B. Decreased liver uptake of the drug

C. Increased gastrointestinal uptake of the drug

D. Increased renal excretion of the drug

Answers

1. **C** (75%) is correct. In this question, a test is performed on people with known coronary artery disease (disease group) and on people who do not have coronary artery disease (control group). People with disease either have a true positive (TP) or a false negative (FN) test result. A TP test result is a positive test in a person with disease. A FN test result is a negative test result in a person with disease. People in a control group, who do not have disease, either have a true negative (TN) or a false positive (FP) test result. A TN test result is a negative test in a person without disease, while a FP test result is a positive test result in a person without disease. The question is asking what is the predictive value (or likelihood) that a positive test result (PV+) is a TP and not a FP. The formula for PV+ is TP/(TP + FP). In this question, the PV+ is 180/(180 + 60) = 180/240 = 75%. In other words, there is a 75% chance that the person has a TP test result and a 25% chance that it is a FP test result.

TABLE 1-3

	Coronary Artery Disease	Control Group	Total
Positive test	True positive 180	False positive 60	240
Negative test	False negative 20	True negative 140	160
Total	200	200	400

A (50%) is incorrect. The prevalence of coronary artery disease is 50%. Prevalence refers to the number of people with a disease in the population under study, which includes all the people with coronary artery disease and all the people in the control group. The formula for prevalence is (TP + FN)/(TP + FN + TN + FP). The prevalence of coronary artery disease is (180 + 20)/(180 + 20 + 140 + 60) = 200/400 = 50%.

B (70%) is incorrect. The specificity of the test is 70%. The specificity of a test refers to the likelihood of having negative test results in people without disease. People without disease have either TN or FP test results; thus, the formula for calculating the specificity of a test is TN/(TN + FP). The specificity of the test in this question is 140/(140 + 60) = 70%.

D (90%) is incorrect. The sensitivity of the test is 90%. The sensitivity of a test refers to the likelihood of having positive test results in people with disease. People with disease have either TP or FN test results, and the formula for calculating the sensitivity of a test is TP/(TP + FN). The sensitivity of the test is 180/(180 + 20) = 90%.

2. **B** (area B) is correct. Using the schematic A in Figure 1-6, note that the cutoff point for the normal range 0–2 is set at the beginning of the disease curve (dotted line). This creates a test with 100% sensitivity. The sensitivity of a test is established by performing the test on people with disease. People with disease have either a true positive (TP) or a false negative (FN) test result; therefore, the formula for the sensitivity of a test is TP/(TP + FN). Note in schematic A that there are no FN test results in the interval between 0 and 2; therefore, the test has a sensitivity of 100%. Using schematic B, the cutoff point for the normal range 0–4 is set at the end of the normal curve (solid line). This creates a test with 100% specificity. The specificity of a test is established by performing the test on people without disease (control group, solid line). People without disease have either a true negative (TN) or a false positive (FP) test result. Note in schematic B that there are no FP test results beyond the cutoff point 4. Area B has normal people without disease. Using the normal range of 0–2 (schematic A), these people are correctly classified as having FP test results (beyond the cutoff point 2). Using the normal range of 0–4 (schematic B), these people are correctly classified as having TN test results.

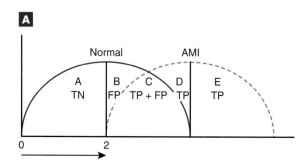
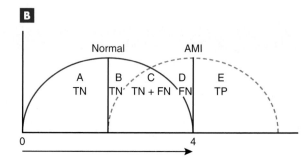

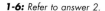
1-6: *Refer to answer 2.*

A (area A) is incorrect. Area A contains normal people without disease. Using the normal range of 0–2 (schematic A), these people have TN test results. However, using the normal range of 0–4 (schematic B), these individuals have TN test results, not FN test results.

C (area C) is incorrect. Area C is an overlap area that has people who are normal and people who have an acute myocardial infarction (AMI). Using the normal range of 0–2 (schematic A), these people have TP and FP test results (not TN and FN test results). Using the normal range of 0–4 (schematic B), these people have TN and FN test results (not TP and FP test results).

D (area D) is incorrect. Area D contains people with an AMI. Using the normal range of 0–2 (schematic A), these people have TP test results (not FP test results). Using the normal range of 0–4 (schematic B), these people have FN test results (not TP test results).

   E (area E) is incorrect. Area E contains people with an AMI. Using the normal range of 0–2 (schematic A) or the normal range of 0–4 (schematic B), these people have TP test results (not FN test results).

3. **C** (false positive, true positive) is correct. A true positive (TP) test result is a positive test result in a person with disease; a false positive (FP) test result is a positive test result in a person without disease. The patient has chest pain for 12 hours with radiation of the pain down the arm and into the jaw and a Q wave in an ECG. These changes are consistent with an acute myocardial infarction (AMI). A hemolyzed blood sample falsely increases the serum potassium (pseudohyperkalemia), because potassium is the major intracellular cation. Further confirmation that it is a FP test result is that the ECG does *not* show peaked T waves, which is a sign of pathologic hyperkalemia. The CK-MB is a true positive test result, because it begins increasing ~6 to 8 hours after an AMI and peaks in 24 hours. It is *not* falsely increased by hemolysis.

   A (false negative, true positive) is incorrect. A false negative (FN) test result is a negative test result in a person with disease. The serum potassium is a FP test result (not a false negative) and the serum CK-MB is correctly classified as a TP test result.

   B (false positive, false positive) is incorrect. The serum potassium is correctly classified as a FP test result; however, the serum CK-MB is a TP test result (not a false positive).

   D (true positive, false positive) is incorrect. The serum potassium is a FP test result (not a true positive), and the serum CK-MB is a TP test result (not a FP).

   E (true positive, true positive) is incorrect. The serum potassium is a FP test result (not a TP), and the serum CK-MB is correctly classified as a TP test result.

4. **C** (increased liver metabolism of the drug) is correct. Alcohol induces the liver microsomal mixed function oxidase system, which is located in the smooth endoplasmic reticulum (SER). This enzyme system is responsible for drug and chemical metabolism. Drugs such as alcohol and chemicals such as polycyclic aromatic hydrocarbons in cigarette smoke "induce" this system by enhancing the rate of synthesis of NADPH-cytochrome P-450 reductase and cytochrome P-450 oxidase, which are the two key enzymes in the system. The increase in enzyme activity increases the metabolism of drugs, in this case, theophylline, leading to a suboptimal concentration of the drug.

   A (decreased gastrointestinal reabsorption of the drug) is incorrect. Although decreased drug reabsorption in the gastrointestinal tract is a potential cause of a suboptimal theophylline level, the most likely cause in this patient with a drinking and smoking history is increased metabolism of the drug in the liver.

B (decreased renal excretion of the drug) is incorrect. Decreased excretion in the kidneys would more likely produce drug toxicity rather than suboptimal levels of the drug.

D (patient noncompliance) is incorrect. Although patient noncompliance is the most common cause of a lack of an appropriate therapeutic response to a drug, the statement by the wife that the patient is taking the medicine as prescribed is sufficient to rule out noncompliance as a possibility.

5. **A** (a negative test result excludes disease X) is correct. People with disease either have a true positive (TP) or a false negative (FN) test result. A TP test result is a positive test in a person with disease, while a FN test result is a negative test result in a person with disease. People in a control group, who do not have disease, either have a true negative (TN) or a false positive (FP) test result. A TN test result is a negative test in a person without disease, while a FP test result is a positive test in a person without disease. The sensitivity of a test is the likelihood of having positive test results in patients who have a selected disease. People with disease have either TP or FN test results, so the formula for calculating the sensitivity of a test is TP/(TP + FN). The less the FN rate, the greater the sensitivity of the test. The sensitivity of the test for disease X is 100/(100 + 0) = 100%. Tests with 100% sensitivity are most often used as screening tests for disease. If the test result is negative, the likelihood (predictive value of a negative test result, PV−) of a TN rather than a FN is 100%, because a test with 100% sensitivity has no FNs. Because tests with 100% sensitivity always have a PV− (TN/TN + FN) of 100%, a negative test result excludes disease. A positive test result includes *all* people with disease but does *not* confirm disease, because the test may be a FP in a person without disease. Other tests are often necessary to distinguish a TP from a FP test result.

TABLE 1-4

	Disease X	Control Group
Positive test	100 TP	20 FP
Negative test	0 FN	80 TN

B (a positive test result confirms disease X) is incorrect. The predictive value of a positive test result (PV+) is the likelihood that a positive test is a TP rather than a FP. The formula for PV+ is TP/(TP + FP). In order for a test to have a positive predictive value (PV+) of 100%, the test must have no FPs. A test with no FPs has 100% specificity. Specificity of a test is the likelihood of having negative test results in people without disease. Because people without disease have test results that are either a TN or a FP, the formula for calculating the specificity is TN/(TN + FP). Tests with 100% specificity always have a PV+ of 100%; therefore, they are most useful for confirming disease. The specificity of this test is 80/(80 + 20) = 80%, and the PV+ is

100/(100 + 20) = ~83%. There is an 83% chance that the test result is a TP and a 17% chance that it is a FP.

C (it is a poor screening test for disease X) is incorrect. Because the test has a sensitivity of 100% and a PV− of 100%, the test is an excellent screening test. A negative test result (PV−) excludes disease, but a positive test result includes all people with disease, but does *not* confirm the presence of disease.

D (the predictive value of a positive test result is 100%) is incorrect. The predictive value of a positive test result (PV+) is ~83%.

E (the prevalence of disease is 60%) is incorrect. Prevalence is the total number of people with disease in the population under study, which includes all the people with coronary artery disease and all the people in the control group. The formula is (TP + FN)/(TP + FN + TN + FP). The prevalence of disease in this study is (100 + 0)/(100 + 0 + 80 + 20) = 100/200 = 50% (not 60%).

6. **B** (a positive test result confirms disease Y) is correct. People with disease either have a true positive (TP) or a false negative (FN) test result. A TP test result is a positive test result in a person with disease, and a FN test result is a negative test result in a person with disease. People in a control group, who do not have disease, either have a true negative (TN) or a false positive (FP) test result. A TN test result is a negative test in a person without disease, and a FP test result is a positive test in a person without disease. Specificity of a test refers to the likelihood of having negative test results in people without disease. Because people without disease have test results that are either TN or FP, the formula for calculating the specificity of a test is TN/(TN + FP). A test with no FPs has 100% specificity. The predictive value of a positive test result (PV+) is the likelihood that a positive test result is a TP rather than a FP; therefore, the formula for calculating the PV+ is TP/(TP + FP). Tests with 100% specificity always have a PV+ of 100%; therefore, they are most useful for confirming disease. The specificity of the test for disease Y is 100/(100 + 0) = 100%, and the PV+ is 70/(70 + 0) = 100%.

TABLE 1-5

	Disease Y	Control Group
Positive test	70 TP	0 FP
Negative test	30 FN	100 TN

A (a negative test result excludes disease Y) is incorrect. The sensitivity of a test is the likelihood of having positive test results in patients who have a selected disease. Because people with disease either have TP or FN test results, the formula for calculating the sensitivity of a test is TP/(TP + FN). The less the FN rate, the greater the sensitivity of the test. Tests with 100% sensitivity are most often used as screening tests for disease. If the test result is negative, the likelihood (predictive value of a negative test result, PV−) of a TN rather than a FN is 100%, because a test with 100% sensitivity has no FNs. Because tests with 100% sensitivity always have a PV− (TN/TN + FN) of

100%, a negative test result excludes disease. The sensitivity of the test for disease Y is $70/(70 + 30) = 70\%$, and the PV− is $100/(100 + 30) = {\sim}77\%$; therefore, a negative test result does *not* exclude disease Y (likelihood of a FN is 23%).

C (it is a poor test for confirming disease Y) is incorrect. The test is an excellent test to confirm disease, because the specificity is 100% and the PV+ is 100%.

D (the predictive value of a negative test result is 100%) is incorrect. The PV− is $100/(100 + 30) = {\sim}77\%$ (not 100%).

E (the prevalence of disease is 60%) is incorrect. Prevalence is the total number of people with disease in the population under study. The formula is $(TP + FN)/(TP + FN + TN + FP)$. The prevalence of disease in this study is $(70 + 30)/(70 + 30 + 100 + 0) = 100/200 = 50\%$ (not 60%).

7. **C** (42–58 mg/dL) is correct. Most normal ranges are established by adding and subtracting 2 standard deviations (SD) from the mean of the test. The standard deviation for the test is 4 mg/dL; therefore, 2 SD is 8 mg/dL. The mean of the test is obtained by adding up the test values for normal people and dividing the sum by the number of people. The mean of the test is $48 + 52 + 50 + 49 + 51 = 250$ mg/dL divided by $5 = 50$ mg/dL. Therefore, the lower limit of the normal range is $50 − 8 = 42$ mg/dL, and the upper limit is $50 + 8 = 58$ mg/dL.

A, B, and D are incorrect.

8. **C** (23%) is correct. Most normal ranges are established by adding and subtracting 2 standard deviations (SD) from the mean of the test, which encompasses 95% of the normal population. Therefore, 5% of the normal population will be outside the normal range (outlier). The likelihood of an outlier increases as the number of tests ordered increases. The likelihood of an outlier $= 100 − (0.95^n \times 100)$, where n is the number of tests ordered. In this patient, five tests were ordered: $100 − (0.95^5 \times 100) = 100 − (0.77 \times 100) = 23\%$ chance of an outlier in one of the five tests.

A, B, D, and E are incorrect.

9. **D** (increases the predictive value of a negative test result) is correct. People with disease either have a true positive (TP) or a false negative (FN) test result. A TP test result is a positive test in a person with disease. A FN test result is a negative test result in a person with disease. People in a control group, who do not have disease, either have a true negative (TN) or a false positive (FP) test result. A TN test result is a negative test in a person without disease, while a FP test result is a positive test result in a person without disease. The sensitivity of a test is the likelihood of having positive test results in patients who have a selected disease. Because people with disease either have TP or FN test results, the formula for calculating the sensitivity of a test is $TP/(TP + FN)$. The less the FN rate, the greater the sensitivity of the test. Tests with 100% sensitivity are most often used as screening tests for disease. The predictive value of a negative test result (PV−) is the likelihood that a negative test result is a TN rather than a FN; therefore, the formula for calculating the PV− is TN/(TN + FN). Tests with 100% sensitivity always have a 100% PV−; therefore, a negative test result excludes disease. The specificity of a test is the likelihood of having a negative test result in a person without disease. Because people without disease have test results that are either a TN or a FP, the formula for calculating the specificity of a test is TN/(TN + FP). The less the FP rate, the greater the specificity of a test. A test with no FPs has 100% specificity. The predictive value of a positive test result (PV+) is the likelihood that a positive test result is a TP rather than a FP; therefore, the formula for PV+ is TP/(TP + FP). Tests with 100% specificity always have a PV+ of 100%; therefore, they are most useful for confirming disease. Assume that the original cutoff point for diagnosing diabetes mellitus is set for 100% specificity (schematic A in Fig. 1-7). The normal population is under the solid curve, but the population with diabetes mellitus is under the curve with the dotted line. Note that beyond a 140 mg/dL cutoff point, all people have TP test results for diabetes. Also note that in the normal range, the number of FNs is increased, which decreases the sensitivity and the PV− of the test. Assume that the new cutoff point for diagnosing diabetes mellitus (126 mg/dL) is set for 100% sensitivity (schematic B in Fig. 1-7). Note that there are no FNs in the normal range; however, beyond the cutoff point of 126 mg/dL there is an increase in the number of FPs, which decreases the specificity and PV+ of the test. Therefore, creating a test with 100% sensitivity and PV− automatically decreases specificity and PV+, while creating a test with 100% specificity and PV+ automatically decreases sensitivity and PV−.

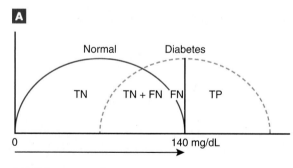
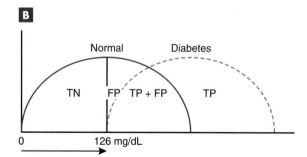

1-7: *Refer to answer 9.*

A (decreases the number of false positive diagnoses of diabetes) is incorrect. In schematic B, the number of FPs *increases* (not decreases). Whenever the sensitivity of a test is increased by altering the normal range, the specificity of the test and the PV+ is automatically decreased.

B (decreases the sensitivity and increases the specificity of the test) is incorrect. Lowering the cutoff point to 126 mg/dL *increases* the sensitivity of the test, and *decreases* the specificity of the test.

C (increases the number of false negative test results) is incorrect. Lowering the cutoff point to 126 mg/dL *decreases* the number of FN test results, which increases sensitivity and PV−.

E (increases the predictive value of a positive test result) is incorrect. Lowering the cutoff point to 126 mg/dL increases the number of FP test results, which *decrease* specificity and PV+.

10. **E** (a 20-year-old woman has a positive rapid plasma reagin test and a negative fluorescent treponemal antibody absorption test) is correct. The antigen used in the RPR test system is beef cardiolipin, which reacts with the reagin antibodies of syphilis as well as anti-cardiolipin antibodies, which are most often present in patients with systemic lupus erythematosus. Because the FTA-ABS has high specificity for diagnosing syphilis, it should be positive if the patient has syphilis. However, the test is negative, which means that the RPR is most likely a false positive test for syphilis and suggests the presence of anti-cardiolipin antibodies.

A (a 7-year-old child, with a healing Colles' fracture, has an increased serum alkaline phosphatase that is beyond the age-adjusted reference interval) is incorrect. The serum alkaline phosphatase (ALP) is normally increased in children owing to increased bone growth corresponding with an increase in osteoblastic activity, which is the source of the ALP. The patient has a Colles' fracture. In the normal repair of a fracture, there is increased osteoblastic activity, which explains the increase in ALP. This is a true positive.

B (a 35-year-old man has an increased serum cholesterol over previous baseline levels ~6 hours after eating bacon and eggs for breakfast) is incorrect. Cholesterol that is derived from food is packaged in chylomicrons, which circulate in the blood stream. The percentage of cholesterol in chylomicrons is <3%; therefore, fasting is not required for obtaining an accurate serum cholesterol. In this patient, the increased serum cholesterol is a true positive.

C (a 45-year-old man, who is an alcoholic, has an increased anion gap metabolic acidosis, and the physician suspects lactic acidosis and ketoacidosis, but lactic acid levels are increased and the serum and urine test for ketone bodies is negative) is incorrect. An increased anion gap metabolic acidosis in an alcoholic is due to lactic acidosis and ketoacidosis, the latter due to an increase in β-hydroxybutyric (β-OHB) acid. The increase in lactic acid relates to the conversion of pyruvate to lactate by an increase in NADH that occurs in alcohol metabolism. The increase in ketoacids is due to the conversion of acetyl CoA, the metabolic end product of alcohol metabolism, into ketone bodies. Acetoacetic acid is converted to β-OHB acid due the presence of NADH as a cofactor. The standard serum and urine tests for ketone bodies detect acetone and acetoacetic acid; however, they do not detect β-OHB acid. Therefore, the negative test result for ketone bodies is a false negative.

D (a 70-year-old man with a normal serum blood urea nitrogen and creatinine level has a creatinine clearance of 65 mL/minute) is incorrect. The creatinine clearance normally decreases with advancing age. The presence of a normal blood urea nitrogen and creatinine level indicates that the decrease in the creatinine clearance is normal and represents a true negative.

11. **B** (increase in the synthesis of thyroid-binding globulin) is correct. The increase in estrogen in pregnancy causes increased synthesis of many proteins in the liver including thyroid-binding globulin (TBG). Because the total serum thyroxine represents the thyroid hormone bound to TBG plus the free unbound thyroid hormone, the total serum thyroxine is increased. The free, unbound metabolically active hormone remains normal; therefore, the serum thyroid-stimulating hormone (TSH) remains normal.

A (increase in the free thyroxine concentration) is incorrect. An increase in the free thyroxine concentration would be associated with signs of thyrotoxicosis and a decrease in the serum TSH concentration (negative feedback). The patient has no signs of thyrotoxicosis.

C (laboratory error in reporting the test) is incorrect. The presence of an increase in serum thyroxine and normal TSH is a normal finding in pregnancy.

D (the patient is taking excess thyroid hormone) is incorrect. Because the patient has no signs of thyrotoxicosis and the serum TSH is normal, the patient cannot be taking an excessive amount of thyroid hormone, which would decrease the serum TSH.

12. **D** (increased erythropoietin) is correct. Smokers with chronic bronchitis (CB) have respiratory acidosis (retention of CO_2). Retention of CO_2 raises the alveolar Pco_2, which automatically decreases the alveolar Po_2. A decrease in alveolar Po_2 decreases arterial Po_2, which is called hypoxemia. Hypoxemia is a stimulus for the renal release of erythropoietin (EPO). EPO stimulates the bone marrow erythroid stem cells to divide, which increases the hemoglobin, hematocrit, and red blood cell count producing secondary polycythemia.

A (decreased arterial Pco_2) is incorrect. Smokers with CB have respiratory acidosis (retention of CO_2), which increases the arterial Pco_2. A decrease in arterial Pco_2 is present in respiratory alkalosis.

B (increased arterial pH) is incorrect. Smokers with CB have respiratory acidosis (retention of CO_2), which increases the arterial Pco_2 and decreases the arterial pH. An increased arterial pH is present in alkalotic conditions.

C (increased serum aspartate aminotransferase, AST) is incorrect. Smokers with CB have normal serum transaminases. An increase in serum AST is a characteristic finding in alcoholics. Alcohol is a mitochondrial toxin and damages hepatocyte mitochondria causing the release of AST. Alanine aminotransferase (ALT) is present in the cytosol and is not increased to the same degree as AST.

E (normal oxygen saturation) is incorrect. Smokers with chronic bronchitis (CB) have respiratory acidosis (retention of CO_2). Retention of CO_2 raises the alveolar Pco_2, which automatically decreases the alveolar Po_2. A decrease in alveolar Po_2 decreases arterial Po_2, which is called hypoxemia. A decrease in arterial Po_2 always decreases the oxygen saturation in red blood cells, which represents the percentage of heme groups in hemoglobin that are occupied by oxygen. An oxygen saturation <80% produces cyanosis (blue discoloration of the skin and mucous membranes).

13. C (decreased plasma hemoglobin) is correct. In pregnancy the plasma volume is disproportionately increased over an increase in red blood cell mass (absolute increase in the number of red blood cells in mL/kg). This has a dilutional effect on the hemoglobin, hematocrit, and red blood cell count (number of RBCs/mm^3).

   A (decreased arterial pH) is incorrect. In pregnancy, estrogen and progesterone stimulate the CNS respiratory center causing respiratory alkalosis (increase in arterial pH and decrease in arterial Pco_2).

   B (decreased creatinine clearance) is incorrect. In pregnancy, the increase in plasma volume increases the glomerular filtration rate, causing an increase in the creatinine clearance.

   D (decreased serum cortisol) is incorrect. In pregnancy, the increase in estrogen causes increased synthesis of transcortin, the binding protein for cortisol. Because the serum cortisol represents cortisol that is bound to transcortin plus cortisol that is free (metabolically active), the serum cortisol is increased. Serum adrenocorticotropic hormone levels are normal, because the free cortisol levels are normal. There are no signs of hypercortisolism.

   E (increased serum blood urea nitrogen) is incorrect. In pregnancy, the increase in plasma volume causes increased clearance of urea in the urine, which causes the serum blood urea nitrogen concentration to be on the low side of the normal range.

14. A (decreased liver metabolism of the drug) is correct. Cimetidine, an imidazole compound that blocks histamine receptors, inhibits cytochrome enzymes in the liver microsomal mixed function oxidase system. This system is located in the smooth endoplasmic reticulum (SER) and is responsible for drug and chemical metabolism. Inhibition of the system produces drug toxicity.

   B (decreased liver uptake of the drug) is incorrect. Cimetidine inhibits the metabolism of the drug in the liver microsomal mixed function oxidase system and does not affect the uptake of the drug into hepatocytes.

   C (increased gastrointestinal uptake of the drug) is incorrect. Increased drug reabsorption in the gastrointestinal tract is a very uncommon cause of drug toxicity, especially if the patient is taking a normal dose of the drug.

   D (increased renal excretion of the drug) is incorrect. Increased excretion in the kidneys is more likely to cause decreased levels of the drug in the serum rather than increased levels.

Electrolyte and Acid-Base Disorders

I. Water and Electrolyte Balance

A. Body fluid compartments

1. Total body water (TBW)
   a. TBW accounts for approximately 60% of the body weight in kg (Fig. 2-1).
   b. TBW distribution
      (1) Intracellular fluid compartment (ICF; 40% body weight in kg)
      (2) Extracellular fluid compartment (ECF; 20% body weight in kg)
2. ECF cations and anions
   a. Sodium (Na^+) and chloride (Cl^-), respectively
   b. Na^+/K^+-ATPase pump
      (1) Na^+ is pumped out of the ICF.
      (2) K^+ is pumped into the ICF.
3. ICF cations and anions
   • Potassium (K^+) and phosphorus (PO_4^{3-}), respectively
4. ECF compartment divisions
   a. Interstitial fluid compartment
   b. Vascular compartment
5. Solutes limited to ECF
   a. Na^+ and glucose
   b. Changes in their concentration produce osmotic gradients.
      (1) Water movements occur between the ECF and ICF.
      (2) Water moves from a low to high solute concentration.
   c. Effect of hyponatremia
      • Water shifts from the ECF to the ICF (expands; Fig. 2-2A).
   d. Effect of hypernatremia or hyperglycemia
      • Water shifts out of the ICF (contracted) into the ECF (Fig. 2-2B).

B. Isotonic, hypotonic, and hypertonic disorders

1. Plasma osmolality (POsm)
   a. Osmolality is the number of solutes in plasma (tonicity of plasma).
   b. POsm formula
      • POsm = 2 (serum Na^+) + serum glucose/18 + serum blood urea nitrogen (BUN)/2.8 = 275–295 mOsm/kg
   c. POsm approximates the serum Na^+ concentration.
   d. Urea equilibrates between ECF and ICF.
      • Water shifts do *not* occur with alterations in urea concentration.

Na^+ and K^+: major ECF and ICF cations, respectively

Solutes causing water movements: Na^+ and glucose

POsm: approximates serum Na^+

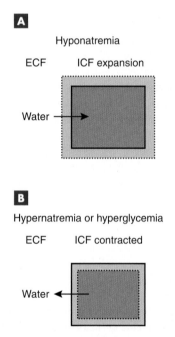

2-1: *Body fluid compartments. See text for description.*

A

Hyponatremia

ECF   ICF expansion

B

Hypernatremia or hyperglycemia

ECF   ICF contracted

2-2: *Effect of serum sodium (**A**) and glucose concentration (**B**) on fluid shifts. See text for description.*

    e. Effective osmolality (EOsm)
      (1) Osmolality that produces water shifts
      (2) EOsm = 2 (serum Na$^+$) + glucose/18
  2. Serum Na$^+$ concentration (mEq/L)
    a. Approximates the ratio of total body Na$^+$ (TBNa$^+$) to total body water (TBW)
      (1) Serum Na$^+$ ~ TBNa$^+$/TBW
      (2) TBNa$^+$
        • Amount of Na$^+$ in the ECF compartment in mg/kg body weight
      (3) TBW is distributed in the ECF and ICF compartments.
    b. Decreased TBNa$^+$ produces signs of volume depletion (Fig. 2-3).

↓TBNa$^+$: signs of volume depletion

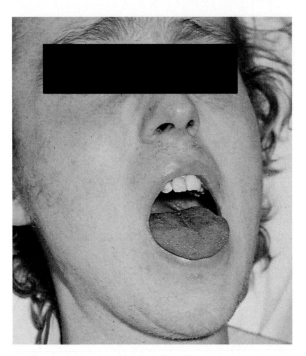

2-3: *This patient with volume depletion has a dry tongue. Additional findings included tenting of the skin and a positive tilt test. (From Forbes C, Jackson W: Color Atlas and Text of Clinical Medicine, 2nd ed. St. Louis, Mosby, 2003, Fig. 7.90.)*

      (1) Dry mucous membranes
      (2) Decreased skin turgor
         • Skin tenting when the skin is pinched
      (3) Positive tilt test
         • Drop in blood pressure and increase in pulse when sitting up
           from a supine position
   c. Signs of increased TBNa$^+$
      (1) Dependent pitting edema
         • Pressure-induced skin indentation due to excess sodium-
           containing interstitial fluid (Fig. 2-4)
      (2) Body cavity effusions (e.g., ascites)
      (3) Increase in weight
      (4) Pathogenesis of pitting edema and body cavity effusions
         • Requires an alteration in Starling's pressures and renal retention
           of sodium

↑ TBNa$^+$: pitting edema, body cavity effusions

> **Fluid movement** across a capillary/venule wall into the interstitial space is driven by Starling's pressures. The plasma oncotic pressure (correlates with the serum albumin concentration) keeps fluid in the vessels, while plasma hydrostatic pressure forces fluid out of the vessels. The net

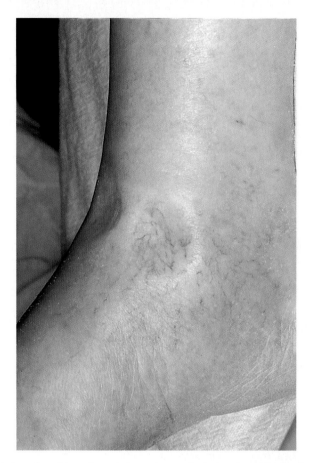

2-4: *Patient with dependent pitting edema. A depression remains in the edema after firm fingertip pressure is applied. (From Forbes C, Jackson W: Color Atlas and Text of Clinical Medicine, 2nd ed. St. Louis, Mosby, 2003, Fig. 5.8.)*

direction of fluid movement can be either out of the vessel or into the vessel depending upon which Starling's pressure is dominant. An increase in plasma hydrostatic pressure or a decrease in plasma oncotic pressure causes fluid to diffuse out of the vessel into the interstitial space resulting in dependent pitting edema and body cavity effusions. Renal retention of sodium increases plasma hydrostatic pressure. Pitting edema and body effusions are unlikely if renal function is normal and Starling's pressure abnormalities are not present.

    d. Normal TBNa$^+$
       (1) Normal skin turgor and hydration of mucous membranes
       (2) Normal blood pressure and pulse

TABLE 2-1
Isotonic and Hypotonic Disorders

Fluid Alteration	Serum Na⁺	ECF Volume	ICF Volume	Disorders
Isotonic loss Na⁺ $\downarrow$TBNa⁺/$\downarrow$TBW	Normal	Contracted Signs of volume depletion	Normal	Adult diarrhea Loss of plasma: e.g., third-degree burn Loss of whole blood
Isotonic gain Na⁺ $\uparrow$TBNa⁺/$\uparrow$TBW	Normal	Expanded Pitting edema, body effusions	Normal	Excessive infusion of isotonic saline
Hypertonic loss Na⁺ $\downarrow\downarrow$TBNa⁺/$\downarrow$TBW	Decreased	Contracted Signs of volume depletion	Expanded	Diuretics: e.g., loop diuretics Addison's disease: Na⁺ loss due to decrease in aldosterone 21-OHase deficiency: Na⁺ loss due to decrease in mineralocorticoids
Gain of water TBNa⁺/$\uparrow\uparrow$TBW	Decreased	Expanded Normal examination	Expanded	Syndrome of inappropriate ADH secretion
Hypotonic gain Na⁺ $\uparrow$TBNa⁺/$\uparrow\uparrow$TBW	Decreased	Expanded Pitting edema, body effusions	Expanded	Right-sided heart failure: increased venous hydrostatic pressure Cirrhosis: increased portal vein hydrostatic pressure, decreased plasma oncotic pressure Nephrotic syndrome: massive proteinuria; decreased plasma oncotic pressure

ADH, antidiuretic hormone; OHase, hydroxylase.

3. Isotonic fluid disorders
   a. Isotonic loss of fluid (Table 2-1)
      (1) Serum Na⁺ remains normal ($\downarrow$TBNa⁺/$\downarrow$TBW)
         • There is *no* osmotic gradient.
      (2) ECF contracts and the ICF is normal.
      (3) Signs of volume depletion
      (4) Examples
         • Adult diarrhea, loss of plasma (e.g., third-degree burns), loss of whole blood

> **Normal (isotonic) saline** (0.9%) approximates plasma tonicity. It is infused in patients to maintain the blood pressure when there is a significant loss of sodium-containing fluid (e.g., blood loss, diarrhea, sweat). Hypotonic saline solutions (e.g., 0.45 normal saline) *cannot* raise the blood pressure.

0.9% normal saline: primary crystalloid used to $\uparrow$ blood pressure

b. Isotonic gain of fluid
   (1) Normal serum Na^+ ($\uparrow$TBNa$^+$/$\uparrow$TBW)
       • There is *no* osmotic gradient.
   (2) ECF expands and ICF is normal.
   (3) Pitting edema and body cavity effusions may occur.
   (4) Example—excessive infusion of isotonic saline
4. Hypotonic fluid disorders (Table 2-1)
   a. Always associated with hyponatremia
   b. Osmotic gradient is present.
       • Water shifts out of the ECF into the ICF compartment (expands).
   c. Hyponatremia due to a hypertonic loss of Na^+
       (1) $\downarrow\downarrow$TBNa$^+$/$\downarrow$TBW
       (2) ECF contracts and the ICF expands.
       (3) Signs of volume depletion
       (4) Examples
           • Loop diuretics, Addison's disease, 21-hydroxylase deficiency

> **Rapid intravenous fluid correction of hyponatremia** with saline in an alcoholic may result in central pontine myelinolysis, an irreversible demyelinating disorder. As a general rule, all intravenous replacement of Na^+-containing fluid should be given slowly over the first 24 hours.

   d. Hyponatremia due to a gain of water
       (1) TBNa$^+$/$\uparrow\uparrow$TBW
       (2) Expansion of the ECF and ICF compartments
       (3) Normal physical examination
       (4) Example—syndrome of inappropriate secretion of antidiuretic hormone (SIADH, e.g., caused by small cell carcinoma of the lung)
   e. Hyponatremia due to a hypotonic gain of Na^+
       (1) $\uparrow$TBNa$^+$/$\uparrow\uparrow$TBW
       (2) Expansion of the ECF and ICF compartments
       (3) Pitting edema states
       (4) Examples
           • Right-sided heart failure, cirrhosis, nephrotic syndrome

> In the **pitting edema states** listed above, the cardiac output is decreased, which causes the release of catecholamines, activation of the renin-angiotensin-aldosterone system, stimulation of ADH release, and increased renal retention of Na^+. The kidney reabsorbs a slightly hypotonic, Na^+-containing fluid ($\uparrow$TBNa$^+$/$\uparrow\uparrow$TBW). Because all of the pitting edema states have alterations in Starling pressures, the Na^+-containing fluid is redirected into the interstitial space causing pitting edema and body cavity effusions.

Loop/thiazide diuretics: most common cause of hyponatremia

Hyponatremia + pitting edema: right-sided heart failure, cirrhosis, nephrotic syndrome

TABLE 2-2
Hypertonic Disorders

Fluid Alteration	Serum Na⁺	ECF Volume	ICF Volume	Disorders
Hypotonic loss Na⁺ $\downarrow$TBNa⁺/$\downarrow\downarrow$TBW	Increased	Contracted Signs of volume depletion	Contracted	Osmotic diuresis: glucose, mannitol Sweating Infant diarrhea
Loss of water TBNa⁺/$\downarrow\downarrow$TBW	Increased	Contracted (mild) Normal examination	Contracted	Insensible water loss: e.g., fever Diabetes insipidus: due to decreased ADH or refractoriness of collecting tubules to ADH
Hypertonic gain Na⁺ $\uparrow\uparrow$TBNa⁺/$\uparrow$TBW	Increased	Expanded Pitting edema, body effusions	Contracted	Na⁺-containing antibiotic Excessive infusion of NaHCO₃ 3% Hypertonic saline
Diabetic ketoacidosis	Decreased Dilutional effect of ICF water	Contracted Signs of volume depletion	Contracted	Lack of insulin in type 1 diabetes mellitus

5. Hypertonic fluid disorders
   a. Most often associated with hypernatremia or hyperglycemia (Table 2-2)
   b. Osmotic gradient is present.
      • Water shifts out of the ICF (contracts) into the ECF.
   c. Hypernatremia due to a hypotonic loss of Na⁺
      (1) $\downarrow$TBNa⁺/$\downarrow\downarrow$TBW
      (2) Contraction of the ECF and ICF compartments
      (3) Signs of volume depletion
      (4) Examples
         • Sweating, osmotic diuresis (glucosuria, mannitol), infant diarrhea
   d. Hypernatremia due to a loss of water
      (1) TBNa⁺/$\downarrow\downarrow$TBW
      (2) Slight contraction of the ECF and ICF

> Nephrologists use the term **dehydration** for a loss of water lacking Na⁺. Loss of water does *not* produce any signs of volume depletion, because there is no loss of Na⁺.

      (3) Normal physical examination
      (4) Examples
         • Diabetes insipidus (due to a loss of ADH or refractoriness of the collecting tubules to ADH), insensible water loss (e.g., fever)
   e. Hypernatremia due to a hypertonic gain in Na⁺
      (1) $\uparrow\uparrow$TBNa⁺/$\uparrow$TBW
      (2) ECF expands and the ICF contracts.
      (3) Pitting edema and body cavity effusions may occur.
      (4) Examples
         • Infusion of NaHCO₃, Na⁺-containing antibiotics, or 3% hypertonic saline

Hypertonic state + hyponatremia: DKA

f. Hypertonic state due to diabetic ketoacidosis (DKA)
   (1) Hyperglycemia causes water to shift from the ICF to the ECF.
      • Produces a dilutional effect on serum Na^+
   (2) Glucosuria produces an osmotic diuresis.
      • Hypotonic loss of water and Na^+ produces volume depletion.
   (3) Correction for the dilutional effect hyperglycemia has on serum Na^+
      (a) Corrected serum Na^+ = serum Na^+ + (glucose/100 × 1.6)
      (b) Example—serum Na^+ 130 mEq/L, serum glucose 1000 mg/dL
         • Corrected serum Na^+ = 130 + (1000/100 × 1.6) = 146 mEq/L (136–145 mEq/L). Hypernatremia will be present once glucose is restored to the normal range by insulin therapy.

II. **Correlation of Nephron Function with Electrolyte Disorders**
   A. **Proximal renal tubule**
      1. Primary site for Na^+ reabsorption
         a. Na^+ reabsorption is increased when cardiac output is decreased.
            • Examples—congestive heart failure, cirrhosis, hypovolemia
         b. Na^+ reabsorption is decreased when cardiac output is increased.
            • Examples—mineralocorticoid excess, isotonic gain in fluid
      2. Primary site for reclamation of bicarbonate (HCO_3^-)
         a. Normal reclamation (Fig. 2-5, steps 1 through 6)
            (1) Hydrogen ions (H^+) in tubular cells are exchanged for Na^+ (step 1).
            (2) H^+ combines with filtered HCO_3^- to form H_2CO_3 (step 2).

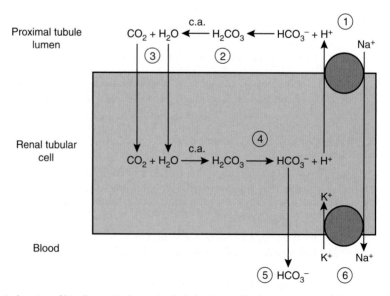

2-5: Reclamation of bicarbonate in the proximal tubule. See text for description. c.a., carbonic anhydrase.

      (3) Carbonic anhydrase (c.a.) dissociates H_2CO_3 to H_2O and CO_2
- CO_2 and H_2O are reabsorbed into proximal renal tubular cells (step 3).

      (4) H_2CO_3 is re-formed in the proximal renal tubular cells.
- H_2CO_3 dissociates into H^+ and HCO_3^- (step 4).

      (5) HCO_3^- is reabsorbed into the blood (step 5).

      (6) A Na^+/K^+-ATPase pump moves Na^+ into the blood (step 6).

  b. Clinical effect of lowering the renal threshold for reclaiming HCO_3^-

      (1) Example—normal threshold is lowered from 24 mEq/L to 15 mEq/L.

      (2) Filtered HCO_3^- is lost in the urine.

        (a) Urine pH > 5.5

        (b) Urine loss occurs until serum HCO_3^- matches the renal threshold.

      (3) Carbonic anhydrase inhibitor (e.g., acetazolamide)

        (a) Lowers the renal threshold for reclaiming HCO_3^-

        (b) HCO_3^- combines with Na^+ to form $NaHCO_3$, which is excreted.
- Proximal tubule diuretic

        (c) Loss of HCO_3^- produces metabolic acidosis (see below).

> *Carbonic anhydrase inhibitor: causes proximal renal tubular acidosis*

  c. Clinical effect of raising the renal threshold for reclaiming HCO_3^-

      (1) Example—volume depletion associated with vomiting

      (2) Increased threshold maintains increased serum HCO_3^- in metabolic alkalosis (see below).

> In **heavy metal poisoning** with lead or mercury, the proximal tubule cells undergo coagulation necrosis, which produces a nephrotoxic acute tubular necrosis. All the normal proximal renal tubule functions are destroyed resulting in a loss of sodium (hyponatremia), glucose (hypoglycemia), uric acid (hypouricemia), phosphorus (hypophosphatemia), amino acids, bicarbonate (type II proximal renal tubular acidosis), and urea in the urine. This is called the Fanconi syndrome.

> *Heavy metal poisoning: produces Fanconi syndrome*

B. **Thick ascending limb (TAL medullary segment)**

  1. Generation of free water (fH_2O)

    a. Occurs via the active Na^+-K^+-$2Cl^-$ cotransporter (Fig. 2-6, steps 1 through 4)

    b. Water proximal to the cotransporter is obligated (o, step 1).

      (1) Water is bound to Na^+ (oNa^+), K^+ (oK^+), and Cl^- (oCl^-).

      (2) Obligated water must accompany every Na^+, K^+, or Cl^- excreted in urine.

      (3) Obligated water is *not* reabsorbed out of the urine.

      (4) Only free H_2O (fH_2O) is reabsorbed out of the urine.

        (a) fH_2O is entirely free of electrolytes.

        (b) Reabsorption of fH_2O concentrates the urine.

        (c) Loss of fH_2O in the urine dilutes urine.

    c. Cotransporter separates oH_2O from Na^+, K^+, and Cl^- (step 2).

> *Na^+-K^+-$2Cl^-$ cotransporter: generates free water*

2-6: Sodium, potassium, chloride cotransporter in the medullary segment of the thick ascending limb. See text for description. ATP, adenosine triphosphate; fH_2O, free water; oH_2O, obligated water.

(1) Water left behind in the urine is fH_2O.

(2) Urine Osm (UOsm) is ~150 mOsm/kg distal to the TAL medullary segment.

d. A Na^+/K^+-ATPase pump moves reabsorbed Na^+ into the interstitium (step 3).

e. Reabsorbed Cl^- and K^+ diffuse through channels into the interstitium (step 4).

2. Loop diuretics (e.g., furosemide)

a. Mainstay in the treatment of congestive heart failure and hypercalcemia

(1) Decrease $TBNa^+$ and TBW (see I.B.2)

(2) Decrease reabsorption of Ca^{2+}

b. Drug attaches to the Cl^- binding site of the cotransporter.

(1) Inhibits reabsorption of Na^+, K^+, and Cl^-.

(2) Impairs generation of fH_2O

(3) oNa^+, oK^+, oCl^- are lost in the urine.

c. Hyponatremia may occur.

(1) Hypertonic loss of Na^+ in the urine (see I.B.4.c)

(2) Impaired excretion of fH_2O impairs normal dilution.

(a) Excess intake of water cannot be excreted as fH_2O.

(b) Excess water remains in the ECF causing hyponatremia.

(c) Patients cannot have unrestricted H_2O intake.

(3) Additional electrolyte abnormalities

• Hypokalemia and metabolic alkalosis (see II.D.1.b)

d. Calcium (Ca^{2+}) is also reabsorbed by the cotransporter.

• Loop diuretics are used in the treatment of hypercalcemia.

C. **Na^+-Cl^- cotransporter in the early distal tubule**

1. Na^+ and Ca^{2+} share the same site for reabsorption (Fig. 2-7, step 1).

• Parathyroid hormone (PTH)-enhanced Ca^{2+} reabsorption

2. Na^+/K^+-ATPase pump moves Na^+ into the blood (step 2).

• Cl^- diffuses through a channel into the blood.

Cl^- binding site in Na^+-K^+-$2Cl^-$ co-transporter: inhibited by loop diuretics

Loop diuretic: hyponatremia, hypokalemia, metabolic alkalosis

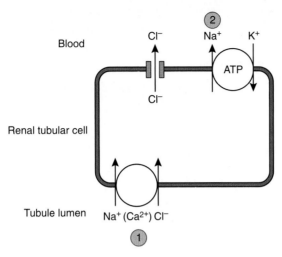

2-7: *Sodium-chloride cotransporter in the early distal tubule. See text for the description. ATP, adenosine triphosphate.*

3. Thiazides
   a. Clinical uses
      (1) Mainstay in the treatment of hypertension in black Americans and the elderly
         • Both patient populations have renal retention of Na^+.
      (2) Treatment of hypercalciuria in Ca^{2+} renal stone formers
   b. Drug attaches to the Cl^- site.
      • Inhibits NaCl reabsorption
   c. Hyponatremia may occur
      (1) Hypertonic loss of sodium (see I.B.2)
      (2) Additional electrolyte abnormalities
         • Hypokalemia and metabolic alkalosis (see II.D.1.b)
   d. Hypercalcemia may occur.
      • Inhibition of Na^+ increases PTH-enhanced reabsorption of Ca^{2+}.
   e. Thiazides are used in the treatment of Ca^{2+} stone formers.
      (1) Hypercalciuria is present in Ca^{2+} stone formers.
      (2) Thiazides increase Ca^{2+} reabsorption out of the urine.
D. **Aldosterone-enhanced channels and pumps**
   1. Na^+ and K^+ channels in the late distal tubule and collecting ducts
      a. Na^+ diffuses into the cell (Fig. 2-8A, step 1)
      b. K^+ diffuses out of the cell to maintain electroneutrality.
         • Primary site for K^+ secretion
      c. Na^+/K^+-ATPase pump moves Na^+ into the blood (step 2).
      d. Effect of K^+ depletion (hypokalemia, Fig. 2-8B)
         (1) Hydrogen (H^+) ions are secreted into the lumen in exchange for Na^+ (step 3).
         (2) HCO_3^- is reabsorbed into the ECF causing metabolic alkalosis (step 4).

Cl^- site in Na^+-Cl^- cotransporter: inhibited by thiazides

Thiazide diuretic: hyponatremia, hypokalemia, metabolic alkalosis, hypercalcemia

Hypokalemia: increased risk for metabolic alkalosis

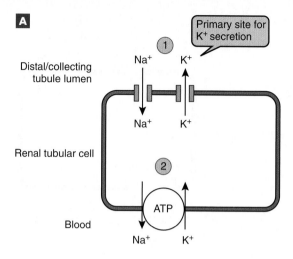

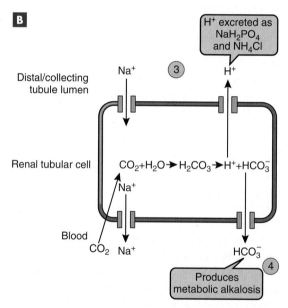

2-8: *Sodium-potassium channels (**A**) and sodium-hydrogen ion channels (**B**) in the late distal tubule and collecting duct. See text for description. ATP, adenosine triphosphate.*

    e. Amiloride and triamterene
      (1) Diuretics with K^+-sparing effect
      (2) Bind to the luminal membrane Na^+ channels
        • Inhibit Na^+ reabsorption and K^+ secretion
    f. Effect of increased distal delivery of Na^+ from loop/thiazide diuretics
      (1) Augmented Na^+ reabsorption and K^+ secretion
      (2) May produce hypokalemia, if K^+ supplements are not taken
      (3) May produce metabolic alkalosis if H^+ exchanges with Na^+ (see II.D.1.d).

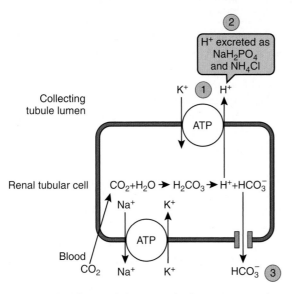

2-9: *H^+/K^+-ATPase pump in the collecting tubule. See text for description. ATP, adenosine triphosphate.*

2. H^+/K^+-ATPase pump (Fig. 2-9)
   a. Located in the α-intercalated cell of the collecting tubule
   b. Primary site for the secretion of H^+ ions
      (1) H^+ ions are secreted into the lumen and K^+ is reabsorbed (step 1).
      (2) H^+ combines with HPO_4^{2-} to produce NaH_2PO_4 (titratable acidity, step 2).
      (3) H^+ also combines with NH_3 and Cl^- to produce NH_4Cl (step 2).
      (4) Both titratable acid and NH_4Cl acidify the urine.
      (5) HCO_3^- is synthesized and reabsorbed into the ECF (step 3).
3. Spironolactone
   a. Diuretic with K^+-sparing effect
   b. Inhibits aldosterone
      (1) Na^+ is lost in the urine (Fig. 2-8A).
      (2) K^+ is retained in the blood (K^+-sparer).
      (3) Hyperkalemia may occur.

Spironolactone: aldosterone inhibitor; K^+ sparer

> An **angiotensin-converting enzyme (ACE) inhibitor** is important in the treatment of congestive heart failure. Inhibition of the enzyme causes a decrease in angiotensin II (ATII) and aldosterone. ATII is normally a vasoconstrictor of peripheral resistance arterioles, which increases afterload (resistance the heart must contract against). Aldosterone normally reabsorbs sodium and increases preload (volume in the left ventricle). Therefore, an ACE inhibitor decreases both afterload and preload. The inhibition of aldosterone is short-lived and is counterbalanced by the use of spironolactone.

   (4) H^+ is retained, which produces metabolic acidosis (Fig. 2-9).

Addison's disease: hyponatremia, hyperkalemia, metabolic acidosis

4. Addison's disease
   a. Most often due to autoimmune destruction of the adrenal cortex
   b. Pathogenesis of electrolyte abnormalities
      • Deficiency of aldosterone and other mineralocorticoids
   c. Clinical findings
      (1) Hyponatremia and hyperkalemia
          (a) Due to inhibition of Na^+ reabsorption and K^+ secretion (Fig. 2-8A)
          (b) Signs of volume depletion
              • Hypertonic loss of Na^+
      (2) Retention of H^+ ions, which produces metabolic acidosis
          • Due to dysfunction of the H^+/K^+-ATPase pump (Fig. 2-9)

Primary aldosteronism: hypernatremia, hypokalemia, metabolic alkalosis

Primary aldosteronism: low plasma renin type of hypertension

5. Primary aldosteronism (Conn's syndrome)
   a. Epidemiology
      • Benign adenoma arising in the zona glomerulosa
   b. Pathogenesis of electrolyte abnormalities
      (1) Enhanced activity of aldosterone channels and pumps
          • Increased Na^+ reabsorption and H^+ and K^+ secretion
      (2) Increased reabsorption of Na^+ causes hypernatremia.
      (3) Increased secretion of K^+ causes hypokalemia.
          • Hypokalemia produces severe muscle weakness (see II.C.2).
      (4) Increased secretion of H^+
          • Causes increased synthesis and reabsorption of HCO_3^- (metabolic alkalosis)
   c. Effect of excess Na^+ in the ECF
      (1) Increases plasma volume
          (a) Increases stroke volume, which increases systolic blood pressure
          (b) Increases peritubular capillary hydrostatic pressure
              • Prevents the proximal tubule from reabsorbing Na^+
          (c) Increases renal blood flow
              • Inhibits the renin-angiotensin-aldosterone system causing a decrease in plasma renin activity (PRA)
      (2) Excess Na^+ enters smooth muscle cells of peripheral resistance arterioles.
          (a) Na^+ opens up Ca^{2+} channels causing vasoconstriction of smooth muscle cells.
          (b) Increased total peripheral resistance increases the diastolic blood pressure.
   d. Summary of clinical findings
      (1) Hypertension
      (2) Polyuria and muscle weakness
          • Complication of hypokalemia (see II.C.2.c)
      (3) Hypernatremia, hypokalemia, metabolic alkalosis
      (4) Decreased PRA
      (5) Absence of pitting edema and effusions

- Due to excessive loss of Na^+ in the urine from inhibition of proximal tubule reabsorption
  e. Treatment is surgery.
6. Bartter's syndrome
   a. Epidemiology
      - Majority of cases occur in children
   b. Pathogenesis
      (1) Renal defect in Cl^- reabsorption in the Na^+-K^+-$2Cl^-$ cotransporter
          - Similar to the mechanism of a loop diuretic
      (2) Loss of Na^+, K^+, and Cl^- ions in the urine
          - Hypertonic loss of Na^+ causes hyponatremia.
      (3) Augmented exchange of Na^+ and secretion of K^+ in distal/collecting tubules
          - Causes hypokalemia and metabolic alkalosis (see II.D.2.b)
      (4) Hypokalemia stimulates increased prostaglandin synthesis in the kidneys
          (a) Stimulates hyperplasia of the juxtaglomerular apparatus
          (b) Increased renin causes hyperaldosteronism.
   c. Clinical findings
      (1) Patients are normotensive (not hypertensive).
          - Due to vasodilation of peripheral resistance arterioles by prostaglandin
      (2) Muscle weakness due to hypokalemia
      (3) Increased PRA
          - Decreased PRA in primary aldosteronism
   d. Treatment
      (1) K^+-sparing diuretic
          - Corrects K^+ loss
      (2) Nonsteroidal anti-inflammatory drug
          - Decreases prostaglandin synthesis

> Bartter's syndrome: hypokalemia, metabolic alkalosis; ↑ aldosterone and PRA

E. **Dilution and concentration of urine**
1. Normal dilution
   a. UOsm in the late distal tubule/collecting ducts is ~150 mOsm/kg.
      (1) Most of the water is fH_2O.
      (2) Small amount of water is obligated water accompanying solute.
   b. Decreased POsm inhibits ADH release from the posterior pituitary.
      - Absence of ADH results in a loss of fH_2O in the urine.
   c. Positive free water clearance (CH_2O)
      (1) $CH_2O = V - COsm$
          - V is the volume of urine in mL/minute and COsm is obligated water.
      (2) $COsm = UOsm \times V/POsm$
      (3) Positive CH_2O indicates dilution.
          - Loss of fH_2O is greater than obligated water.
      (4) Example—urine volume 10 mL, POsm 250 mOsm/kg, UOsm 150 mOsm/kg
          - $COsm = 150 \times 10/250 = 6$ mL, $CH_2O = 10 - 6 = +4$ mL

> +CH_2O: indicates dilution; absence of ADH

d. Syndrome of inappropriate ADH secretion (SIADH)
   (1) Epidemiology
       (a) Ectopic production of ADH
           • Small cell carcinoma of lung is the most common cause of SIADH.

SIADH: small cell carcinoma of lung most common cause

       (b) Drugs that enhance ADH effect
           • Chlorpropamide, cyclophosphamide
       (c) CNS injury, lung infections (e.g., tuberculosis)
   (2) Pathophysiology of electrolyte abnormalities
       (a) Urine is always concentrated (never diluting), because ADH is always present.
           • Negative CH_2O (see II.E.2.c)
       (b) Hypotonic gain of water produces a dilutional hyponatremia.

SIADH: serum $Na^+ < 120$ mEq/L

           • Serum Na^+ is usually <120 mEq/L (136–145 mEq/L)
       (c) Increased plasma volume increases peritubular capillary hydrostatic pressure
           • Decreased proximal tubular cell reabsorption of Na^+ with random urine $Na^+ > 40$ mEq/L
   (3) Clinical findings
       (a) Mental status abnormalities from cerebral edema
       (b) Treatment is to restrict water.

Treatment of SIADH: restrict water

> **Demeclocycline** is often used when a patient has a small cell carcinoma of the lung. The drug inhibits the effect of ADH on the collecting tubules (acquired nephrogenic diabetes insipidus) causing loss of fH_2O in the urine. It is unnecessary to restrict water while the patient is taking the drug.

2. Normal concentration
   a. Increased POsm stimulates ADH synthesis and release
   b. ADH reabsorbs fH_2O and concentrates the urine.

$-CH_2O$: concentration; presence of ADH

   c. Negative CH_2O clearance
      (1) fH_2O is reabsorbed back into the blood.
          • Loss of obligated water is greater than fH_2O.
      (2) Example—urine volume 10 mL, POsm 300 mOsm/kg, UOsm 900 mOsm/kg
          • COsm = $900 \times 10/300 = 30$ mL, $CH_2O = 10 - 30 = -20$ mL
   d. Diabetes insipidus
      (1) Epidemiology
          (a) Central diabetes insipidus (CD) is absence of ADH.
              • Causes: CNS trauma and tumors
          (b) Nephrogenic diabetes insipidus (NDI) is refractoriness to ADH.
              • Causes: drugs (e.g., demeclocycline, lithium) and hypokalemia (see III.C.2.c)

(2) Pathogenesis of electrolyte abnormalities
  (a) Urine is always diluted, causing a loss of fH_2O.
  (b) Positive CH_2O

CDI and NDI: hypernatremia, polyuria

(3) Clinical findings
  (a) Increased thirst and polyuria
  (b) Hypernatremia due to a loss of water.

CDI and NDI: always diluting, never concentrating

(4) Treatment
  (a) CDI is treated with desmopressin acetate.
  (b) NDI is treated with diuretics.
    • Volume depletion decreases polyuria.

III. Potassium (K^+) Disorders
A. Functions of potassium
1. Regulation of neuromuscular excitability and muscle contraction
2. Regulation of insulin secretion
   a. Hypokalemia inhibits insulin secretion.
   b. Hyperkalemia stimulates insulin secretion.
B. Control of potassium
1. Aldosterone
   a. Increases secretion of K^+ in the distal/collecting tubules.
   b. Increases reabsorption of K^+ by the H^+/K^+-ATPase pump.
2. Arterial pH
   a. Alkalosis

Alkalosis/acidosis: potential for hypokalemia or hyperkalemia, respectively

   (1) H^+ moves out of cells and K^+ into cells (Fig. 2-10A).
   (2) Potential for hypokalemia
   b. Acidosis
   (1) H^+ moves into cells (for buffering) and K^+ out of cells (Fig. 2-10B).
   (2) Potential for hyperkalemia

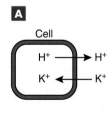

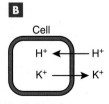

2-10: *Effect of alkalosis (**A**) and acidosis (**B**) on potassium. See text for description.*

**TABLE 2-3
Causes of
Hypokalemia**

Pathogenesis	Causes
Decreased intake	Elderly patients, eating disorders
Transcellular shift	Alkalosis Drugs enhancing Na^+/K^+-ATPase pump: insulin, β_2-agonists (e.g., albuterol)
Gastrointestinal loss	Diarrhea (~30 mEq/L) Laxatives Vomiting (~5 mEq/L) Villous adenoma (mucus rich in K^+)
Renal loss	Loop and thiazide diuretics (most common cause) Osmotic diuresis: glucosuria, mannitol Mineralocorticoid excess: primary aldosteronism, 11-hydroxylase deficiency, Cushing's syndrome, Bartter's syndrome

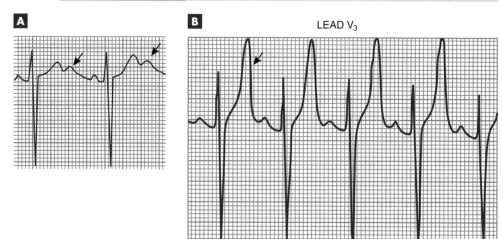

2-11: *Electrocardiogram showing hypokalemia (**A**) and hyperkalemia (**B**). The electrocardiogram in A shows characteristic U waves (arrows) after the T waves. This is a sign of hypokalemia. The electrocardiogram in B shows peaked T waves (arrow) with a normal sinus rhythm. Peaked T waves are a sign of hyperkalemia. (A, adapted from Forbes C, Jackson W: Color Atlas and Text of Clinical Medicine, 2nd ed. St. Louis, Mosby, 2003, Fig. 7.43. B, adapted from Goldman, Bennet: Cecil Textbook of Medicine, 21st ed. Philadelphia, WB Saunders, 1999, Fig.102-8.)*

Enhance Na^+/K^+-ATPase pump: albuterol, insulin
Inhibit Na^+/K^+-ATPase pump: β-blocker, digitalis, succinylcholine

3. Drugs enhancing the Na^+/K^+-ATPase pump
   • Examples—insulin, β_2-agonists (e.g., albuterol)
4. Drugs inhibiting the Na^+/K^+-ATPase pump
   • Examples—β-antagonists (e.g., propranolol), digitalis toxicity, succinylcholine

C. **Hypokalemia (serum $K^+ < 3.5$ mEq/L)**
   1. Causes of hypokalemia (Table 2-3)
   2. Clinical findings
      a. Muscle weakness
         • Due to changes in the intracellular/extracellular K^+ membrane potential

Loop/thiazide diuretics: most common cause of hypokalemia

      b. U waves on an electrocardiogram (ECG; Fig. 2-11A)

TABLE 2-4
Causes of
Hyperkalemia

Pathogenesis	Causes
Tissue breakdown	Iatrogenic (e.g., venipuncture) Rhabdomyolysis (rupture of muscle)
Transcellular shift	Acidosis Drugs inhibiting Na^+/K^+-ATPase pump: β-blocker (e.g., propanolol), digitalis toxicity, succinylcholine.
Decreased renal excretion	Renal failure (most common cause) Mineralocorticoid deficiency: Addison's disease, 21-hydroxylase deficiency, hyporeninemic hypoaldosteronism (destruction of juxtaglomerular apparatus) Drugs: spironolactone, triamterene, amiloride

    c. Polyuria
       (1) Tubular refractoriness to ADH
         • Collecting tubules have vacuoles (called vacuolar nephropathy)
       (2) Acquired nephrogenic diabetes insipidus.
    d. Paralytic ileus (absent bowel sounds)
    e. Rhabdomyolysis
       (1) Hypokalemia inhibits insulin, which decreases muscle glycogenesis
       (2) Decreased muscle glycogen leads to rhabdomyolysis with exercise.
  3. Treatment
    • Oral replacement (safest) or intravenous replacement
 D. **Hyperkalemia (serum $K^+ > 5.0$ mEq/L)**
  1. Causes of hyperkalemia (Table 2-4)
  2. Clinical findings
    a. Ventricular arrhythmias
      • Severe hyperkalemia (e.g., 7–8 mEq/L) causes the heart to stop in diastole.
    b. Peaked T waves on an ECG (Fig. 2-11B)
      • Due to accelerated repolarization of cardiac muscle
    c. Muscle weakness
      • Hyperkalemia partially depolarizes the cell membrane which interferes with membrane excitability.
  3. Treatment
    a. Infuse calcium gluconate, which decreases membrane excitability
      • Protects the heart
    b. Redistribute K^+ to the ICF
      • Example—insulin plus glucose infusion
    c. Eliminate K^+
      • Example—loop diuretics or stool binding agents (e.g., sodium polystyrene)

IV. **Acid-Base Disorders**
 A. **Respiratory acidosis**
  1. Epidemiology
    • Causes of respiratory acidosis (Table 2-5)

Renal failure: most common cause of hyperkalemia

ECG: U wave hypokalemia; peaked T wave hyperkalemia

Loop diuretic: treatment of hyperkalemia

**TABLE 2-5
Causes of
Respiratory
Acidosis and
Respiratory
Alkalosis**

Anatomic Site	Respiratory Acidosis	Respiratory Alkalosis
CNS respiratory center	Depression of center: trauma, barbiturates	Overstimulation: anxiety, high altitude, normal pregnancy (estrogen/progesterone effect), salicylate poisoning, endotoxic (septic) shock, cirrhosis
Upper airway	Obstruction: acute epiglottitis (*Haemophilus influenzae*), café coronary (food obstruction), croup (parainfluenza virus)	
Muscles of respiration	Paralysis: ALS, phrenic nerve injury, Guillain-Barré syndrome, hypokalemia, hypophosphatemia ($\downarrow$ ATP)	Rib fracture: hyperventilation from pain
Lungs	Obstructive disease: chronic bronchitis, cystic fibrosis Other: pulmonary edema, ARDS, RDS, severe bronchial asthma	Restrictive disease: sarcoidosis, asbestosis Others: pulmonary embolus, mild bronchial asthma

ALS, amyotrophic lateral sclerosis; ARDS, acute respiratory distress syndrome; ATP, adenosine triphosphate; RDS, respiratory distress syndrome.

2. Pathogenesis of respiratory acidosis
   a. Alveolar hypoventilation with retention of CO_2
   b. Arterial P_{CO_2} (Pa_{CO_2}) > 45 mm Hg (normal 33–45 mm Hg)
      • $\downarrow$ pH ~ $\uparrow$ HCO_3^- $\uparrow\uparrow P_{CO_2}$
   c. Metabolic alkalosis is compensation.
      (1) Acute respiratory acidosis, serum HCO_3^- ≤ 30 mEq/L
      (2) Chronic respiratory acidosis, serum HCO_3^- > 30 mEq/L
         • Indicates renal compensation

Respiratory acidosis: acute, HCO_3^- ≤ 30 mEq/L; chronic, HCO_3^- > 30 mEq/L

> **Compensation** refers to respiratory and renal mechanisms that bring the arterial pH close to but *not* into the normal pH range (7.35–7.45). In primary respiratory acidosis and alkalosis, compensation is metabolic alkalosis and metabolic acidosis, respectively. In primary metabolic acidosis and alkalosis, compensation is respiratory alkalosis and respiratory acidosis, respectively. When the expected compensation remains in the normal range, it is called an uncompensated disorder. When the expected compensation moves outside the normal range but does not bring the pH into the normal range, a partially compensated disorder is present. When the expected compensation brings the pH into the normal range, a fully compensated disorder is present. This rarely occurs in clinical medicine.

3. Calculation of expected compensation in acute respiratory acidosis
   a. Expected $\Delta HCO_3^- = 0.10 \times \Delta P_{CO_2}$ (difference from normal of 40 mm Hg)

     b. Example—pH 7.20, P_{CO_2} 74 mm Hg, HCO_3^- 27 mEq/L
       (1) Expected $\Delta HCO_3^- = 0.10 \times (74 - 40) = 3.4$ mEq/L
       (2) Expected $HCO_3^- = 24$ mEq/L (mean HCO_3^-) $+ 3.4 = 27.4$ mEq/L
         • Note that measured and expected calculated HCO_3^- are similar.

  4. Calculation of expected compensation in chronic respiratory acidosis
     a. Expected $\Delta HCO_3^- = 0.40 \times \Delta P_{CO_2}$
     b. Example—pH 7.34, P_{CO_2} 60 mm Hg, HCO_3^- 32 mEq/L
       (1) Expected $\Delta HCO_3^- = 0.40 \times (60 - 40) = 8$ mEq/L
       (2) Expected $HCO_3^- = 24 + 8 = 32$ mEq/L
         • Note that measured and expected calculated HCO_3^- are similar.

  5. Clinical findings in respiratory acidosis
     a. Somnolence
     b. Cerebral edema
       • Due to vasodilation of cerebral vessels

B. **Respiratory alkalosis**
  1. Epidemiology
     • Causes of respiratory alkalosis (see Table 2-5)
  2. Pathogenesis of respiratory alkalosis
     a. Alveolar hyperventilation with elimination of CO_2
     b. $Pa_{CO_2} < 33$ mm Hg (normal 33–45 mm Hg)
       • ↑ pH ~ ↓ HCO_3/↓↓ P_{CO_2}
     c. Metabolic acidosis is compensation.
       (1) Acute respiratory alkalosis, serum $HCO_3^- \geq 18$ mEq/L
       (2) Chronic respiratory alkalosis, serum $HCO_3^- < 18$ mEq/L but > 12 mEq/L
  3. Calculation of expected compensation in acute respiratory alkalosis
     a. Expected $\Delta HCO_3^- = 0.20 \times \Delta Pa_{CO_2}$ (difference from normal of 40 mm Hg)
     b. Example—pH 7.56, Pa_{CO_2} 24 mm Hg, HCO_3^- 21 mEq/L
       (1) Expected $\Delta HCO_3^- = 0.20 \times (40 - 24) = 3.2$ mEq/L
       (2) Expected $HCO_3^- = 24$ mEq/L (mean HCO_3^-) $- 3.2 = 20.8$ mEq/L
         • Note that measured and expected calculated HCO_3^- are similar.
  4. Calculation of expected compensation in chronic respiratory alkalosis
     a. Expected $\Delta HCO_3^- = 0.50 \times \Delta Pa_{CO_2}$
     b. Example—pH 7.47, Pa_{CO_2} 18 mm Hg, HCO_3^- 13 mEq/L
       (1) Expected $\Delta HCO_3^- = 0.50 \times (40 - 18) = 11$ mEq/L
       (2) Expected $\Delta HCO_3^- = 24 - 11 = 13$ mEq/L
         • Note that measured and expected calculated HCO_3^- are similar.
  5. Clinical findings in respiratory alkalosis
     a. Alkalosis increases the number of negative charges on albumin.
       (1) Additional calcium is bound by albumin.
       (2) Ionized calcium level is decreased causing tetany.
     b. Signs of tetany
       (1) Thumb adduction into the palm (carpopedal spasm)
       (2) Perioral twitching when the facial nerve is tapped (Chvostek sign)
       (3) Perioral numbness and tingling

Respiratory alkalosis: anxiety most common cause

Respiratory alkalosis: signs of tetany

C. **Metabolic acidosis**
1. Serum $HCO_3^- < 22$ mEq/L (normal 22–28 mEq/L)
   - $\downarrow$ pH ~ $\downarrow\downarrow$ HCO_3^-/$\downarrow$ P_{CO_2}
2. Respiratory alkalosis is compensation.
3. Calculation of the expected compensation
   a. Expected $\Delta Paco_2 = 1.2 \times \Delta HCO_3^- \pm 2$
      - ΔHCO_3^- is measured HCO_3^- subtracted from the mean HCO_3^- of 24 mEq/L.
   b. Example—pH 7.27, $\Delta Paco_2$ 27 mm Hg, HCO_3^- 12 mEq/L
      (1) Expected $\Delta Paco_2 = 1.2 \times (24 - 12) = 14.4$ mm Hg
      (2) Expected $Paco_2 = 40$ (mean $Paco_2$) $- 14.4 = 25.6$ mm Hg (23.6–27.6)
         - Note that measured $Paco_2$ is within the calculated range.
4. Anion gap (AG)

Anion gap: detects anions of acids (e.g., lactate anions)

   (1) Distinguishes increased AG metabolic acidosis from normal AG metabolic acidosis
   (2) $AG = $ serum $Na^+ - $ (serum $Cl^- + $ serum HCO_3^-) $= 12$ mEq/L ± 2
      (a) *Not all* analytes with a positive and negative charge are in the formula.
      (b) AG of 12 mEq/L represents anions *not* accounted for in the formula.
         - Examples—albumin, phosphorus, sulfate, organic acids

> **Another approach to calculating the AG** is to add up all the unmeasured anions (UA) that are *not* in the formula—albumin (15 mEq/L), organic acids (5 mEq/L), phosphate (2 mEq/L), sulfate (1 mEq/L)—and to subtract the sum of the unmeasured cations (UC)—calcium (5.0 mEq/L), potassium (4.5 mEq/L), magnesium (1.5 mEq/L). The AG (UA – UC) is equal to 12 mEq/L. Using this concept, an increase in the AG may be due to an increase in UAs that are *not* normally present (e.g., lactate, salicylate) or a decrease in UAs that are normally present (e.g., hypoalbuminemia). A decrease in the AG may be due to an increase in UCs that are normally present (e.g., hypercalcemia, hyperkalemia) or an increase in UCs that are *not* normally present (e.g., increase in immunoglobulins in multiple myeloma).

5. Increased anion gap metabolic acidosis
   a. Epidemiology

↑ Anion gap metabolic acidosis: lactic acidosis most common cause

      - Causes of increased AG metabolic acidosis (Table 2-6)

> **Calculation of the osmolal gap** is useful in evaluating causes of an increased AG metabolic acidosis. The plasma osmolality (POsm) is calculated: POsm = 2 (serum Na^+) + serum glucose/18 + serum blood urea nitrogen/2.8 + serum ethanol (mg/dL)/4.6 (if the patient is drinking ethanol) and is then

TABLE 2-6
Causes of Increased Anion Gap Metabolic Acidosis

Causes	Pathogenesis
Lactic acidosis	Most common type
	Any cause of tissue hypoxia with concomitant anaerobic glycolysis: e.g., shock, CN poisoning, CO poisoning, severe hypoxemia ($PaO_2 < 35$ mm Hg), CHF, severe anemia (Hb < 6 g/dL)
	Alcoholism: pyruvate is converted to lactate from the excess of NADH in alcohol metabolism
	Liver disease: liver normally converts lactate to pyruvate; liver disease (e.g., hepatitis, cirrhosis) causes lactate to accumulate in the blood
	Drugs: e.g., phenformin
Ketoacidosis	Diabetic ketoacidosis (type 1 diabetes mellitus): accumulation of AcAc and β-OHB
	Alcoholism: acetyl CoA in alcohol metabolism is converted to ketoacids
	Increase in NADH causes AcAc to convert to β-OHB, which is not detected with standard tests for ketone bodies
	Starvation
Renal failure	Retention of organic acids: e.g., sulfuric and phosphoric acids
Salicylate poisoning	Salicylic acid is an acid; it is also a mitochondrial toxin that uncouples oxidative phosphorylation leading to tissue hypoxia and lactic acidosis; in some cases, excess salicylate overstimulates the CNS respiratory center producing a primary respiratory alkalosis
Ethylene glycol poisoning	Ethylene glycol is in antifreeze; it is converted to glycolic and oxalic acid by alcohol dehydrogenase; oxalate anions combine with calcium to produce calcium oxalate crystals that obstruct the renal tubules causing renal failure; IV infusion of ethanol decreases the metabolism of ethylene glycol, because alcohol dehydrogenase is preferentially metabolizing alcohol; unmetabolized ethylene glycol is removed by hemodialysis; another treatment is the use of 4-methylpyrazole, which inhibits alcohol dehydrogenase
	Osmolal gap >10 mOsm/kg
Methyl alcohol poisoning	Methyl alcohol is present in window shield washer fluid, Sterno, and solvents for paints; it is converted into formic acid by alcohol dehydrogenase; formic acid damages the optic nerve causing optic neuritis and the potential for permanent blindness; IV infusion of ethanol decreases the metabolism of methyl alcohol, because alcohol dehydrogenase is preferentially metabolizing alcohol; another treatment is the use of 4-methylpyrazole, which inhibits alcohol dehydrogenase
	Osmolal gap >10 mOsm/kg

AcAc, acetoacetate; β-OHB, β-hydroxybutyrate; CHF, congestive heart failure; CN, cyanide; CO, carbon monoxide; Hb, hemoglobin; IV, intravenous.

subtracted from the measured POsm. A difference of <10 mOsm/kg is normal. A difference of >10 mOsm/kg is highly suspicious for methanol or ethylene glycol poisoning.

   b. Pathogenesis of increased AG metabolic acidosis
      (1) Excess H^+ ions are buffered by HCO_3^-, which decreases the serum HCO_3^-.
      (2) Every HCO_3^- lost is replaced by an anion of the acid (e.g., lactate) to maintain electroneutrality (Fig. 2-12A).

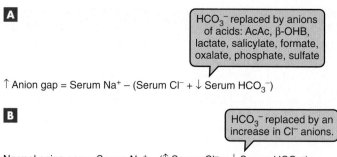

A

> HCO_3^- replaced by anions of acids: AcAc, β-OHB, lactate, salicylate, formate, oxalate, phosphate, sulfate

↑ Anion gap = Serum Na^+ − (Serum Cl^- + ↓ Serum HCO_3^-)

B

> HCO_3^- replaced by an increase in Cl^- anions.

Normal anion gap = Serum Na^+ − (↑ Serum Cl^- + ↓ Serum HCO_3^-)

2-12: *Increased anion gap metabolic acidosis (**A**) and normal anion gap metabolic acidosis (**B**). See text for description. AcAc, acetoacetate, β-OHB, β-hydroxybutyrate.*

(3) Example—serum Na^+ 130 mEq/L (136–145), serum Cl^- 88 mEq/L (95–105), serum HCO_3^- 10 mEq/L (22–28)

    (a) AG = 130 − (88 + 10) = 32 mEq/L (12 mEq/L ± 2)

    (b) Drop in HCO_3^- from 24 mEq/L to 10 mEq/L is balanced by a 14 mEq/L increase in anions of the acid (e.g., lactate, salicylate).

6. Normal anion gap metabolic acidosis

  a. Epidemiology

    • Causes of a normal AG metabolic acidosis (Table 2-7)

  b. Pathogenesis

    (1) Decrease in HCO_3^- due to

      (a) Loss of HCO_3^- from the gastrointestinal tract or urinary tract

      (b) Inability to regenerate HCO_3^- in the H^+/K^+-ATPase pump

    (2) Decreased HCO_3^- is counterbalanced by a corresponding increase in Cl^- anions (Fig. 2-12B).

      • Hyperchloremic normal AG metabolic acidosis

  c. Example—serum Na^+ 136 mEq/L, serum Cl^- 110 mEq/L, serum HCO_3^- 14 mEq/L.

    (1) AG = 136 − (110 + 14) = 12 mEq/L

    (2) 10 mEq/L drop of HCO_3^- from normal (24 − 14 = 10)

    (3) 10 mEq/L increase in Cl^- ions from normal (100 + 10 = 110)

7. Clinical findings in metabolic acidosis

  a. Hyperventilation (Kussmaul breathing)

  b. Warm skin

    • Acidosis vasodilates peripheral resistance arterioles.

  c. Osteoporosis

    • Bone buffers the excess H^+ ions.

D. **Metabolic alkalosis**

  1. $HCO_3^- > 28$ mEq/L

    • ↑ pH ~ ↑↑ HCO_3^-/↑Pco_2

  2. Respiratory acidosis is compensation.

  3. Calculation of expected compensation

Normal anion gap metabolic acidosis: diarrhea most common cause

TABLE 2-7
Causes of Normal
Anion Gap
Metabolic Acidosis

Causes	Pathogenesis
Diarrhea	Most common type in children Loss of HCO_3^- in stool: HCO_3^- is secreted from the pancreas to alkalinize the gastric meal
Cholestyramine	Binds HCO_3^- as well as bile salts, vitamins, and some drugs
Drainage of bile or pancreatic secretions	Bile and pancreatic secretions contain large amounts of HCO_3^-
Type I distal renal tubular acidosis	Inability to regenerate HCO_3^- in the H^+/K^+-ATPase pump in the collecting tubules Excess H^+ ions in the blood combine with Cl^- anions; hypokalemia is severe Inability to secrete H^+ ions decreases titratable acidity and NH_4Cl causing the urine pH to be >5.5 Causes: amphotericin, light chains in multiple myeloma Rx: oral administration of HCO_3^-
Type II proximal renal tubular acidosis	Renal threshold for reclaiming HCO_3^- is lowered from a normal of ~24 mEq/L to ~15 mEq/L Urine pH is initially >5.5 due to loss of filtered HCO_3^- in the urine; when the serum HCO_3^- is equal to the renal threshold, the proximal tubules reclaim HCO_3^- causing the urine pH to drop to <5.5. Hypokalemia may occur due to K^+ binding to HCO_3^- Causes: carbonic anhydrase inhibitors (most common cause), primary hyperparathyroidism ($\uparrow$ PTH, $\downarrow$ proximal tubule HCO_3^- reclamation), proximal tubule nephrotoxic drugs/chemicals (e.g., aminoglycosides, heavy metals) Rx: thiazides to produce volume depletion, which increases the renal threshold for reclaiming HCO_3^-
Type IV renal tubular acidosis	Due to destruction of the JG apparatus: e.g., hyaline arteriolosclerosis of afferent arterioles in DM, acute or chronic tubulointerstitial inflammation (e.g., legionnaires' disease) Produces hyporeninemic hypoaldosteronism Only RTA with hyperkalemia: due to hypoaldosteronism

DM, diabetes mellitus; JG, juxtaglomerular; PTH, parathyroid hormone; RTA, renal tubular acidosis; Rx, treatment.

a. Expected $\Delta Paco_2 = 0.7 \times \Delta HCO_3^- \pm 2$
b. Example—pH 7.58, $Paco_2$ 49 mm Hg, HCO_3^- 39 mEq/L
  (1) Expected $\Delta Paco_2 = 0.7 \times (39 - 24) = 10.5$
  (2) Expected $Paco_2 = 40 + 10.5 = 50.5$ mm Hg (48.5–52.5)
     • Note that measured $Paco_2$ is within the calculated range.
 4. Epidemiology
   • Causes of metabolic alkalosis (Table 2-8)
 5. Pathogenesis of metabolic alkalosis
  a. Generation phase of metabolic alkalosis
    (1) Loss of H^+ ions (e.g., vomiting)
    (2) Addition of HCO_3^- (e.g., aldosterone excess)
  b. Maintenance phase of metabolic alkalosis in vomiting
    (1) Volume depletion from vomiting raises renal threshold for reclaiming HCO_3^-.

Metabolic alkalosis: vomiting most common cause

TABLE 2-8
Causes of Metabolic Alkalosis

Causes	Pathogenesis
Vomiting	Volume depletion increases proximal tubule reabsorption of Na^+, which increases the reclamation of HCO_3^-. Correction of volume depletion with 0.9% normal saline corrects the alkalosis (chloride-responsive).
Mineralocorticoid excess	There is enhanced function of aldosterone-mediated channels (Na^+-H^+) and pumps (H^+/K^+-ATPase), both of which increase the synthesis of HCO_3^-, leading to metabolic alkalosis. Infusion of 0.9% normal saline does *not* correct the metabolic alkalosis (chloride-resistant). Causes: primary aldosteronism, Bartter's syndrome, 11-hydroxylase deficiency, Cushing's syndrome
Thiazide and loop diuretics	There is augmented late distal and collecting tubule reabsorption of Na^+ and secretion of H^+, the latter increasing synthesis of HCO_3^- leading to metabolic alkalosis. Volume depletion also increases the proximal tubule reclamation of HCO_3^-, which maintains the metabolic alkalosis. Replacing volume deficits with normal saline corrects the alkalosis (chloride responsive).
Milk-alkali syndrome	There is chronic ingestion of milk or calcium carbonate antacids leading to hypercalcemia and metabolic alkalosis. Hypercalcemia causes calcium to deposit in the renal tubule basement membranes (nephrocalcinosis), which produces renal failure.
Conversion of precursors to HCO_3^-	Acetate (in volume expanders), lactate (in Ringer's lactate), and citrate (in blood transfusions) are metabolic precursors for HCO_3^-.
High-dose carbenicillin or penicillin	IV administration of high doses of Na^+-carbenicillin or other penicillin derivatives produces hypokalemia and metabolic alkalosis. Carbenicillin acts as a nonabsorbable anion and increases luminal negativity, which increases the loss of H^+ and K^+ ions. Loss of K^+ causes hypokalemia. Loss of H^+ produces a corresponding increase in the synthesis of HCO_3^- causing metabolic alkalosis.

IV, intravenous.

- Volume depletion is the key factor affecting the maintenance phase.
  (2) Most of the excess HCO_3^- filtered is reclaimed in the proximal tubule.
  (3) Infusion of 0.9% NaCl corrects alkalosis by correcting volume depletion.
     (a) Renal threshold for reclaiming HCO_3^- returns to normal.
     (b) Chloride-responsive type of metabolic alkalosis
  c. Maintenance phase of metabolic alkalosis in mineralocorticoid excess
     - Excess aldosterone increases synthesis of HCO_3^- (see IV.D.5)
     - Infusion of 0.9% NaCl does *not* correct the alkalosis.
        - Chloride-resistant metabolic alkalosis

TABLE 2-9
Mixed Acid-Base Disorders

A. Primary metabolic acidosis + Primary respiratory alkalosis

	pH	$PaCO_2$	HCO_3^-
Metabolic acidosis	↓	↓	↓↓
Respiratory alkalosis	↑	↓↓	↓
Final blood gas	↔	↓↓↓	↓↓↓

B. Primary respiratory acidosis + Primary metabolic alkalosis

	pH	$PaCO_2$	HCO_3^-
Respiratory acidosis	↓	↑↑	↑
Metabolic alkalosis	↑	↑	↑↑
Final blood gas	↔	↑↑↑	↑↑↑

C. Primary metabolic acidosis + Primary metabolic alkalosis

	pH	$PaCO_2$	HCO_3^-
Metabolic acidosis	↓	↓	↓↓
Metabolic alkalosis	↑	↑	↑↑
Final blood gas	↔	↔	↔

D. Primary metabolic acidosis + Primary respiratory acidosis

	pH	$PaCO_2$	HCO_3^-
Metabolic acidosis	↓	↓	↓↓
Respiratory acidosis	↓	↑↑	↑
Final blood gas	↓↓	↑	↓

E. Primary metabolic alkalosis + Primary respiratory alkalosis

	pH	$PaCO_2$	HCO_3^-
Metabolic alkalosis	↑	↑	↑↑
Respiratory alkalosis	↑	↓↓	↓
Final blood gas	↑↑	↓	↑

Arrows represent degrees of magnitude.

6. Clinical findings
    a. Increased risk for ventricular arrhythmias; due to
        (1) Metabolic alkalosis, which left-shifts the oxygen-binding curve
        (2) Respiratory acidosis (compensation), which decreases PaO_2
    b. Tetany (see respiratory alkalosis discussion, Section IVB)

E. **Mixed acid-base disorders**
    1. Multiple acid-base disorders occurring at the same time
    2. Clues suggesting a mixed disorder
        a. Mixed primary acidosis and primary alkalosis produces a normal pH
          (Table 2-9A); examples follow:
          (1) Primary metabolic acidosis + primary respiratory alkalosis
            • Examples—endotoxic shock or salicylate intoxication
            (a) Shock produces lactic acidosis and salicylic acid produces an
               increased AG metabolic acidosis.
            (b) Endotoxins and salicylate anions overstimulate the CNS
               respiratory center causing respiratory alkalosis.
          (2) Primary respiratory acidosis + primary metabolic alkalosis (see
            Table 2-9B)
            • Example—patient with chronic bronchitis who is taking a loop
              diuretic

Mixed acid-base disorder: combination of two or more acid-base disorders

TABLE 2-10
Examples of Electrolyte Disorders

Serum Na⁺ (136–145 mEq/L*)	Serum K⁺ (3.5–5.0 mEq/L*)	Serum Cl⁻ (95–105 mEq/L*)	Serum HCO₃⁻ (22–28 mEq/L*)	Discussion
118	3.0	84	22	SIADH: dilutional effect on all electrolytes
128	5.9	96	20	Addison's disease: electrolyte effects due to ↓ aldosterone
				Normal AG metabolic acidosis
138	4.8	90	10	↑ AG metabolic acidosis (e.g., lactic acidosis)
				DKA: dilutional hyponatremia would be present from hyperglycemia
				K⁺ may be normal to increased (shift of K⁺ for H⁺)
146	5.5	104	18	Renal failure: tubular function in all parts of the nephron are dysfunctional
				↑ AG metabolic acidosis (e.g., organic acids)
138	2.2	114	14	Normal AG metabolic acidosis
				Causes: adult diarrhea, type I and II RTA. Type IV RTA has hyperkalemia
130	2.9	80	36	Hyponatremia, hypokalemia, metabolic alkalosis
				Causes: thiazides, loop diuretics, vomiting
152	2.8	110	33	Hypernatremia, hypokalemia, metabolic alkalosis
				Mineralocorticoid excess: primary aldosteronism, Cushing's syndrome, 11-hydroxylase deficiency

*Range of normal values.
AG, anion gap; DKA, diabetic ketoacidosis; RTA, renal tubular acidosis; SIADH, syndrome of inappropriate antidiuretic hormone.

   (a) Chronic obstructive lung disease produces respiratory acidosis.
   (b) Loop diuretics produce metabolic alkalosis.
 (3) Primary metabolic acidosis + primary metabolic alkalosis (see Table 2-9C)
   • Example—diabetic in ketoacidosis who is vomiting

TABLE 2-11
Examples of Acid-Base Disorders

pH (7.35–7.45*)	Paco₂ (33–45 mm Hg*)	HCO₃⁻ (22–28 mEq/L*)	Discussion
7.00	52	13	Mixed disorder: primary metabolic acidosis + primary respiratory acidosis Example: cardiogenic shock with respiratory arrest
7.20	74	28	Uncompensated acute respiratory acidosis Examples: CNS respiratory center depression, severe bronchial asthma, upper airway obstruction
7.33	60	31	Partially compensated chronic respiratory acidosis Examples: chronic bronchitis, cystic fibrosis, bronchiectasis
7.28	28	12	Partially compensated metabolic acidosis Examples: disorders associated with increased and normal AG metabolic acidosis
7.38	70	40	Mixed disorder: primary respiratory acidosis + primary metabolic alkalosis. Example: CB + loop diuretic/vomiting
7.38	40	23	Normal or mixed disorder with primary metabolic acidosis + primary metabolic alkalosis Example: patient with DKA who is vomiting
7.42	22	14	Mixed disorder: primary metabolic acidosis + primary respiratory alkalosis Examples: salicylate poisoning, endotoxic shock
7.50	47	35	Partially compensated metabolic alkalosis Causes: loop/thiazide diuretics, vomiting, mineralocorticoid excess
7.56	24	21	Partially compensated acute respiratory alkalosis Causes: anxiety, pulmonary embolus, normal pregnancy

*Range of normal values.
AG, anion gap; CNS, central nervous system; CB, chronic bronchitis; DKA, diabetic ketoacidosis.

      (a) Ketoacidosis causes an increased AG metabolic acidosis
      (b) Vomiting produces a metabolic alkalosis
  b. Mixed primary metabolic acidosis + primary respiratory acidosis causing extreme acidemia (see Table 2-9D)
    • Example—cardiogenic shock causing respiratory arrest
    (1) Cardiogenic shock produces lactic acidosis.
    (2) Respiratory arrest produces respiratory acidosis.
  c. Mixed primary metabolic alkalosis + primary respiratory alkalosis producing extreme alkalemia (see Table 2-9E)
    • Example—pregnant woman who is vomiting
    (1) Pregnancy produces respiratory alkalosis.
    (2) Vomiting produces metabolic alkalosis.
F. **Examples of electrolyte disorders** (Table 2-10)
G. **Examples of acid-base disorders** (Table 2-11)

Questions

Each numbered item is followed by options arranged in alphabetical or logical order. Select the best answer to each question. Some options may be partially correct, but there is only *one best* answer.

1. A 50-year-old man complains of muscle weakness. An electrocardiogram (ECG) shows prominent U waves in lead V_3. Which of the following drugs is most likely responsible for these findings?
   A. Aldosterone blocker
   B. β-Blocker
   C. Digitalis
   D. Loop diuretic

2. A 55-year-old woman complains of muscle weakness. An electrocardiogram (ECG) shows peaked T waves in lead V_3. Which of the following is most likely responsible for these findings?
   A. Chronic renal failure
   B. Diarrhea
   C. Primary aldosteronism
   D. Type I renal tubular acidosis
   E. Vomiting

3. A 40-year-old man develops increased thirst and frequency of urination 6 weeks after hitting his head on the windshield in an automobile accident. Which of the following laboratory findings is expected if the patient is deprived of water?

	POsm	Serum ADH
A.	Decreased	Decreased
B.	Decreased	Increased
C.	Increased	Decreased
D.	Increased	Increased

ADH, antidiuretic hormone; POsm, plasma osmolality.

4. A 40-year-old man is found unconscious under a bridge. An empty container of antifreeze is found next to the man. Initial laboratory test findings in the emergency room show the following:
   Serum bicarbonate: 14 mEq/L (22–28 mEq/L)
   Serum blood urea nitrogen (BUN): 40 mg/dL (7–18 mg/dL)
   Serum creatinine: 4 mg/dL (0.6–1.2 mg/dL)
   Urine dipstick test: negative for ketone bodies and glucose
   Sediment examination: calcium oxalate crystals
   Osmolal gap = 25 mOsm/kg (<10 mOsm/kg)

What is the most likely diagnosis?
A. Diabetic ketoacidosis
B. Ethylene glycol poisoning
C. Isopropyl alcohol poisoning
D. Methyl alcohol poisoning

Use the following chart to answer questions 5 through 13:

	pH 7.35–7.45	$PaCO_2$ 33–45 mm Hg	HCO_3^- 22–28 mEq/L
A.	7.00	52	13
B.	7.20	74	28
C.	7.33	60	31
D.	7.28	28	12
E.	7.38	70	40
F.	7.38	40	23
G.	7.42	22	14
H.	7.50	47	35
I.	7.56	24	21

Each lettered entry in the chart indicates a set of options relating to arterial blood gas disorders. For questions 5 through 13, select the *one* lettered option that is most closely associated with it. Each lettered option may be selected once, more than once, or not at all.

5. A 52-year-old man has a history of smoking two packs of cigarettes a day for the past 35 years. He has coughed up a tablespoon or more of yellow-green sputum almost every morning for the past 10 years. Physical examination shows cyanosis of the skin and mucous membranes and scattered coarse inspiratory crackles in the lungs that clear with coughing.

6. A 49-year-old woman complains of muscle weakness and increased frequency of urination. Physical examination reveals hypertension. A random urine potassium is increased. An electrocardiogram (ECG) shows prominent U waves. A CT scan shows a nodular mass in the right adrenal gland.

7. An obese, 43-year-old woman develops fever, tachypnea, dyspnea, and right lower lobe pleuritic type chest pain 4 days after removal of an acutely inflamed gallbladder. Her right calf is swollen and tender to compression.

8. A comatose 32-year-old woman is brought to the emergency room. An empty bottle of barbiturates was found next to her bed along with a suicide note.

9. A 72-year-old man is in hypovolemic shock secondary to blood loss from a ruptured abdominal aortic aneurysm.

10. A 52-year-old man with a 35-year history of smoking cigarettes has chronic bronchitis and right-sided heart failure secondary to pulmonary hypertension. He is currently taking a loop diuretic for the right-sided heart failure and is not receiving any potassium supplements.

11. A 62-year-old woman develops cardiogenic shock and respiratory arrest while in the emergency room. An arterial blood gas is drawn prior to resuscitation.

12. A 46-year-old woman with rheumatoid arthritis, who takes aspirin for pain, develops ringing in her ears.

13. A 25-year-old man with type 1 diabetes mellitus presents to a local emergency room with vomiting and ketoacidosis. Physical examination reveals dry mucous membranes, poor skin turgor, and hypotension. A urine dipstick for glucose and ketone bodies is strongly positive.

Refer to the following chart for questions 14 though 21:

	Serum Na$^+$	TBNa$^+$
A.	Decreased	Decreased
B.	Decreased	Increased
C.	Decreased	Normal
D.	Increased	Decreased
E.	Increased	Increased
F.	Increased	Normal
G.	Normal	Decreased
H.	Normal	Increased

Each letter in the chart describes a set of options relating serum sodium (Na$^+$) and total body sodium (TBNa$^+$) to different volume disorders. For questions 14 through 21, select the *one* lettered option that is most closely associated with it. In answering these questions, each lettered option may be selected once, more than once, or not at all.

14. A 49-year-old man has alcoholic cirrhosis, ascites, and dependent pitting edema.

15. A 24-year-old man collapses at the end of a marathon. His running partner states that his friend was sweating profusely throughout the race and did not replenish his fluid losses. The physical examination shows dry mucous membranes and poor skin turgor. His blood pressure is 110/70 mm Hg and pulse rate is 120 beats/minute when lying down. When sitting up, the blood pressure drops to 80/60 mm Hg and the pulse rate increases to 150 beats/minute.

16. A 48-year-old woman with type 2 diabetes mellitus is receiving chlorpropamide. She develops headaches and problems with memory. The skin turgor is normal.

17. A 78-year-old man with a history of chronic ischemic heart disease requires a prostate transurethral resection for urinary retention secondary to prostate hyperplasia. During the procedure, he is infused with an excessive amount of 0.9% normal saline. Following surgery he develops dyspnea. Physical examination demonstrates bibasilar crackles.

18. A 72-year-old man with a history of chronic renal disease develops neck vein distention, bibasilar crackles, and dependent pitting edema within 24 hours after receiving multiple ampules of intravenous sodium bicarbonate (hypertonic saline) during a cardiorespiratory arrest.

19. A 19-year-old man with type 1 diabetes mellitus develops ketoacidosis. Physical examination shows dry mucous membranes and poor skin turgor. The blood pressure lying down and sitting up is decreased and the pulse rate is increased. The serum glucose is 800 mg/dL and ketone bodies are increased in plasma and urine.

20. An afebrile 28-year-old medical student who spent spring break in Tijuana, Mexico, develops travelers' diarrhea. Physical examination demonstrates dry mucous membranes, poor skin turgor, and hypotension.

21. An 82-year-old man in a nursing home has 105°F temperature from a lobar pneumonia due to *Klebsiella pneumoniae.* The mucous membranes are well hydrated and the blood pressure is normal.

Use the following chart to answer questions 22 though 27:

	Serum Na$^+$ (136–145 mEq/L)	Serum K$^+$ (3.5–5.0 mEq/L)	Serum Cl$^-$ (95–105 mEq/L)	Serum HCO$_3^-$ (22–28 mEq/L)
A.	118	3.0	84	22
B.	128	5.9	96	20
C.	146	5.5	104	18
D.	138	2.2	114	14
E.	130	2.9	80	36
F.	152	2.8	110	33

Each letter in the chart describes a set of options relating to acid-base disorders. For questions 22 through 27, select the *one* lettered option that is most closely associated with it. In answering these questions each lettered option may be selected once, more than once, or not at all.

22. A 65-year-old woman who has smoked cigarettes for the past 45 years develops a cough, weight loss, and diffuse cerebral edema. Physical examination reveals coarse inspiratory crackles in both lungs. A chest radiograph shows a centrally located mass in the left hilum. A sputum cytology report states that small, hyperchromatic malignant cells are present consistent with a small cell carcinoma.

23. A 49-year-old man has fatigue and postural hypotension. Physical examination reveals dry mucous membranes, an increase in heart rate, and drop in blood pressure when moved from the supine to sitting position, and increased pigmentation of the buccal mucosa and skin. Laboratory studies show a decrease in serum cortisol and an increase in serum adrenocorticotropic hormone (ACTH). A peaked T wave is present on an electrocardiogram (ECG).

24. A 48-year-old man with essential hypertension has muscle weakness and clinical evidence of volume depletion. He is currently taking a thiazide diuretic. An ECG shows prominent U waves.

25. A 36-year-old woman with focal segmental glomerulosclerosis secondary to intravenous heroin abuse has chronic renal failure. The serum blood urea nitrogen (BUN) is 60 mg/dL (7–18) and serum creatinine is 6.0 mg/dL (0.6–1.2). An ECG shows peaked T waves.

26. A 34-year-old missionary in India develops cholera. Physical examination shows dry mucous membranes, poor skin turgor, and hypotension.

27. A 35-year-old woman who is a painter in a pottery factory complains of recurrent abdominal pain, diarrhea, and muscle weakness. A urinalysis reveals a positive dipstick for glucose and an alkaline urine pH. A blood lead level is increased.

Answers

1. **D** (loop diuretic) is correct. Loop diuretics commonly produce hypokalemia (decreased serum K^+ concentration). Hypokalemia produces muscle weakness due to changes in the intracellular and extracellular K^+ membrane potential. The characteristic ECG pattern of hypokalemia is a U wave following the T wave. Loop diuretics cause hypokalemia by blocking the chloride binding site in the Na^+-K^+-$2Cl^-$ cotransporter in the medullary segment of the thick ascending limb. This leads to increased exchange of Na^+ for K^+ in the aldosterone-dependent Na^+-K^+ channels of the late distal and collecting tubules causing increased urinary loss of K^+. If the patient was taking K^+ supplements, hypokalemia would not have occurred.

A (aldosterone blocker) is incorrect. An aldosterone blocker (e.g., spironolactone) interferes with the normal exchange of Na^+ for K^+ in the late distal and collecting tubules causing increased urinary loss of Na^+ and retention of K^+ (hyperkalemia). Hyperkalemia produces peaked T waves on an ECG.

B (β-blocker) is incorrect. β-Blockers inhibit the Na^+/K^+-ATPase pump, causing Na^+ to move into cells and K^+ out of cells causing hyperkalemia.

C (digitalis) is incorrect. Digitalis inhibits the Na^+/K^+-ATPase pump in cardiac muscle, which causes Na^+ to move into the muscle and K^+ out of the muscle. Hyperkalemia is a potential complication of digitalis toxicity.

2. **A** (chronic renal failure) is correct. In chronic renal failure, the aldosterone-dependent Na^+ and K^+ channels in the late distal and collecting ducts are dysfunctional. This causes retention of K^+ (hyperkalemia). The characteristic electrocardiogram finding of hyperkalemia is the presence of peaked T waves, which are caused by accelerated repolarization of cardiac muscle. Any increase or decrease in K^+ concentration produces conduction disturbances in muscle that culminate in muscle weakness.

B (diarrhea) is incorrect. Diarrhea is associated with a loss of Na^+-containing fluid, loss of HCO_3^- (metabolic acidosis), and loss of K^+ (hypokalemia). The characteristic ECG pattern of hypokalemia is a U wave following the T wave.

C (primary aldosteronism) is incorrect. An increase in aldosterone enhances the activity of the Na^+-K^+ channels in the late distal and collecting ducts causing a gain in Na^+ (hypernatremia) and a loss of K^+ (hypokalemia).

D (type I renal tubular acidosis) is incorrect. Type I (distal) renal tubular acidosis is due to dysfunction of the aldosterone-dependent H^+/K^+-ATPase pump in the collecting tubules. This causes retention of H^+ ions (metabolic acidosis) and loss of K^+ in the urine leading to hypokalemia. H^+ ions combine with Cl^- ions, which produces a normal anion gap type of metabolic acidosis.

E (vomiting) is incorrect. Vomiting causes metabolic alkalosis due to the loss of acid and retention of HCO_3^-. Alkalosis causes a transcellular shift of H^+ ions out of cells in exchange for K^+ causing hypokalemia.

3. **C** (POsm increased, serum ADH decreased) is correct. The patient has central diabetes insipidus (absence of ADH) caused by transection of the pituitary stalk from a previous automobile accident. ADH is synthesized in the hypothalamus and travels through the pituitary stalk to the posterior pituitary, where it is stored and secreted. ADH is required to concentrate urine by reabsorbing electrolyte free water from the collecting tubules of the kidneys. Therefore, absence of ADH causes polyuria (increased urinary frequency) due to a loss of free water in the urine. When the patient is deprived of water, the urine osmolality (UOsm) decreases and the serum plasma osmolality (POsm) increases, due to the loss in water. An increase in POsm corresponds with an increase in serum Na^+ (hypernatremia). An increase in POsm stimulates thirst.

A (POsm decreased, serum ADH decreased) is incorrect. A decrease in POsm and a decrease in serum ADH occurs in normal dilution of urine. A decrease in POsm inhibits the release of ADH, causing a loss of free water in the urine.

B (POsm decreased, serum ADH increased) is incorrect. A decrease in POsm and an increase in serum ADH occurs when there is inappropriate secretion of ADH. This is most often caused by ectopic secretion of ADH by a primary small cell carcinoma of the lung in a patient who is a cigarette smoker. An excess of ADH causes increased reabsorption of electrolyte free water causing a dilutional hyponatremia and a corresponding decrease in POsm.

D (POsm increased, serum ADH increased) is incorrect. An increase in POsm and an increase in ADH occurs in normal concentration of urine. An increase in POsm stimulates the release of ADH, which increases reabsorption of electrolyte free water.

4. **B** (ethylene glycol poisoning) is correct. Ethylene glycol is present in antifreeze. It is converted by alcohol dehydrogenase to oxalic acid, which forms calcium oxalate crystals in the kidney tubules and other tissues. Obstruction of the renal tubules produces renal failure (increased serum blood urea nitrogen and creatinine) and metabolic acidosis (decreased serum bicarbonate), because bicarbonate is used up in buffering excess hydrogen ions. The metabolic acidosis is of the increased anion gap type with oxalate anions replacing the lost bicarbonate anions. The osmolal gap is increased in ethylene glycol poisoning. It is calculated by subtracting the calculated POsm—2 (serum Na^+) + serum glucose/18 + serum blood urea nitrogen/2.8—from the measured POsm.

A (diabetic ketoacidosis) is incorrect. Although diabetic ketoacidosis produces a metabolic acidosis, the urine dipstick test is negative for ketone bodies and glucose, which excludes that diagnosis.

C (isopropyl alcohol poisoning) is incorrect. Isopropyl alcohol, or rubbing alcohol, is converted to acetone, which gives a fruity odor to the breath. Calcium oxalate crystals and metabolic acidosis are *not* produced in this type of poisoning.

D (methyl alcohol poisoning) is incorrect. Methyl alcohol (methanol) is present in solvents such as window washing fluid. When ingested, it is converted to formic acid by alcohol dehydrogenase. Formic acid damages the optic nerve causing optic neuritis and the potential for blindness. Unlike ethylene glycol poisoning, it does *not* produce renal failure. An increase in formic acid produces an increased anion gap metabolic acidosis, since formate is an anion and bicarbonate is used up in buffering excess hydrogen ions. The osmolal gap is increased in methyl alcohol poisoning.

5. **C** (pH 7.33, $Paco_2$ 60, HCO_3^- 31) is correct. The patient has chronic bronchitis (productive cough for 10 years) caused by smoking cigarettes. Hypoxemia (decreased Pao_2) causes a decrease in O_2 saturation, which accounts for the patient's cyanosis. Chronic bronchitis is characterized by obstruction of airflow out of the lung due to inflammation and increased mucus production in the terminal bronchioles. During expiration, CO_2 is trapped behind mucus plugs causing retention of CO_2 and respiratory acidosis (pH 7.33, $Paco_2$ 60 mm Hg). Compensation for respiratory acidosis is metabolic alkalosis (HCO_3^- 31 mEq/L). Because the bronchitis is chronic, the kidney is involved in the compensation process, which explains why the HCO_3^- is >30 mEq/L.

6. **H** (pH 7.50, $Paco_2$ 47, HCO_3^- 35) is correct. The hypertension is caused by an adrenal adenoma that is secreting aldosterone (primary aldosteronism). Hyperaldosteronism leads to an increased exchange of Na^+ for K^+ in the late distal and collecting tubules, causing an increase in serum Na^+ and a decrease in serum K^+ (hypokalemia) from urinary loss of K^+. Hypokalemia produces prominent U waves (positive wave after the T wave) on an ECG and causes muscle weakness due to a lack of muscle repolarization. Once K^+ is depleted, Na^+ exchanges for H^+ ions, which causes increased synthesis and reabsorption of HCO_3^- (metabolic alkalosis; pH 7.50, serum HCO_3^- 35 mEq/L). The compensation for metabolic alkalosis is respiratory acidosis ($Paco_2$ 47 mm Hg). Increased frequency of urination is due to vacuolar nephropathy of the collecting tubules, which is a complication of hypokalemia. The tubules become resistant to antidiuretic hormone producing an acquired nephrogenic diabetes insipidus.

7. **I** (pH 7.56, $Paco_2$ 24, HCO_3^- 21) is correct. The patient has acute respiratory alkalosis due to a pulmonary embolus originating from a thrombus in the deep veins of the right leg. Tachypnea (rapid shallow breathing) is produced by reflexes in the lung and stimulation of peripheral chemoreceptors by a decrease in Pao_2. Rapid breathing blows off CO_2 causing respiratory alkalosis (pH 7.56, $Paco_2$ 24 mm Hg). Compensation for respiratory alkalosis is metabolic acidosis (HCO_3^- 21 mEq/L).

8. **B** (pH 7.20, $Paco_2$ 74, HCO_3^- 28) is correct. The patient has acute respiratory acidosis due to a barbiturate overdose. Barbiturates depress the medullary center in the medulla causing hypoventilation with subsequent retention of CO_2 leading to respiratory acidosis (pH 7.20, $Paco_2$ 74 mm Hg). The compensation for respiratory acidosis is metabolic alkalosis. However, there has not been enough time for renal compensation; therefore, the serum HCO_3^- remains in the normal range (HCO_3^- 28 mEq/L, uncompensated respiratory acidosis).

9. **D** (pH 7.28, $Paco_2$ 28, HCO_3^- 12) is correct. Hypovolemic shock produces inadequate oxygenation of tissue leading to anaerobic glycolysis and lactic acidosis. Lactic acidosis is an increased anion gap type of metabolic acidosis (pH 7.28, HCO_3^- 12 mEq/L) where lactate anions replace the HCO_3^- anions that are used up in buffering excess hydrogen ions. The compensation for metabolic acidosis is respiratory alkalosis ($Paco_2$ 28 mm Hg).

10. **E** (pH 7.38, $Paco_2$ 70, HCO_3^- 40) is correct. The patient has a mixed acid-base disorder with a combination of chronic respiratory acidosis ($Pco_2 > 45$ mm Hg, $HCO_3^- > 30$ mEq/L) from chronic bronchitis and metabolic alkalosis caused by a loop diuretic that is being used to treat right-sided heart failure. The pH is normal (7.38), because the two primary disorders have opposing effects. Although a normal pH implies that there is full compensation, this rarely occurs and is most often due to a primary acidosis and a primary alkalosis. The $Paco_2$ is increased ($Paco_2$ 70 mm Hg), because of the additive effect of CO_2 retention due to chronic bronchitis plus respiratory acidosis as compensation for metabolic alkalosis. To document the existence of two primary disorders, the formulas for calculating the compensation for either metabolic alkalosis or chronic respiratory acidosis can be used. For example, using the formula for metabolic alkalosis (expected $\Delta Paco_2 = 0.7 \times \Delta HCO_3^- \pm 2$), the calculation is as follows: expected $\Delta Paco_2 = 0.7 \times (40 - 24) = 11.2$. Expected $Paco_2 = 40 + 11.2 = 51.2$ mm Hg (49.2 – 53.2). Because the measured $Paco_2$ is 70 mm Hg, an additional component of primary respiratory acidosis must be present to explain the higher than expected $Paco_2$.

11. A (pH 7.00, $Paco_2$ 52, HCO_3^- 13) is correct. The patient has a mixed acid-base disorder with a combination of a primary acute respiratory acidosis and a primary metabolic acidosis. The two acidoses have produced a extreme acidemia (pH 7.00). Because the patient has respiratory arrest, CO_2 is retained causing respiratory acidosis with an increased $Paco_2$ (52 mm Hg). Cardiogenic shock produces lactic acidosis secondary to anaerobic glycolysis. This produces an increased anion gap metabolic acidosis causing a decreased HCO_3^- (13 mEq/L). Calculation of the expected compensation is unnecessary, because an acidosis cannot be a compensation for another acidosis.

12. G (pH 7.42, $Paco_2$ 22, HCO_3^- 14) is correct. The patient has a mixed acid-base disorder due to salicylate poisoning (ringing in her ears). The pH is normal, because there is a primary metabolic acidosis (salicylic acid, HCO_3^- 14 mEq/L) and a primary respiratory alkalosis ($Paco_2$ 22 mm Hg) due to overstimulation of the medullary center in the brain by salicylates. In order to document the presence of a mixed disorder, calculation of the expected compensation for either chronic respiratory alkalosis or metabolic acidosis can be used. Using the metabolic acidosis formula (expected $\Delta Paco_2 = 1.2 \times \Delta HCO_3^- \pm 2$), the calculation is as follows. Expected $\Delta Paco_2 = 1.2 \times (24 - 14) = 12$. Expected $Paco_2 = 40 - 12 = 28$ mm Hg (26–30). Because the measured $Paco_2$ (22 mm Hg) is less than the calculated $Paco_2$ (26–30 mm Hg), an additional component of primary respiratory alkalosis must be present.

13. F (pH 7.38, $Paco_2$ 40, HCO_3^- 23) is correct. The patient has a mixed acid-base disorder due to a primary metabolic acidosis (ketoacidosis) and a primary metabolic alkalosis (vomiting). The pH, $Paco_2$, and HCO_3^- are all in the normal range, because the two acid-base disorders are exact opposites. Ketoacidosis is documented by the positive dipstick for ketone bodies and glucose, however, the metabolic alkalosis is documented by history. The patient has signs of volume depletion (dry mucous membranes, poor skin turgor, hypotension) due to the loss of Na^+-containing fluid by osmotic diuresis secondary to glucosuria. The calculations for expected compensation are not helpful in this clinical situation.

14. **B** (serum Na^+ decreased, $TBNa^+$ increased) is correct. Patients with cirrhosis have alterations in Starling's pressures. Decreased liver synthesis of albumin reduces the plasma oncotic pressure, which normally retains fluid in the vascular compartment. Decreased plasma oncotic pressure contributes to the development of ascites and is the primary cause of the patient's dependent pitting edema. Portal hypertension secondary to cirrhosis is associated with an increase in hydrostatic pressure, which is a force that drives fluid out of the vascular compartment into the interstitial space and body cavities. An increase in portal vein hydrostatic pressure, along with hypoalbuminemia, contributes to the development of ascites. The cardiac output is decreased in cirrhosis, because fluid is trapped in the interstitial space and body cavities by the Starling's pressure abnormalities. Decreased renal blood flow causes the kidney to reabsorb a slightly hypotonic salt-containing fluid, which produces hyponatremia ($\downarrow$ serum $Na^+ = \uparrow TBNa^+/\uparrow\uparrow TBW$). The fluid is redirected into the interstitial space (decreased plasma oncotic pressure) and body cavities (decreased plasma oncotic pressure and increased portal vein hydrostatic pressure).

15. **D** (serum Na^+ increased, $TBNa^+$ decreased) is correct. Excessive sweating without fluid replacement is associated with a loss of hypotonic salt-containing fluid, which produces hypernatremia ($\uparrow$ serum $Na^+ = \downarrow TBNa^+/\downarrow\downarrow$ TBW). The patient has signs of volume depletion ($\downarrow TBNa^+$) from the loss of sodium, mainly dry mucous membranes and a positive tilt test (blood pressure dropped and pulse rate increased when sitting up).

16. **C** (serum Na^+ decreased, $TBNa^+$ normal) is correct. The patient has the syndrome of inappropriate secretion of antidiuretic hormone (ADH) due to excessive stimulation of ADH release by chlorpropamide, a oral hypoglycemic agent. ADH reabsorbs electrolyte-free water from the collecting tubules causing a dilutional hyponatremia ($\downarrow$ serum $Na^+ = TBNa^+/\uparrow\uparrow TBW$). Because Na^+ is not reabsorbed by ADH, the $TBNa^+$ is normal; therefore, there are no signs of pitting edema. The mental status abnormalities are due to hyponatremia, which creates an osmotic gradient that favors the movement of water into the cells in the brain.

17. **H** (serum Na^+ normal, $TBNa^+$ increased) is correct. Due to the patient's chronic ischemic heart disease, he is unable to handle the excess gain of isotonic saline and develops left-sided heart failure (bibasilar crackles). An isotonic gain of fluid does *not* alter the serum Na^+ ($\leftrightarrow$serum $Na^+ = \uparrow TBNa^+/\uparrow TBW$); however, the excess salt-containing fluid is directed into the alveoli in the lungs owing to an increase in plasma hydrostatic pressure from the increase in plasma volume.

18. E (serum Na^+ increased, $TBNa^+$ increased) is correct. The patient received a hypertonic salt solution (intravenous sodium bicarbonate) during treatment for a cardiorespiratory arrest. Owing to chronic renal disease, he cannot excrete the excess Na^+ load and develops hypernatremia ($\uparrow$serum $Na^+ = \uparrow\uparrow$ $TBNa^+/\uparrow TBW$) and signs of left-sided heart failure (bibasilar crackles) and right-sided heart failure (dependent pitting edema) due to an increase in plasma hydrostatic pressure from an increase in plasma volume related to the sodium bicarbonate infusions.

19. A (serum Na^+ decreased, $TBNa^+$ decreased) is correct. In diabetic ketoacidosis (DKA), hyperglycemia is the major osmotically active solute in the vascular compartment and causes water to move out of the intracellular fluid compartment into the extracellular fluid compartment producing a dilutional hyponatremia. However, glucosuria is also present in DKA which produces an osmotic diuresis causing loss of a hypotonic salt-containing fluid in the urine. The loss of Na^+ is responsible for the signs of volume depletion (dry mucous membranes, poor skin turgor, hypotension).

20. G (serum Na^+ normal, $TBNa^+$ decreased) is correct. Travelers' diarrhea is most often due to enterotoxigenic *Escherichia coli*, which produces a toxin that activates adenylate or guanylate cyclase in enterocytes in the small intestine causing an isotonic loss of diarrheal fluid (secretory type of diarrhea). Loss of isotonic fluid does *not* alter the serum Na^+ concentration ($\leftrightarrow$serum $Na^+ = \downarrow TBNa^+/\downarrow TBW$); however, the decrease in $TBNa^+$ causes signs of volume depletion (dry mucous membranes, poor skin turgor, hypotension).

21. F (serum Na^+ increased, $TBNa^+$ normal) is correct. Fever causes a loss of pure water due to evaporation of water from warm skin and mucous membranes. A loss of pure water produces hypernatremia ($\uparrow$serum $Na^+ = TBNa^+/\downarrow\downarrow TBW$); however, the $TBNa^+$ remains unchanged. The normal $TBNa^+$ accounts for the lack of signs of volume depletion in this patient, mainly dry mucous membranes and hypotension. Clinicians use the term dehydration for this type of fluid loss.

22. A (serum Na^+ 118, serum K^+ 3.0, serum Cl^- 84, serum HCO_3^- 22) is correct. The patient has the syndrome of inappropriate secretion of antidiuretic hormone (SIADH). It is most often caused by ectopic secretion of ADH by a primary small cell carcinoma of the lung (left hilar mass; small, hyperchromatic cells in the sputum) in a patient with a smoking history. Excess ADH causes increased reabsorption of electrolyte-free water, which produces a severe dilutional hyponatremia and cerebral edema.

23. **B** (serum Na^+ 128, serum K^+ 5.9, serum Cl^- 96, serum HCO_3^- 20) is correct. The patient has Addison's disease, which is most often due to autoimmune destruction of the adrenal cortex. Destruction of the zona glomerulosa produces a deficiency of aldosterone, which is responsible for the electrolyte abnormalities. There is inhibition of Na^+ reabsorption and K^+ secretion by the aldosterone-dependent Na^+ and K^+ channels located in the distal tubule and collecting ducts causing a hypertonic loss of Na^+ in the urine (hyponatremia) and retention of K^+ (hyperkalemia with peaked T waves). Due to dysfunction of the aldosterone-dependent H^+/K^+-ATPase pump in the collecting tubules, there is retention of H^+ ions and a subsequent lack of synthesis of HCO_3^-, which produces metabolic acidosis. The excess H^+ ions combine with Cl^- anions producing a normal anion gap type of metabolic acidosis—anion gap = serum Na^+ 128 − (serum Cl^- 96 + serum HCO_3^- 20) = 12 mEq/L. The decrease in serum cortisol causes an increase in serum ACTH due to the loss of a negative feedback on ACTH by cortisol. Because ACTH has melanocyte-stimulating properties, there is diffuse pigmentation of the buccal mucosa and skin.

24. **E** (serum Na^+ 130, serum K^+ 2.9, serum Cl^- 80, serum HCO_3^- 36) is correct. Thiazide diuretics inhibit the Cl^- channel in the Na^+-Cl^- cotransporter located in the early distal tubule. This causes an increase in the urinary loss of Na^+ (hyponatremia) and Cl^- (hypochloremia). Increased delivery of Na^+ to the late distal and collecting tubules results in augmented exchange of Na^+ for K^+ in the aldosterone-dependent Na^+ channels resulting in increased urinary loss of K^+ (hypokalemia with U waves on an ECG). When K^+ is depleted, Na^+ exchanges with H^+ ions causing increased synthesis and reabsorption of HCO_3^- causing metabolic alkalosis.

25. **C** (serum Na^+ 146, serum K^+ 5.5, serum Cl^- 104, serum HCO_3^- 18) is correct. In chronic renal failure there is tubular cell dysfunction resulting in retention of K^+ (hyperkalemia with peaked T waves on an ECG) and an increased anion gap type of metabolic acidosis due to retention of organic acids such as sulfuric and phosphaturic acid. The anion gap in this case is calculated as follows: anion gap = serum Na^+ 146 − (serum Cl^- 104 + serum HCO_3^- 18) = 24 mEq/L (12 mEq/L ± 2). Focal segmental glomerulosclerosis is the most common cause of chronic renal failure in intravenous heroin abusers.

26. **D** (serum Na^+ 138, serum K^+ 2.2, serum Cl^- 114, serum HCO_3^- 14) is correct. Cholera is caused by *Vibrio cholerae,* which produces a toxin that activates adenylate cyclase in enterocytes causing a secretory diarrhea with the loss of isotonic fluid. Loss of isotonic fluid does *not* alter the serum Na^+

concentration. Diarrheal fluid is rich in K^+ and HCO_3^-, the former resulting in hypokalemia and the latter a normal anion gap type of metabolic acidosis. The anion gap calculation is as follows: anion gap = serum Na^+ 138 − (serum Cl^- 114 + serum HCO_3^- 14) = 10 mEq/L (12 mEq/L ± 2). The serum Cl^- is increased, because it replaces the HCO_3^- anions that are lost in the diarrheal fluid in order to maintain electroneutrality.

27. **D** (serum Na^+ 138, serum K^+ 2.2, serum Cl^- 114, serum HCO_3^- 14) is correct. The patient has a type II proximal renal tubular acidosis due to lead poisoning. Lead produces coagulation necrosis of the proximal tubule cells, which interferes with all of the proximal tubule functions. Because the proximal tubule is important in the reclamation of HCO_3^-, the filtered HCO_3^- is lost in the urine producing an alkaline urine pH and a normal anion gap type of metabolic acidosis (calculated anion gap is 10 mEq/L). Potassium, phosphate, glucose, amino acids, and uric acid are also lost in the urine. The serum Cl^- is increased, because it replaces the HCO_3^- anions that are lost in the urine in order to maintain electroneutrality.

Pulmonary Function Tests

I. **Spirometry**
  A. **Purpose of spirometry**
     • Evaluates ventilation function, or the process of exchange of air between the lungs and the environment

  B. **Test descriptions**
     1. Measurements (Fig. 3-1)
        a. Static volumes
           • Example—tidal volume (TV)
        b. Capacities
           (1) Two or more volumes
           (2) Example—vital capacity (VC)
        c. Dynamic functions
           (1) Forced expiratory flow rates
           (2) Example—forced expiratory volume 1 second, $FEV_{1 \text{ sec}}$
     2. Normal lung volumes and capacities
        a. Vary according to gender, age, height, and ethnic group
        b. Normal values are between 80% and 120% of the predicted value.
           • Based on data obtained from nonsmoking individuals without lung disease
     3. Tidal volume (TV)
        a. Volume of air that enters or leaves the lungs during normal quiet respiration
        b. Normal TV is 0.5 L.
     4. Expiratory reserve volume (ERV)
        a. Amount of air forcibly expelled at the end of a normal expiration
        b. Normal ERV is 1.2 L.
     5. Volumes and capacities that are *not* directly measured by spirometry
        a. Total lung capacity (TLC)
           (1) Total amount of air in a fully expanded lung
           (2) Normal TLC is 6.0 L.

        b. Residual volume (RV)
           (1) Volume of air left over in the lung after maximal expiration
           (2) Normal RV is 1.2 L.

        c. Functional residual capacity (FRC)
           (1) Total amount of air in the lungs at the end of normal expiration (end of TV)
           (2) Normal FRC is 2.4 L.

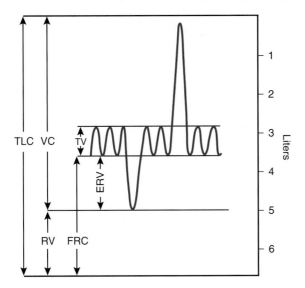

3-1: *Measurement of lung volumes and capacities by spirometry. See text for discussion. ERV, expiratory reserve volume; FRC, functional residual capacity; RV, residual volume; TLC, total lung capacity; TV, tidal volume; VC, vital capacity.*

      (3) Most reproducible test
         • Measurement is independent of patient effort.
      (4) Commonly used to calculate residual volume
         • RV = FRC − ERV
    d. Measurement of TLC, RV, FRC
      • Helium-dilution or total body plethysmography
  6. Forced vital capacity and $FEV_{1\ sec}$ (Fig. 3-2, curve A)
    a. Best tests of ventilatory function
    b. Forced vital capacity (FVC)
      (1) Total amount of air expelled after a maximal inspiration
      (2) Normal FVC is 5.0 L.
    c. $FEV_{1\ sec}$
      (1) Total amount of air expelled in 1 second after a maximal inspiration
         • Normal $FEV_{1\ sec}$ is 4 L.
      (2) Nonsmokers show a normal decline in $FEV_{1\ sec}$
         • Rate of decline is 20 to 30 mL a year.

> There is no improvement in the $FEV_{1\ sec}$ after cessation of smoking. However, the rate of decline of the $FEV_{1\ sec}$ is similar to that of a nonsmoker.

    d. Preoperative evaluation using $FEV_{1\ sec}$ and FVC
      • Increased risk for pulmonary complications if these parameters are <50% of predicted value
    e. Ratio of $FEV_{1\ sec}$/FVC

FVC, $FEV_{1\ sec}$: best tests of ventilatory function

3-2: *Measurement of forced expiratory volume at 1 second (FEV$_{1\text{ sec}}$) and forced vital capacity (FVC) by spirometry. See text for discussion.*

FEV$_{1\text{ sec}}$/FVC ratio: differentiates obstructive vs. restrictive disorders

(1) Useful in differentiating obstructive from restrictive lung disorders

(2) Normal FEV$_{1\text{ sec}}$/FVC is 75% to 80%.

> The **peak expiratory flow meter** is an outpatient method of evaluating FVC. It is commonly used by asthmatics to evaluate their airway function in response to bronchodilators.

7. Flow-volume loop
   a. Plot of inspiratory and expiratory flow rate (L/second) versus lung volume (L)
      • Patient takes a maximal inspiration followed by a maximal expiration
   b. Loop consists of an inspiration curve and an expiration curve (Fig. 3-3).
      (1) Maximal inspiration
         • Begins at point A (RV) and extends to point B (TLC)
      (2) Maximal expiration

TLC and RV: TLC end of maximal inspiration; RV end of maximal expiration

      (a) Extends from point B to point C (peak expiratory flow, PEF) and then trails off back to point A
      (b) PEF occurs early in expiratory phase of the loop (point B to C)
         • Due to elastic recoil of the lungs into low-resistance large-caliber airways
      (c) Flow rate becomes linear from point C to A.
         • Encounters increased resistance in the small airways

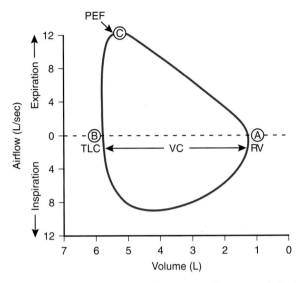

3-3: *Flow-volume loop. See text for discussion. PEF, peak expiratory flow; RV, residual volume; TLC, total lung capacity; VC, vital capacity.*

      (3) Volume of air in liters between points A and B is the vital capacity (VC).

C. **Patterns of abnormal ventilatory function**
    1. Obstructive pattern
      a. Limitation of expiratory air flow (i.e., increased airway resistance on expiration)
        • Some air remains in the lungs after maximal expiration (increased RV).
      b. Causes of obstruction
        (1) Plugging of the small airways (e.g., mucus plugs)
          • Occurs in chronic bronchitis, bronchiectasis, asthma
        (2) Destruction of elastic tissue support in alveoli and airway walls
          • Example—emphysema
      c. Spirometry findings
        (1) Increased TLC
          • Due to an increase in RV from air trapped in the distal airways
        (2) Decreased FVC
          • Example—3 L (Fig. 3-2, curve C)
        (3) Decreased $FEV_{1\ sec}$
          • Example—1 L (Fig. 3-2, curve C)

Obstructive disorder: ↑ airway resistance on expiration

> The magnitude of functional impairment in obstructive lung disease correlates closely with the $FEV_{1\ sec}$. A $FEV_{1\ sec}$ around 4 L indicates that there is no significant exercise impairment in the patient. A $FEV_{1\ sec}$ between 2 and 3 L/second is consistent with mild exercise impairment;

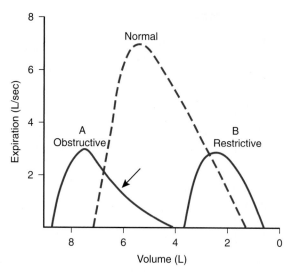

3-4: *Flow-volume loops in normal person, in obstructive disorder (A), and in restrictive disorder (B). See text for discussion.*

1 to 2 L/second indicates moderate exercise impairment; and <1 L/second indicates severe exercise impairment.

Obstructive pattern: ↑ TLC, RV, FRC; ↓ FVC, $FEV_{1\ sec}$, $FEV_{1\ sec}$/FVC ratio

    (4) Decreased $FEV_{1\ sec}$/FVC ratio
- Example—1 L/3 L = 33%

    (5) Increased FRC, due to the increase in RV

  d. Flow-volume loop findings (Fig. 3-4A)

    (1) TLC is increased (e.g., ~8.5 L) and RV is increased (e.g., 4 L)
- Expiratory curve is shifted to the left of the normal curve.

Obstructive pattern: nonuniform emptying; expiratory curve shift to left of normal curve

    (2) Decreased PEF

    (3) Nonuniform emptying of the airways
- Concave configuration of the curve (arrow) due to mucus plugs or collapsed small airways

2. Restrictive pattern

Restrictive disorder: ↓ filling of lungs

  a. Limited filling of the lungs (i.e., decreased compliance, "stiff lungs")
- All lung volumes and capacities are equally decreased.

  b. Types of restriction

    (1) Pulmonary parenchymal with inspiratory dysfunction

      (a) Increased elastic recoil of the lungs

      (b) Examples—idiopathic pulmonary fibrosis, sarcoidosis

    (2) Extraparenchymal with inspiratory dysfunction
- Examples—obesity, kyphoscoliosis

    (3) Extraparenchymal with inspiratory and expiratory dysfunction
- Examples—neuromuscular disorders such as myasthenia gravis, amyotrophic lateral sclerosis

  c. Spirometry findings in restrictive parenchymal disease

    (1) All volumes and capacities are equally decreased.

TABLE 3-1
**Spirometer
Findings in
Obstructive and
Restrictive
Disorders**

Measurement	Restrictive Parenchymal Disorders	Obstructive Disorders
TLC	↓	↑
RV	↓	↑
FRC	↓	↑
FVC	↓	↓
$FEV_{1\ sec}$	↓	↓↓
$FEV_{1\ sec}$/FVC	Normal to ↑	↓↓

    (2) Decreased FVC—e.g., 3 L (Fig. 3-2, curve B)
    (3) Decreased $FEV_{1\ sec}$—e.g., 3 L (Fig. 3-2, curve B)

> The $FEV_{1\ sec}$ value, though decreased in restrictive lung disease, is greater than in obstructive disease. This is due to increased elastic recoil in restrictive parenchymal disorders and decreased elastic recoil in obstructive disease (e.g., emphysema).

    (4) Normal to increased $FEV_{1\ sec}$/FVC ratio
      • Example—3 L/3 L = 100% (normal is 0.75–0.80%)

> Increased elastic recoil often results in similar values for the $FEV_{1\ sec}$ and FVC causing the ratio to be normal to increased. The ratio is *always* decreased in obstructive disease.

    (5) Decreased FRC due to a decrease in ERV and RV
    (6) Comparison of obstructive versus restrictive lung disorders (Table 3-1)
  d. Spirometry findings in extraparenchymal disease
    (1) Inspiratory dysfunction
      (a) Underlying lungs are normal.
      (b) Lungs inspire against a stiff chest wall (e.g., kyphoscoliosis) or excess weight in the chest wall (e.g., obesity).
      (c) TLC is decreased.
        • Inspiratory dysfunction *always* decreases TLC.
      (d) RV is preserved, because expiratory function is preserved.
      (e) FVC and $FEV_{1\ sec}$ are normal.
    (2) Inspiratory and expiratory dysfunction (e.g., neuromuscular disease)
      (a) Underlying lungs are normal.
      (b) Lack of inspiratory effort to expand the lungs decreases TLC.
      (c) Lack of expiratory effort to exhale all the air increases RV and decreases FVC and $FEV_{1\ sec}$
        • Inability to fully expire all the air *always* increases RV.
  e. Flow-volume loop findings in restrictive parenchymal disease (Fig. 3-4B)
    (1) TLC is decreased (e.g., ~4 L).

Restrictive parenchymal: ↓ volumes/capacities; normal to ↑ $FEV_{1\ sec}$/FVC ratio

Extraparenchymal inspiratory dysfunction: ↓ TLC, normal RV

Extraparenchymal inspiratory/expiratory dysfunction: ↓ TLC, FVC, $FEV_{1\ sec}$; ↑ RV

Restrictive parenchymal: expiratory curve shifted to right of normal curve

(2) RV is decreased (e.g., ~0.3 L).

(3) Expiratory curve is shifted to the right of the normal curve.
- Expiratory curve is narrow due to decreased lung volumes.

II. **Arterial Blood Gases (ABG)**
   A. **Purpose**
      - Evaluates O_2 and CO_2 exchange in the lungs
   B. **Sample collection and measurement**
      1. ABG is collected in heparinized syringes.
      2. Exposure of ABG to ambient air
         a. Falsely increases partial pressure of O_2 in arterial blood (P_aO_2)
            (1) Gases diffuse from areas of high pressure to areas of low pressure
            (2) Ambient Po_2 is higher than Pao_2.
         b. Falsely decreases partial pressure of CO_2 in arterial blood ($Paco_2$)
            - Ambient Pco_2 is lower than $Paco_2$.
         c. Partial pressure of a gas
            (1) Driving pressure that keeps a gas dissolved in blood
            (2) The actual quantity of a gas in blood is dependent on the following:
               (a) Solubility in plasma
               (b) Ability to bind to hemoglobin (Hb) and amount of available Hb in red blood cells (RBCs)
      3. Parameters directly measured by ABG analyzer
         - Arterial pH, Pao_2, and $Paco_2$
      4. Parameters calculated by ABG analyzer
         a. O_2 saturation (Sao_2)
            - Calculated from Pao_2
         b. Bicarbonate
            - Calculated from $Paco_2$
   C. **ABG measurements evaluating gas exchange**

ABG analyzer: measures pH, PaO_2, $PaCO_2$; calculates SaO_2, bicarbonate

      1. Alveolar Po_2 (Pao_2)
         a. Depends on
            (1) Percent of inspired O_2 (Fio_2)
               (a) Decreased Fio_2 (gas mixture <21%) decreases Pao_2.
                  - Example—person trapped in a mine
               (b) Increased Fio_2 (gas mixture >21%) increases Pao_2.
                  - Example—person breathing 100% O_2
            (2) Atmospheric pressure (AP)
               (a) Decreased AP decreases Pao_2.
                  - Example—at high altitude, AP is decreased but the %O_2 is 21%
               (b) Increased AP increases Pao_2.
                  - Example—hyperbaric chamber
            (3) Alveolar Pco_2
               (a) Increased $Paco_2$ (i.e., respiratory acidosis) decreases Pao_2.
               (b) Decreased $Paco_2$ (i.e., respiratory alkalosis) increases Pao_2.
         b. Calculation of Pao_2

(1) $P_{AO_2} = F_{IO_2} \times (PB - P_{H_2O}) - P_{aCO_2}/R$

(2) F_{IO_2} is the fractional concentration of inspired O_2

    (a) F_{IO_2} is ~21% when breathing ambient air, or

    (b) Percent O_2 being delivered to the patient via assisted ventilation

(3) PB is the atmospheric pressure at sea level (760 mm Hg).

(4) P_{H_2O} is the water vapor pressure (47 mm Hg).

(5) P_{aCO_2} is equivalent to P_{ACO_2}.

(6) R is the respiratory quotient.

    • Ratio of CO_2 production to O_2 consumption (usually 0.8)

(7) Example calculation using normal values

    • $P_{AO_2} = 0.21 (760 - 47) - 40/0.8 = 100$ mm Hg

2. P_{aO_2}

  a. P_{aO_2} is the best measure of effective oxygenation.

    (1) Normal P_{aO_2} is 80 to 100 mm Hg.

    (2) It normally decreases with age.

    (3) Decreased P_{aO_2} is called hypoxemia.

  b. P_{aO_2} is dependent on

    (1) F_{IO_2}

      (a) P_{aO_2} decreases if a gas mixture is <21% O_2.

      (b) P_{aO_2} increases if a gas mixture is >21% O_2.

    (2) AP

      (a) P_{aO_2} decreases with a decrease in AP.

      (b) P_{aO_2} increases with increased AP.

    (3) P_{aCO_2}

      (a) Increased P_{aCO_2} (i.e., respiratory acidosis) produces a corresponding decrease in P_{AO_2} and P_{aO_2}.

      (b) Decreased P_{aCO_2} (i.e., respiratory alkalosis) produces a corresponding increase in P_{AO_2} and P_{aO_2}.

    (4) Diffusion of O_2 through the alveolar-capillary septum

      • Disorders decreasing diffusion include pulmonary edema, interstitial fibrosis

    (5) Ventilation (V) and perfusion (Q)

      (a) V/Q ratio is highest in the apices of the lungs.

        • Blood flow is lowest; P_{aCO_2} is lowest (e.g., 28 mm Hg); P_{AO_2} pressure is highest; and P_{aO_2} is highest (e.g., 130 mm Hg).

      (b) V/Q ratio is lowest at the bases of the lungs.

        • Blood flow is highest; P_{aCO_2} is highest (e.g., 42 mm Hg); P_{AO_2} pressure is lowest; and P_{aO_2} is lowest (e.g., 89 mm Hg).

      (c) Blood leaving the different lung regions is mixed.

        • Average P_{aO_2} is 95 to 100 mm Hg and average P_{aCO_2} is 40 mm Hg (Fig. 3-5A).

3. V/Q defects

  a. Compromise gas exchange leading to alterations in P_{aO_2} and P_{aCO_2}

  b. Ventilation defects

Margin notes:

$P_{AO_2} = O_2\% \times (PB - P_{H_2O}) - P_{aCO_2}/0.8$

P_{aO_2}: best measure of oxygenation

Hypoxemia: $\downarrow P_{aCO_2}$

$\uparrow P_{aCO_2} = \downarrow P_{AO_2}$ and P_{aO_2}; $\downarrow P_{aCO_2} = \uparrow P_{AO_2}$ and P_{aO_2}

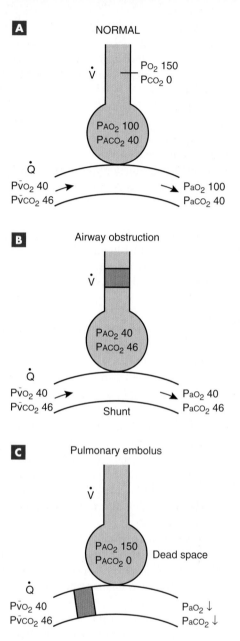

3-5: *Ventilation (V)-perfusion (Q) defects. See text for discussion. PvCO₂, partial pressure of carbon dioxide in mixed venous blood; PvO₂, partial pressure of oxygen in mixed venous blood.*

(1) Impaired delivery of O_2 to alveoli
  - Perfusion of alveoli *without* gas exchange
(2) Causes
  (a) Airway obstruction (e.g., tumor blocking bronchus)
  (b) Alveolar collapse (e.g., atelectasis)
(3) Produces intrapulmonary shunting (Fig. 3-5B)
  - Decreased Pao_2 (hypoxemia) and increased $Paco_2$ (respiratory acidosis)

> The decreased PaO_2 is relatively refractory to supplemental O_2, because blood is bypassing oxygenation at the alveolar-capillary level. Intracardiac defects with right-to-left shunts (e.g., tetralogy of Fallot) have findings that are similar to intrapulmonary shunts.

Atelectasis/right-to-left cardiac shunt: intrapulmonary shunt; ↓ PaO_2, ↑ $PaCO_2$

c. Perfusion defects (Fig. 3-5C)
  (1) Absence of blood flow to alveoli
  (2) Pulmonary embolism is an example of a perfusion defect.
  (3) Produces increased dead space (i.e., O_2 present but *no* gas exchange)
    (a) Decreased Pao_2 stimulates the aortic and carotid bodies causing hyperventilation.
    (b) Hyperventilation decreases $Paco_2$ (respiratory alkalosis)
      - Clearance of CO_2 is increased in alveoli where perfusion is present.

> Assisted ventilation increases the PaO_2, because other areas of the lungs that have perfusion compensate with increased oxygenation of blood.

Pulmonary embolus: ↑ dead space; ↓ PaO_2, ↓ $PaCO_2$

4. Arterial O_2 saturation (Sao_2)
  a. Average percentage of O_2 bound to Hb
    (1) Normal Sao_2 is 94% to 98%.
    (2) Sao_2 <80% produces cyanosis.
      - Dusky blue-colored skin and mucous membranes
  b. Sao_2 is dependent on
    (1) Pao_2
      - Sao_2 is *always* decreased if Pao_2 is decreased.
    (2) Valence of heme iron
      (a) Ferrous iron (Fe^{2+}) binds to O_2.
      (b) Ferric iron (Fe^{3+}) does *not* bind to O_2.
        - Iron in the ferric state is called methemoglobin (metHb).

SaO_2: %O_2 bound to Hb; ↓ SaO_2 causes cyanosis

Methemoglobin: heme iron +3 valence

> Pulse oximetry is a noninvasive alternative for measuring SaO_2. It utilizes a probe that is usually clipped over a patient's finger. Oximetry emits red and infrared light at specified wavelengths that identify oxyhemoglobin (oxyHb) and deoxyhemoglobin (deoxyHb), respectively.

Pulse oximeter: noninvasive measurement of SaO_2

The oximeter calculates the SaO_2 using the following equation: oxyHb/oxyHb + deoxyHb. Less reliable measurements are obtained if there is decreased perfusion of cutaneous vessels (e.g., use of vasoconstrictors, decrease in cardiac output). In addition, the wavelengths emitted by a pulse oximeter *cannot* identify dyshemoglobins such as metHb and carboxyhemoglobin (i.e., carbon monoxide bound to Hb, COHb), which normally decrease the SaO_2 (see below). In the presence of these dyshemoglobins, the oximeter calculates a falsely high SaO_2, because metHb or COHb are *not* included in the calculation of SaO_2 (Fig. 3-6). However, a co-oximeter, which emits multiple wavelengths, calculates the decrease in SaO_2, because it identifies metHb and COHb and includes them in the calculation of SaO_2: oxyHb/oxyHb + deoxyHb + MetHb or COHb.

5. O_2 content
   a. Total amount of O_2 in blood
   b. Calculation: $1.34 \times Hb \times SaO_2 + 0.003 \times PaO_2$
      (1) O_2 content of blood in an adult is ~20.0 mL O_2/100 mL of blood.
      (2) Hb fully saturated with O_2 is the most important carrier of O_2.
         • Hb is the primary determinant for the total amount of O_2 delivered to tissue.

Hb concentration: determines amount of O_2 delivered to tissue

PULSE OXIMETRY

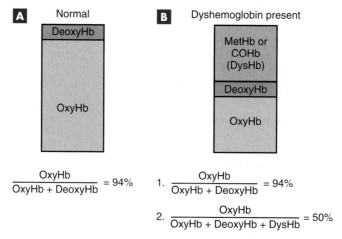

3-6: *Schematic of pulse oximetry measurement in normal blood (**A**) and blood containing dyshemoglobins (**B**). A pulse oximeters measures oxyhemoglobin (OxyHb) and deoxyhemoglobin (DeoxyHb) directly and calculates O_2 saturation as shown in A. However, if a dyshemoglobin (DysHb) is present such as methemoglobin (MetHb) or carboxyhemoglobin (COHb), it will not be detected and is left out of the calculation for O_2 saturation resulting in an erroneously high reading (**B**, equation 1). A co-oximeter detects the presence of a dyshemoglobin and calculates the true O_2 saturation, as shown in equation 2.*

In anemia, the Hb is decreased; therefore, less O_2 is delivered to tissue. However, the PaO_2 and SaO_2 are normal, because gas exchange is normal.

(3) $0.003 \times PaO_2$ is the amount of O_2 (volume %) dissolved in plasma.

The PaO_2 is the driving force for diffusion of O_2 into tissue at the level of the capillaries. If the PaO_2 is decreased (i.e., hypoxemia), less O_2 diffuses into tissue.

PaO_2: driving force for O_2 diffusion

6. $PaCO_2$
   a. Best indicator of the adequacy of elimination of CO_2 in the lungs
   b. Interpretation of $PaCO_2$ alterations (see Chapter 2)
      (1) Increased $PaCO_2$
         (a) Primary respiratory acidosis if arterial pH is decreased
         (b) Compensation for metabolic alkalosis if arterial pH is increased
      (2) Decreased $PaCO_2$
         (a) Primary respiratory alkalosis if arterial pH is increased
         (b) Compensation for metabolic acidosis if arterial pH is decreased
7. Alveolar-arterial O_2 gradient (A-a gradient)
   a. Formula: A-a gradient = $PAO_2 - PaO_2$
      (1) PAO_2 and PaO_2 are *not* the same.
         • Ventilation and perfusion are *not* evenly matched throughout the lungs.
      (2) A-a gradient increases with age.
         (a) A-a gradient in young individuals is usually <15 mm Hg.
         (b) A-a gradient in elderly may be as high as 30 mm Hg.
         (c) A-a gradient >30 mm Hg is *always* medically significant.

A-a gradient: $PAO_2 - PaO_2$; >30 mm Hg medically significant

   b. Use of A-a gradient in evaluating hypoxemia (Table 3-2)
      (1) Increased A-a gradient plus hypoxemia
         (a) Primary lung disease (e.g., ventilation, perfusion, diffusion defects)
         (b) Right-to-left cardiac shunts (e.g., tetralogy of Fallot)
         (c) Example: patient breathing 0.30 O_2, $PaCO_2$ 80 mm Hg (33–45 mm Hg), PaO_2 40 mm Hg
            • $PAO_2 = 0.30 (713) - 80/0.8 = 114$ mm Hg; A-a = $114 - 40 = 74$ mm Hg

↑ A-a, ↓ PaO_2: V/Q defect, cardiac right-to-left shunts

      (2) Normal A-a gradient plus hypoxemia
         (a) Hypoventilation (i.e., respiratory acidosis) due to extrapulmonary disease
            • Depression of the respiratory center, extraparenchymal restrictive lung disease
         (b) Example: patient breathing room air, $PaCO_2$ 80 mm Hg, PaO_2 40 mm Hg
            • $PAO_2 = 0.21 (713) - 80/0.8 = 50$ mm Hg; A-a gradient = $50 - 40 = 10$ mm Hg

Normal A-a, ↓ PaO_2: hypoventilation due to extrapulmonary disease

**TABLE 3-2
Evaluation of
Hypoxemia**

Type of Hypoxemia	Causes/Discussion

Increased A-a gradient	Intrapulmonary shunt
	    Atelectasis: RDS, ARDS, post-surgery
	    Alveolar consolidation: pulmonary edema, pneumonia
	    Right-to-left cardiac shunt
	    Tetralogy of Fallot, reversal of VSD, ASD, or PDA
	V/Q mismatch
	    Obstructive lung disease: chronic bronchitis, emphysema,
	      asthma, bronchiectasis
	    Restrictive lung disease: idiopathic pulmonary fibrosis,
	      pneumoconioses (e.g., asbestosis), sarcoidosis
	    Pulmonary vascular disease: pulmonary embolus, recurrent
	      pulmonary emboli, pulmonary hypertension

Normal A-a gradient	High altitude
	Hypoventilation (respiratory acidosis): depression of respiratory
	    center (e.g., barbiturates), neuromuscular disease (e.g.,
	    paralysis diaphragm, ALS, myasthenia gravis, poliomyelitis)

ALS, amyotrophic lateral sclerosis; ARDS, acute respiratory distress syndrome; ASD, atrial septal defect; PDA, patent ductus arteriosus; RDS, respiratory distress syndrome; VSD, ventricular septal defect.

III. **Diffusing Capacity of the Lung**
  A. **Test characteristics**
    1. Evaluates the ability of a gas to diffuse through the alveolar-capillary septum
    2. Assessed by the diffusion capacity of the lung for carbon monoxide (D$_{LCO}$)
      a. Patient inhales in a single breath a gas mixture containing CO.
      b. During exhalation, the expired gas is analyzed for CO.
        (1) Reported as mL CO/second/mm Hg
        (2) Typical normal value is 0.42 mL CO/second/mm Hg.

D$_{LCO}$: evaluates alveolar-capillary septum function

  B. **Parameters affecting D$_{LCO}$** (Fig. 3-7)
    1. CO reaching the alveolus; decreased D$_{LCO}$
      a. Airway obstruction (e.g., mucus plugs)
      b. Atelectasis (e.g., collapse of alveoli in respiratory distress syndrome)
    2. CO crossing the alveolar-capillary septum; decreased D$_{LCO}$
      a. Interstitial lung disease (e.g., idiopathic pulmonary fibrosis)
      b. Destruction of alveoli (e.g., emphysema)
      c. Decreased volume in the pulmonary vascular bed
        • Examples—recurrent pulmonary emboli, emphysema
      d. Decrease in alveolar-capillary surface area
        • Examples—pneumonectomy, pneumothorax, emphysema

↓ D$_{LCO}$: airway obstruction, atelectasis; interstitial, alveolar, capillary disease

    3. CO crossing the alveolar-capillary septum; increased D$_{LCO}$
      a. Increase in the alveolar-capillary surface area
        • Hyperinflation of the lung due to bronchial asthma
      b. Hyperinflation of the lung in emphysema is offset by destruction of the alveoli and the volume of the pulmonary capillary bed.
    4. CO binding to Hb in RBCs in the pulmonary capillary; decreased D$_{LCO}$

DIFFUSING CAPACITY (DLCO$_2$)

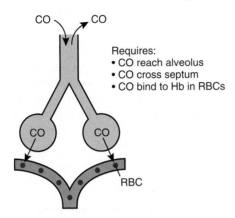

Requires:
• CO reach alveolus
• CO cross septum
• CO bind to Hb in RBCs

3-7: *Measurement of pulmonary diffusion capacity for carbon monoxide (DLCO). See text for discussion. Hb, hemoglobin; RBCs, red blood cells.*

• Anemia, where decreased RBC mass means less binding of CO to RBCs (more is exhaled)

5. CO binding to Hb in RBCs in the pulmonary capillary; increased DLCO
   a. Polycythemia, where increased RBC mass means greater binding of CO to RBCs (less is exhaled)
   b. Intra-alveolar hemorrhage, where CO binds to Hb in alveoli
      • Example—Goodpasture's syndrome

> In the laboratory, the DLCO is usually corrected for the Hb concentration; therefore, the above changes related to anemia and polycythemia reflect changes that would only occur if the correction was not made.

↑DLCO: ↓CO in expired air

↓DLCO: ↑CO in expired air

IV. Selected Disorders
A. Pulmonary infarction
1. Epidemiology and pathogenesis
   a. Risk factors
      (1) Stasis of blood flow
         • Examples—postoperative state, long airplane ride, scuba diving
      (2) Hypercoagulable states
         • Examples—oral contraceptives (estrogen component), antithrombin III deficiency
   b. Most infarctions are located in the lower lobes.
      • Perfusion is greater than ventilation in the lower lobes.
2. Pathogenesis
   a. Venous thrombi most often develop in the deep veins below the knee
      • Propagation into the femoral vein increases the risk for embolization to medium-sized and small pulmonary arteries.
   b. Consequences of pulmonary artery occlusion

Bronchial arteries: protect lungs from infarction

(1) Increase in pulmonary artery pressure
(2) Decreased blood flow to pulmonary parenchyma
- May cause hemorrhagic infarction

> The lung parenchyma is supplied by both bronchial and pulmonary arteries. Bronchial arteries originate from the thoracic aorta and intercostal arteries; therefore, their blood flow is entirely dependent on the cardiac output. If cardiac output is normal and there are no ventilation/perfusion defects in the lungs, a pulmonary embolus is *not* likely to produce a pulmonary infarction. However, if the cardiac output is decreased (e.g., congestive heart failure) or ventilation/perfusion defects are present (e.g., obstructive lung disease), then occlusion of a pulmonary vessel will likely result in a hemorrhagic infarction, which significantly increases morbidity and mortality risks.

Pulmonary infarction: dyspnea and tachypnea most common symptom and sign, respectively

3. Clinical findings
   a. Sudden onset of dyspnea and tachypnea
   b. Fever
   c. Pleuritic chest pain (pain on inspiration), friction rub, hemorrhagic effusion
4. Laboratory findings with a pulmonary infarction
   a. Respiratory alkalosis ($Paco_2 < 33$ mm Hg)
      - Due to stimulation of peripheral chemoreceptors by hypoxemia
   b. $Pao_2 < 80$ mm Hg (90% of cases)
   c. Increased A-a gradient (100% of cases)
   d. Abnormal perfusion radionuclide scan (Fig. 3-8)

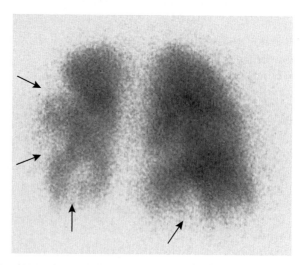

3-8: Radionuclide perfusion scan in the lung. The radionuclide scan shows multiple perfusion defects in both lungs (arrows) due to multiple pulmonary emboli. (From Forbes C, Jackson W: Color Atlas and Text of Clinical Medicine, 2nd ed. St. Louis, Mosby, 2003, Fig. 4.49.)

(1) Ventilation scan is normal, but the perfusion scan is abnormal

(2) Pulmonary angiogram is the gold standard confirmatory test.

   e. Positive D-dimers (see Chapter 7, Hemostasis Disorders)

B. **Sarcoidosis**

1. Epidemiology
   - Accounts for ~25% of restrictive parenchymal lung diseases

2. Pathogenesis
   - CD4 T_H cells interact with an unknown antigen leading to the formation of noncaseating granulomas.

3. Lung disease
   a. Most common noninfectious granulomatous disease of lungs
   b. Location of noncaseating granulomas
      - Interstitium primarily along the lymphatics and around the bronchi and blood vessels
   c. Healing of granulomas results in varying degrees of interstitial fibrosis

4. Laboratory findings
   a. Spirometry and flow-volume loop studies show a restrictive pattern.
   b. Respiratory alkalosis ($Paco_2 < 33$ mm Hg)
   c. Hypoxemia, increased A-a gradient
   d. Decreased D_{LCO}
   e. Increased angiotensin-converting enzyme
      - Excellent marker of disease activity and response to corticosteroid therapy
   f. Hypercalcemia (5% of cases)
      (1) Increased synthesis of $1\text{-}\alpha\text{-hydroxylase}$ by macrophages in the granulomas
      (2) Produces hypervitaminosis D

> Sarcoidosis: most common noninfectious granulomatous disease of lungs

C. **Chronic bronchitis**

1. Epidemiology
   a. Cigarette smoking is the most common cause in adults.
   b. Cystic fibrosis is the most common cause in children.

2. Pathogenesis
   a. Hypersecretion of mucus in bronchi and bronchioles
   b. Obstruction to airflow in the terminal bronchioles

> Turbulent airflow in the bronchi is converted into laminar airflow in the terminal (nonrespiratory) bronchioles. The terminal bronchioles undergo parallel branching, which reduces airflow resistance and spreads air out over a large cross-sectional area. Mucus plugs located in proximal terminal bronchioles prevent the elimination of CO_2 arising from gas exchange in the alveoli. Retention of CO_2 produces respiratory acidosis leading to cyanosis; hence, the term "blue bloater" for patients with chronic bronchitis.

> Chronic bronchitis: affects proximal large and small airways; retention of CO_2

3. Clinical findings
   a. Productive cough for at least 3 months for 2 consecutive years
      - Chronic bronchitis is a clinical diagnosis.

b. Dyspnea is mild and occurs late in the disease.
c. Cyanosis ("blue bloaters")
  • Due to retention of CO_2 causing respiratory acidosis–hypoxemia-decreased Sao_2
d. Cor pulmonale
  (1) Pulmonary hypertension (PH) plus right ventricular hypertrophy (RVH)
  (2) Chronic hypoxemia and respiratory acidosis cause pulmonary artery vasoconstriction leading to PH
  (3) PH imposes an afterload to the right ventricle resulting in RVH.
e. Patients tend to be stocky or obese.
4. Laboratory findings
  a. Spirometry and flow-volume loop studies show an obstructive pattern
  b. Severe hypoxemia (Pao_2 45–60 mm Hg), increased A-a gradient
  c. Chronic respiratory acidosis ($Paco_2$ 50–60 mm Hg)
  d. Normal to slightly decreased D_{LCO}
  e. Increased Hb and RBC count
    • Early onset of hypoxemia stimulates erythropoietin release causing a secondary polycythemia
  f. Chest radiograph
    (1) Large, horizontally oriented heart
    (2) Increased bronchial markings due to inflammation
D. **Emphysema**
  1. Epidemiology
    a. Cigarette smoking is the most common cause
    b. Hereditary α_1-antitrypsin (AAT) deficiency
  2. Pathogenesis
    a. Permanent enlargement of all or part of the respiratory unit
      • Respiratory unit—respiratory bronchioles, alveolar ducts, alveoli (Fig. 3-9A)
    b. Cigarette smoke is chemotactic to neutrophils and inactivates AAT.
      • AAT is an anti-elastase and anti-protease.
    c. Neutrophils release elastases, proteases, and oxidant free radicals.
      (1) Damage elastic tissue support of all or part of the respiratory unit
      (2) Damage elastic tissue support of terminal bronchioles in proximity to the respiratory bronchioles
      (3) Inactivated AAT cannot prevent neutrophil destruction of elastic tissue.
    d. Damaged terminal bronchioles collapse when the lungs are compressed during expiration.
      (1) Air is trapped in the respiratory unit.
      (2) There is distention of those structures that have been damaged.
    e. Centriacinar (centrilobular) emphysema (Fig. 3-9B)
      (1) Involves the upper lobes of the lungs
      (2) Respiratory bronchiole elastic tissue support is damaged and traps air
    f. Panacinar emphysema (Fig. 3-9C)

Emphysema: affects the distal airways (respiratory unit)

A **Normal**

B **Centriacinar emphysema**   **C** **Panacinar emphysema**

3-9: *Types of emphysema. The schematic shows a normal distal airway (**A**), including a terminal bronchiole (TB) leading into the respiratory unit consisting of a respiratory bronchiole (RB), alveolar duct (AD), and alveoli (ALV). Elastic fibers apply radial traction to keep these airways open. Centriacinar emphysema (**B**) is characterized by trapping of air in the respiratory bronchioles. Note how the elastic fibers of the distal TB are destroyed causing obstruction to airflow on expiration. This causes the trapped air to distend the RBs, whose elastic tissue support is destroyed. Panacinar emphysema (**C**) is characterized by trapping of air in the entire respiratory unit behind the collapsed TB. (From Goljan EF: Rapid Review Pathology, 2nd ed. St. Louis, Mosby, 2007, Fig. 16-16.)*

      (1) Involves the lower lobes of the lungs
      (2) Entire respiratory unit elastic tissue support is damaged and
            traps air
   3. Clinical findings
      a. Progressive severe dyspnea and hyperventilation
         (1) Gas exchange is normal until late in the disease.
         (2) Patients work hard at breathing in order to deliver O_2 to the
            alveoli during inspiration and to eliminate CO_2 during expiration
            against increased resistance in the collapsed terminal bronchioles.

> Emphysema patients purse their lips (tensing of the upper and lower lips) in order to increase pressure in the distal airways to prevent their collapse on expiration. Therefore, oxygenation and elimination of CO_2 are well maintained until late in the disease; hence the term "pink puffer" for the emphysema patient.

      b. Scant sputum production, thin body habitus

    c. Breath sounds diminished due to hyperinflation
- Hyperinflation increases the anteroposterior diameter of the chest.

4. Laboratory findings
    a. Spirometry and flow-volume loop studies show an obstructive pattern (see Section IC).
    b. Hypoxemia (Pao_2 65–75 mm Hg)
- Late finding because of matched losses of ventilation (i.e., destruction of alveoli) and perfusion (i.e., destruction of pulmonary capillary bed)

    c. Normal to slightly decreased $Paco_2$ (30–40 mm Hg)
    d. Increased A-a gradient
    e. Decreased D_{LCO}
    f. Chest radiograph (Fig. 3-10)
      (1) Hyperlucent lung fields, increased anteroposterior diameter, and depressed diaphragms due to increased TLC
      (2) Vertically oriented heart

E. **Methemoglobinemia (metHb)**
1. Epidemiology and pathophysiology
    a. Heme group iron is oxidized to the ferric (Fe^{3+}) state.

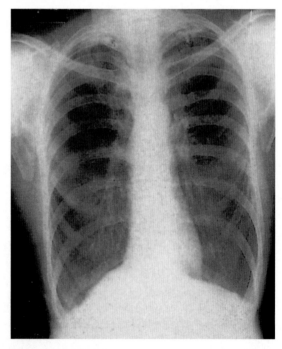

3-10: *Posteroanterior chest radiograph in a patient with emphysema. The chest radiograph shows hyperinflation in both lung fields producing depression of both diaphragms. The heart has a vertical orientation. Multifocal areas of dystrophic calcification are also noted in the apices of both lungs, resulting from healed tuberculosis. (From Forbes C, Jackson W: Color Atlas and Text of Clinical Medicine, 2nd ed. St. Louis, Mosby, 2003, Fig. 4.95.)*

(1) MetHb concentration >1% is called methemoglobinemia.

(2) NADH-methemoglobin reductase reduces ferric iron to ferrous (Fe^{2+}).

(3) NADPH methemoglobin oxidase and ascorbic acid assume a minor role in reducing ferric iron to the ferrous state.

b. Oxidized heme groups cannot bind O_2.

- Sao_2 is decreased, Pao_2 is normal.

c. Left-shifted O_2-binding curve

- Increased affinity of reduced heme for O_2

d. Caused by exogenous oxidant stresses

(1) Drugs and chemicals

- Nitroglycerin, sodium nitrite (used in treatment of cyanide poisoning), nitrites in well water, dapsone (treatment of leprosy), trimethoprim-sulfamethoxazole (treatment of urinary tract infections and *Pneumocystis jiroveci* pneumonia), primaquine (treatment of malaria)

(2) Congenital deficiency of NADH methemoglobin reductase

(3) Congenital methemoglobinemia

- M-hemoglobins stabilize iron in its oxidized form.

2. Clinical findings

a. Cyanosis unresponsive to supplemental O_2

- Methemoglobin levels >1.5 g/dL

b. Chocolate-colored blood (increased deoxyhemoglobin)

c. Headache, tachypnea, tachycardia, coma

3. Laboratory findings

a. Decreased Sao_2, normal Pao_2

(1) ABGs performed *without* a co-oximeter show a normal Sao_2.

- Sao_2 is calculated from the Pao_2.

(2) Pulse oximeter reads a falsely high Sao_2.

- Cannot identify methemoglobin (see Section IIC)

(3) Co-oximeter identifies metHb.

- Correctly calculates Sao_2, because it includes metHb in the calculation for Sao_2 resulting in a decreased Sao_2 (see Section IIC)

b. May produce a hemolytic anemia

(1) Oxidation of Hb produces Heinz bodies (clumps of denatured Hb)

(2) Macrophages remove Heinz bodies close to the RBC membrane and produce bite cells.

- Hemolytic anemia, Heinz bodies, and bite cells are also seen in glucose 6-phosphate deficiency (see Chapter 5).

c. Increased anion gap metabolic acidosis due to lactic acidosis (see Chapter 2)

4. Treatment

a. Methylene blue

(1) Activates NADPH metHb reductase pathway

(2) Methylene blue directly reduces ferric to ferrous heme.

MetHb: ↓Sao_2, normal Pao_2

MetHb: treat with methylene blue

b. Ascorbic acid, which is a reducing agent
- An ancillary treatment that does *not* replace methylene blue.

F. **Carbon monoxide (CO) poisoning**

1. Epidemiology and pathogenesis

a. Produced by incomplete combustion of carbon-containing material.

b. High binding affinity for heme groups in

(1) Hb

(2) Myoglobin

(3) Cytochrome P-450 in the liver microsomal mixed function oxidase system

(4) Cytochrome oxidase in the mitochondrial electron transport chain

c. CO prevents utilization of O_2 by the above pigments and enzymes.

(1) By binding to heme groups in Hb, CO decreases SaO_2 *without* affecting the PaO_2.

(2) By binding to cytochrome oxidase, CO inhibits the generation of ATP by oxidative phosphorylation in the mitochondria.

(3) By binding to myoglobin, CO reduces availability of O_2 for aerobic metabolism in cardiac muscle.

- Decrease in myocardial contractility and cardiac output

(4) By binding to cytochrome P-450 enzymes, CO inhibits the metabolism of drugs in the liver.

- Increases the potential for drug toxicities

d. Left-shifts the O_2-binding curve

- Prevents the release of O_2 to tissue

e. Causes

(1) Automobile exhaust

(2) Smoke inhalation (house fires)

(3) Wood stoves (space heaters) with poor exhaust system

(4) Inhaling methyl chloride vapor

- Component in paint stripping solutions

(5) Cigarette smoking

2. Clinical findings

a. Headache is the most common initial symptom.

b. Cherry-red color of skin

(1) Due to the red coloration of COHb in blood and CO bound to muscle

(2) Skin discoloration masks the presence of cyanosis.

c. Somnolence, seizures, coma leading to death

d. Rhabdomyolysis, necrosis of globus pallidus (parkinsonism), stroke

3. Laboratory findings

a. Decreased SaO_2

(1) ABGs performed *without* a co-oximeter show a normal SaO_2.

- SaO_2 is calculated from the PaO_2.

(2) Pulse oximeter reads a falsely high SaO_2.

- Cannot identify COHb (see Section IIC)

(3) Co-oximeter identifies COHb and correctly calculates SaO_2.

CO: binds heme groups; left-shift OBC

CO: ↓SaO_2, normal PaO_2

- Includes COHb in the calculation for Sao_2 resulting in a decreased Sao_2 (see Section IIC)

b. Normal Pao_2 and A-a gradient

4. Treatment
   - Ventilation with 100% O_2 displaces CO.

Questions

Each numbered item is followed by options arranged in alphabetical or logical order. Select the best answer to each question. Some options may be partially correct, but there is only *one best* answer.

1. A 45-year-old man presents to his physician with dyspnea and cyanosis. He is currently breathing room air. An arterial blood gas reveals the following: pH of 7.20, Pco_2 72 mm Hg, HCO_3^- 28 mEq/L, Po_2 50 mm Hg. Which of the following conditions is most compatible with the history and laboratory findings?
   A. Acute respiratory distress syndrome
   B. Barbiturate overdose
   C. Chronic bronchitis
   D. Emphysema
   E. Pulmonary infarction

2. A 35-year-old man has severe smoke inhalation from a house fire. In the emergency room, the patient complains of a severe headache and has a cherry-red discoloration of his skin and mucous membranes. Which of the following laboratory findings is most likely present?
   A. Decreased arterial O_2 saturation (Sao_2)
   B. Decreased arterial Po_2
   C. Increased alveolar-arterial gradient
   D. Increased serum bicarbonate
   E. Normal O_2 content

3. A 45-year-old cattle farmer who recently dug a well for drinking water presents to his family physician with fatigue, dyspnea, and a headache. Physical examination reveals bluish discoloration of the skin and mucous membranes. Supplemental O_2 does not alleviate his symptoms or alter the skin discoloration. Blood drawn for arterial blood gases has a chocolate brown discoloration. Which of the following laboratory test findings is expected?
   A. Decreased arterial O_2 saturation (Sao_2)
   B. Decreased arterial Po_2
   C. Increased alveolar-arterial gradient
   D. Increased serum bicarbonate
   E. Normal O_2 content

4. A 60-year-old man who has smoked two packs of cigarettes daily for 35 years complains of difficulty with breathing at rest and with exercise. Physical examination reveals a man with an emaciated appearance and pink discoloration

of the skin. It is difficult to hear heart and lung sounds. A chest radiograph shows hyperinflation in both lung fields, depression of both diaphragms, an increase in the anteroposterior diameter, and a vertically oriented cardiac silhouette. Which of the following pulmonary function test results is expected?

A. Decreased functional residual capacity
B. Decreased total lung capacity
C. Increased forced expiratory volume 1 second/forced vital capacity ratio
D. Increased residual volume
E. Increased tidal volume

5. In which of the following clinical scenarios would spirometry dynamic flow studies show an increased forced expiratory volume (FEV) 1 second/forced vital capacity (FVC) ratio?

A. A 12-year-old child has cystic fibrosis and repeated respiratory infections.
B. A 28-year-old nonsmoking man has bilateral lower lobe emphysema.
C. A 30-year-old man has low grade fever, flu-like symptoms, and nonproductive cough.
D. A 39-year-old black American man has dyspnea, bilateral hilar adenopathy, and uveitis.
E. A 56-year-old smoking man has productive cough, dyspnea, and cyanosis.

6. Which of the following clinical disorders most likely produces an increase in the diffusing capacity of the lung for carbon monoxide (D_{LCO})?

A. Acute respiratory distress syndrome
B. Emphysema
C. Polycythemia vera
D. Recurrent pulmonary emboli
E. Sarcoidosis

Answers

1. **B** (barbiturate overdose) is correct. The arterial blood gas reveals an acute, uncompensated respiratory acidosis with hypoxemia: pH 7.20 (acidemia), $Paco_2$ 72 mm Hg (respiratory acidosis), HCO_3^- 28 mEq/L (normal), Po_2 50 mm Hg (hypoxemia). To determine whether the hypoxemia is pulmonary or extrapulmonary in origin, a calculation of the alveolar-arterial (A-a) gradient is required. The alveolar Po_2 is calculated as follows: 0.21 (room air) × 713 mm Hg (atmospheric pressure—water vapor pressure) − 72 mm Hg (arterial $Paco_2$)/0.8 (respiratory quotient) = 60 mm Hg. Because the Pao_2 is 50 mm Hg, the A-a gradient is 60 − 50 = 10 mm Hg. An A-a gradient >30 mm Hg is medically significant. Hypoxemia in the presence of a normal A-a gradient indicates an extrapulmonary cause of hypoxemia that involves hypoventilation (respiratory acidosis) due to depression of the respiratory center in the brain (e.g., barbiturates) or chest wall dysfunction (e.g., neuromuscular disease, kyphoscoliosis, obesity, paralysis of the diaphragms). Hypoxemia in the presence of an increased A-a gradient indicates a primary disease in the lungs (e.g., atelectasis, ventilation-perfusion defect, pulmonary vascular disease) or congenital heart disease with a right-to-left shunt (e.g., tetralogy of Fallot; reversal of a ventricular or atrial septal defect).

A (acute respiratory distress syndrome) is incorrect. ARDS is associated with acute respiratory acidosis leading to severe hypoxemia. It is characterized by neutrophil damage to the alveoli (ventilation-perfusion defect), atelectasis (decreased surfactant from destruction of type II pneumocytes causing intrapulmonary shunting of blood), and noncardiogenic pulmonary edema with hyaline membranes (diffusion defect). All these lung findings cause an increase in the A-a gradient.

C (chronic bronchitis) is incorrect. Chronic bronchitis is an obstructive lung disease associated with chronic respiratory acidosis leading to severe hypoxemia. Inflammation and mucus plugs blocking the terminal bronchioles interferes with clearance of CO_2 causing an increase in alveolar Pco_2 and a corresponding decrease in alveolar Po_2 and Pao_2. The proximal small airway obstruction produces a major ventilation-perfusion mismatch causing an increase in the A-a gradient.

D (emphysema) is incorrect. Emphysema is an obstructive lung disease that produces destruction of the respiratory unit (respiratory bronchioles, alveolar ducts, alveoli) and the pulmonary vascular bed leading to a matched loss of ventilation and perfusion causing hypoxemia and an increased A-a gradient. Arterial blood gases either show a normal $Paco_2$ or slightly decreased $Paco_2$, the latter due to respiratory alkalosis from hyperventilation.

E (pulmonary infarction) is incorrect. Pulmonary infarction is associated with an acute respiratory alkalosis (alkaline pH, decreased P_{CO_2}) and mild hypoxemia. Thromboembolism originating from the femoral vein is the most common cause of a pulmonary infarction. Obstruction of pulmonary vessels produces a perfusion defect leading to an increase in dead space in the lungs causing a mild hypoxemia and an increase in the A-a gradient.

2. **A** (decreased arterial O_2 saturation, Sa_{O_2}) is correct. Carbon monoxide (CO) commonly occurs in house fires. CO is produced by incomplete combustion of carbon-containing materials. CO has a 230 to 270 times greater binding affinity for heme groups than O_2. Sa_{O_2} is the average percentage of O_2 bound to heme groups in hemoglobin (Hb), so it is decreased in CO poisoning. If a co-oximeter attachment is *not* used in measuring the arterial blood gas, the Sa_{O_2} is normal, because it is calculated from the Pa_{O_2}, which is normal in CO poisoning.

B (decrease in arterial P_{O_2}) is incorrect. The arterial P_{O_2} is normal in CO poisoning, because CO does *not* interfere with the concentration of alveolar P_{O_2} or the diffusion of O_2 through the alveolar-capillary septum.

C (increased alveolar-arterial gradient) is incorrect. The A-a gradient is obtained by subtracting the measured arterial P_{O_2} from the calculated alveolar P_{O_2}. Because of a disparity between ventilation and perfusion in different portions of the lung, the arterial P_{O_2} is always less than the alveolar P_{O_2}, which causes the A-a gradient. The gradient is increased when there is a further disparity between alveolar and arterial P_{O_2}. This occurs most often with ventilation-perfusion defects due to primary lung disease (e.g., emphysema, chronic bronchitis, atelectasis) or in congenital heart disease with right-to-left shunts. In CO poisoning, the A-a gradient is normal, because there is no alteration in either the alveolar or the arterial P_{O_2}.

D (increased serum bicarbonate) is incorrect. An increased serum bicarbonate indicates the presence of metabolic alkalosis, either as compensation for respiratory acidosis or as a primary disorder. In CO poisoning, a decrease in Sa_{O_2} causes tissue hypoxia (lack of O_2 in tissue), which results in anaerobic glycolysis. Lactic acid is the end product of anaerobic glycolysis and produces metabolic acidosis with a decrease in serum bicarbonate.

E (normal O_2 content) is incorrect. The O_2 content represents the total amount of O_2 that is being carried in the blood. It is calculated with the following formula: $1.34 \times Hb \times Sa_{O_2} + 0.003 \times Pa_{O_2}$. Because the Sa_{O_2} is decreased in CO poisoning, the O_2 content is decreased and the total amount of O_2 that is available to tissue is decreased.

3. **A** (decreased arterial O_2 saturation, SaO_2) is correct. The patient has methemoglobinemia. Methemoglobinemia results from exposure to chemicals that oxidize heme iron in hemoglobin (Hb) from its ferrous (Fe^{2+}) state to a ferric (Fe^{3+}) state. Oxidizing agents include nitrate and nitrite salts and sulfur-containing drugs or chemicals (e.g., dapsone, trimethoprim-sulfamethoxazole). The patient was most likely exposed to nitrate and nitrite salts in the well water. Because O_2 only binds to heme iron in the ferrous condition, the SaO_2 (percentage of heme groups on Hb occupied by O_2) is decreased. The increase in deoxyhemoglobin (Hb lacking O_2) gives blood a chocolate-colored appearance and causes cyanosis (bluish discoloration of the skin and mucous membranes) that does *not* respond to supplemental O_2. The treatment of choice is methylene blue, which directly reduces iron back to the ferrous state and also enhances NADPH methemoglobin reductase. Ascorbic acid, a reducing agent, is used as adjunctive therapy.

B (decreased arterial PO_2) is incorrect. The arterial PO_2 is normal in methemoglobinemia, because gas diffusion from the lungs into the pulmonary capillaries is normal.

C (increased alveolar-arterial gradient) is incorrect. The A-a gradient is obtained by subtracting the measured arterial PO_2 from the calculated alveolar PO_2. Because of a disparity between ventilation and perfusion in different portions of the lung, the arterial PO_2 is always less than the alveolar PO_2, which causes the A-a gradient. The gradient is increased when there is a further disparity between alveolar and arterial PO_2. This occurs most often with ventilation-perfusion defects due to primary lung disease (e.g., emphysema) or in congenital heart disease with right-to-left shunts. In methemoglobinemia, the A-a gradient is normal, because there is no alteration in either the alveolar or the arterial PO_2.

D (increased serum bicarbonate) is incorrect. An increased serum bicarbonate indicates the presence of metabolic alkalosis, either as compensation for respiratory acidosis or as a primary disorder. In methemoglobinemia, a decrease in SaO_2 causes tissue hypoxia (lack of O_2 in tissue), which results in anaerobic glycolysis. Lactic acid is the end product of anaerobic glycolysis and produces metabolic acidosis with a decrease in serum bicarbonate.

E (normal O_2 content) is incorrect. The O_2 content represents the total amount of O_2 that is being carried in the blood. It is calculated with the following formula: $1.34 \times Hb \times SaO_2 + 0.003 \times PaO_2$. Because the SaO_2 is decreased in methemoglobinemia, the O_2 content is decreased and the total amount of O_2 that is available to tissue is decreased.

4. **D** (increased residual volume, RV) is correct. The patient has emphysema (chronic dyspnea, hyperinflated lungs, depressed diaphragms) related to a long history of smoking cigarettes. Emphysema is a chronic obstructive pulmonary disease that produces permanent enlargement of all or part of the respiratory unit (respiratory bronchioles, alveolar ducts, and alveoli) as well as destruction of the pulmonary capillary bed. Elastic tissue destruction in small airways causes trapping of air and distention of the distal airspace, which increases the RV (volume of air left in the lung after maximal expiration). An increase in RV always increases the total lung capacity (TLC, total amount of air in the lungs after a maximal inspiration). An increase in TLC causes hyperinflation of the lungs, an increase in the anteroposterior diameter, and depression of the diaphragms.

A (decreased functional residual capacity, FRC) is incorrect. The FRC is the total amount of air in the lungs at the end of a normal expiration. It is the sum of the expiratory reserve volume (amount of air forcibly expelled at the end of a normal expiration) and the RV. In emphysema, the RV is increased, which increases (not decreases) the FRC.

B (decreased total lung capacity, TLC) is incorrect. In emphysema, the RV is increased, which increases (not decreases) the TLC.

C (increased forced expiratory volume 1 second/forced vital capacity ratio, $FEV_{1\,sec}$/FVC) is incorrect. In emphysema, lung compliance (ability to fill the lung with air) is increased and elasticity (recoil of the lung) is decreased because of destruction of elastic tissue by elastases and oxidant free radicals released from neutrophils. The $FEV_{1\,sec}$, or the amount of air expelled from the lungs in 1 second after a maximal inspiration, is decreased (e.g., 1 L versus the normal 4 L) because of trapping of air in the distended distal airways. The FVC, or total amount of air expelled after a maximal inspiration, is also decreased (e.g., 3 L versus the normal 5 L) causing the $FEV_{1\,sec}$/FVC ratio to be decreased (not increased).

E (increased tidal volume) is incorrect. In emphysema, the tidal volume (volume of air that enters or leaves the lungs during normal quiet respiration) is decreased (not increased) as the FRC increases and compresses the remaining volumes and capacities.

5. **D** (a 39-year-old black American man has dyspnea, bilateral hilar adenopathy, and uveitis) is correct. An increase in the $FEV_{1\,sec}$/FVC ratio is present in restrictive parenchymal disorders. Restrictive disorders are characterized by limited filling of the lungs causing all the lung volumes to be decreased (i.e., "stiff lungs"). Elastic recoil of the lung is increased, due to an increase of fibrous tissue in the interstitium. Dynamic flow studies in spirometry show a decrease in FVC (total amount of air expelled after a maximal inspiration) and the $FEV_{1\,sec}$ (amount of air expelled from the lungs in 1 second after a maximal inspiration). However, due to an increase in elastic recoil in the lungs, the $FEV_{1\,sec}$ and FVC are frequently the same (e.g., 3 L) causing the ratio of the two to be normal or increased. The patient in the clinical scenario has sarcoidosis, which is a restrictive parenchymal lung disease that is common in the black American population. CD4 T_H cells interact with an unknown antigen leading to the formation of noncaseating granulomas. Granulomas in the interstitium heal with scarring leading to restrictive lung disease.

A (a 12-year-old child has cystic fibrosis and repeated respiratory infections) is incorrect. Patients with cystic fibrosis are prone to frequent bacterial pneumonias that destroy the elastic tissue support of the airways leading to bronchiectasis, a type of chronic obstructive pulmonary disease (COPD). In bronchiectasis, the $FEV_{1\,sec}$ and the FVC are both decreased due to collapse of the airways on expiration, causing the $FEV_{1\,sec}/FVC$ ratio to be decreased.

B (a 28-year-old nonsmoking man has bilateral lower lobe emphysema) is incorrect. Emphysema is a COPD that produces permanent enlargement of all or part of the distal airways as well as destruction of the pulmonary capillary bed. In a nonsmoking individual with lower lobe emphysema, the patient most likely has panacinar emphysema due to a deficiency of α_1-antitrypsin, a protein that normally neutralizes elastases produced by neutrophils. In obstructive lung disease, the $FEV_{1\,sec}/FVC$ ratio is decreased.

C (a 30-year-old man has low-grade fever, flu-like symptoms, and nonproductive cough) is incorrect. Pneumonias with low-grade fever and nonproductive cough are called atypical pneumonias, because they involve the interstitium of the lung and do *not* produce alveolar exudates. *Mycoplasma pneumoniae* is the most common cause of atypical pneumonia. Atypical pneumonias do *not* produce permanent lung disease; therefore, the $FEV_{1\,sec}/FVC$ ratio is normal.

E (a 56-year-old smoking man has productive cough, dyspnea, and cyanosis) is incorrect. Productive cough with dyspnea and cyanosis in a smoker is a classic history for chronic bronchitis, which is a COPD. The $FEV_{1\,sec}/FVC$ ratio is decreased in obstructive lung disease.

6. **C** (polycythemia vera) is correct. The D_{LCO} is dependent on CO reaching the alveolus, CO crossing the alveolar-capillary septum, and CO binding to hemoglobin (Hb) in RBCs in the pulmonary capillary. The D_{LCO} is calculated by measuring the amount of CO remaining in expired air. A decrease in CO in expired air indicates that there is an increase in D_{LCO}, while an increase in CO in expired air indicates a decrease in D_{LCO} and a problem with one of the above parameters. The D_{LCO} is increased in polycythemia, because an increase in RBC mass causes more CO to bind with Hb; therefore, less CO is expired in air. In contrast, the D_{LCO} is decreased in anemia (more CO is present in expired air), because there is a decrease in RBC mass and less binding of CO to Hb.

A (acute respiratory distress syndrome, ARDS) is incorrect. In ARDS, there is destruction of the alveoli and small airways and damage to pulmonary capillaries causing alveolar exudates and hyaline membranes, all of which cause a decrease in the D_{LCO} (increase in CO in expired air).

B (emphysema) is incorrect. Emphysema is associated with destruction of the distal airways and the pulmonary capillary bed, which restricts CO from diffusing through the alveolar-capillary septum, causing a decrease in the D_{LCO} (increase in CO in expired air).

D (recurrent pulmonary emboli) is incorrect. Recurrent pulmonary emboli decrease the volume of the pulmonary capillary bed, which restricts CO from binding to Hb in RBCs in the pulmonary capillaries causing a decrease in the D_{LCO} (increase in CO in expired air).

E (sarcoidosis) is incorrect. Sarcoidosis is a restrictive parenchymal lung disease that is associated with interstitial fibrosis, which restricts CO from diffusing through the alveolar-capillary septum, causing a decrease in the D_{LCO} (increase in CO in expired air).

Renal Disorders

I. **Renal Function Overview**
   A. **Excretion**
      - Removes waste products of metabolism (e.g., urea, creatinine, uric acid)
   B. **Reabsorption**
      - Retains certain electrolytes and solutes (e.g., sodium, glucose, amino acids)
   C. **Acid-base homeostasis**
      - Controls the synthesis and excretion of bicarbonate and hydrogen ions (see Chapter 2)
   D. **Water and sodium metabolism** (see Chapter 2)
      1. Controls water by concentrating and diluting urine
      2. Controls sodium reabsorption in the proximal and distal/collecting tubules
   E. **Vascular tone**
      1. Angiotensin II
         a. Derivative of the renin-angiotensin-aldosterone system
         b. Vasoconstricts peripheral resistance arterioles and efferent arterioles
         c. Stimulates the synthesis and release of aldosterone
      2. Renal-derived prostaglandin
         - Vasodilates the afferent arterioles
   F. **Erythropoiesis**
      - Erythropoietin is synthesized in the endothelial cells in the peritubular capillaries.
   G. **Calcium homeostasis**
      1. 1-α-Hydroxylase
         a. Synthesized in the proximal renal tubule cells
         b. Converts 25-hydroxycholecalciferol to 1,25-dihydroxycholecalciferol, the active form of vitamin D
      2. Vitamin D
         a. Increases gastrointestinal reabsorption of calcium and phosphorus
            - Regulates serum calcium
         b. Promotes bone mineralization
         c. Increases the production of osteoclasts from macrophage stem cells

Kidneys: synthesize erythropoietin and vitamin D

> Vitamin D promotes bone mineralization by stimulating the release of alkaline phosphatase from osteoblasts. Alkaline phosphatase hydrolyzes (dephosphorylates) pyrophosphate and other inhibitors of calcium-phosphate crystallization.

II. **Renal Function Tests**
   A. **Indicators of renal disease**
      1. Increased serum blood urea nitrogen (BUN) and serum creatinine
      2. Decreased creatinine clearance
      3. Loss of urine concentration (most important) and dilution
      4. Proteinuria
      5. Hematuria
      6. Pyuria (i.e., neutrophils in the urine)
      7. Presence of renal tubular casts
   B. **Serum BUN**
      • Normal range is 7 to 18 mg/dL.
      1. End product of amino acid and pyrimidine metabolism
         a. Produced by the liver urea cycle

         > Ammonia derived from amino acid metabolism or from degradation of amino acids in the gastrointestinal tract by bacteria is fed into the urea cycle and excreted as urea.

         Urea cycle: converts ammonia to urea

         b. Filtered in the kidneys and partly reabsorbed in the proximal tubule
         c. Extrarenal sites of excretion
            • Skin, gastrointestinal tract
         d. Serum levels are dependent on the following
            (1) Glomerular filtration rate (GFR)
            (2) Protein content in the diet
            (3) Tissue metabolism
            (4) Proximal tubule reabsorption, which is dependent on the GFR
            (5) Functional status of the hepatic urea cycle

            Urea: filtered and reabsorbed; excreted in extrarenal sites

      2. Causes of increased and decreased serum BUN (Table 4-1)
   C. **Serum creatinine**
      • Normal range is 0.6 to 1.2 mg/dL.
      1. Metabolic end product of creatine in muscle

         Most common cause increased serum BUN: congestive heart failure

         > Creatine phosphate is the main storage depot for energy in muscle. It is a ready source of phosphate for ATP synthesis.

         a. Filtered in the kidneys and *not* reabsorbed or secreted
         b. Serum concentration varies with the following:
            (1) Age (increases after 90 years of age)
            (2) Gender (men > women)
            (3) Muscle mass (parallels creatine concentration in muscle)
         c. Increased in renal disease, hypovolemia, and tissue necrosis
         d. Poor indicator of early renal disease
            • Approximately 50% to 70% of functioning renal tissue must be destroyed before creatinine is increased.
         e. Drug and chemical interference in certain assays
            (1) Falsely increased with certain cephalosporins (e.g., cefoxitin)
            (2) Falsely increased in diabetic ketoacidosis

         Creatinine: end product of creatine metabolism

TABLE 4-1
Causes of Increased and Decreased Serum BUN

Serum Concentration	Discussion
Increased serum BUN	
Decreased cardiac output	Examples: congestive heart failure, shock (e.g., hemorrhage), volume depletion (e.g., diuretics) ↓ Cardiac output → ↓ GFR → ↑ proximal tubule reabsorption urea → ↑ serum BUN
Increased protein intake	Examples: high-protein diet, TPN, blood in gastrointestinal tract ↑ Amino acid degradation → ↑ serum BUN
Increased tissue catabolism	Examples: third-degree burns, postoperative state, tetracycline, wasting disease (HIV) ↑ Amino acid degradation → ↑ serum BUN
Acute glomerulonephritis	Example: poststreptococcal glomerulonephritis ↓ GFR → ↑ serum BUN
Acute or chronic renal failure	Examples: acute tubular necrosis, diabetic glomerulopathy ↓ GFR → ↑ serum BUN
Postrenal disease	Example: urinary tract obstruction (e.g., urinary stone, BPH) ↓ GFR + back-diffusion of urea → ↑ serum BUN
Decreased serum BUN	
Increased plasma volume	Examples: normal pregnancy, SIADH ↑ Plasma volume → ↑ GFR → ↓ serum BUN
Decreased urea synthesis	Examples: cirrhosis, fulminant liver failure Dysfunctional urea cycle → ↓ serum BUN
Decreased protein intake	Examples: kwashiorkor, starvation ↓ Amino acid degradation → ↓ serum BUN

BPH, benign prostatic hyperplasia; BUN, blood urea nitrogen; GFR, glomerular filtration rate; HIV, human immunodeficiency virus; SIADH, syndrome of inappropriate secretion of antidiuretic hormone; TPN, total parenteral nutrition.

Pregnancy: ↓ serum BUN and creatinine

- Due to acetone and acetoacetic acid
    (3) Falsely decreased in hyperbilirubinemia
  2. Causes of increased and decreased serum creatinine (Table 4-2)
D. **Serum BUN:creatinine ratio**
  - Normal ratio is 15 (Fig. 4-1A).
  1. Ratio alterations are subdivided into
    a. Changes occurring before the kidneys (prerenal)
    b. Changes within the kidney parenchyma (renal)
    c. Changes after the kidneys (postrenal)
  2. Prerenal, renal, and postrenal azotemia
    - Azotemia refers to an increase in serum BUN and creatinine.
    a. Prerenal azotemia

Prerenal azotemia:
↓ cardiac output →
↓ renal blood flow →
↓ GFR

    (1) Hypoperfusion of the kidneys (decreased GFR) in the absence of parenchymal damage to the kidneys
    (2) Examples
      (a) Volume depletion (e.g., blood loss, gastrointestinal loss, burns, excessive sweating)
      (b) Congestive heart failure
      (c) Hemorrhagic pancreatitis (loss of protein-rich fluid around the pancreas)

Serum Concentration	Discussion
Increased serum creatinine	
Decreased cardiac output	Examples: congestive heart failure, shock (e.g., hemorrhage), volume depletion (e.g., diuretics).
	↓ Cardiac output → ↓ GFR → ↑ serum creatinine
Increased muscle mass	Example: body builder
	↑ Creatine in muscle → ↑ serum creatinine
Increased tissue necrosis	Examples: third-degree burns, rhabdomyolysis
	↑ Creatine degradation → ↑ serum creatinine
Acute glomerulonephritis	Example: post-streptococcal glomerulonephritis
	↓ GFR → ↑ serum creatinine
Acute or chronic renal failure	Examples: acute tubular necrosis, diabetic glomerulopathy
	↓ GFR → ↑ serum creatinine
Postrenal disease	Examples: urinary tract obstruction (e.g., urinary stone, BPH)
	↓ GFR → ↑ serum creatinine
Creatine supplements	Example: creatine supplements in body builders
	↑ Creatine degradation → ↑ serum creatinine
Drug/chemical interference	Example: some cephalosporins, diabetic ketoacidosis
Decreased serum creatinine	
Increased plasma volume	Examples: normal pregnancy, SIADH
	↑ Plasma volume → ↑ GFR → ↓ serum creatinine
Emaciated patient	Examples: wasting disease, marasmus
	↓ Creatine in muscle → ↓ serum creatinine
Chemical interference	Example: hyperbilirubinemia

TABLE 4-2
Causes of Increased and Decreased Serum Creatinine

BPH, benign prostatic hyperplasia; GFR, glomerular filtration rate; SIADH, syndrome of inappropriate secretion of antidiuretic hormone.

In prerenal azotemia (Fig. 4-1B), there is a decrease in GFR, which causes both the creatinine and urea to back up in the blood; however, the BUN:Cr ratio remains the same. In addition, the decrease in GFR and renal plasma flow causes an increased glomerular filtration fraction (more urea and Cr are filtered than normal). After urea and Cr are filtered, creatinine is lost in the urine; however, an excessive amount of urea is reabsorbed out of the proximal tubule into the blood causing the ratio to be > 15. For example: serum BUN 80 mg/dL and serum creatinine 4 mg/dL produce a ratio of 20.

Prerenal azotemia: BUN:creatinine ratio >15

b. Renal azotemia (uremia)
   (1) Azotemia is due to damage of the proximal tubules in the kidneys.
   (2) Examples—acute tubular necrosis, chronic renal failure

In renal azotemia (Fig. 4-1C), the GFR is decreased causing a back-up of urea and creatinine in the blood. However, some urea is also lost in extrarenal sites (e.g., skin, gastrointestinal tract) causing a disproportionate increase in creatinine and a

Renal azotemia: BUN:creatinine ratio <15

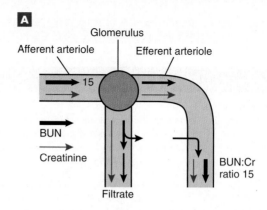

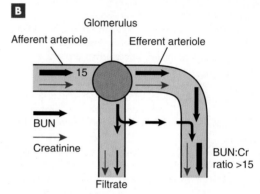

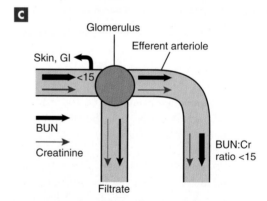

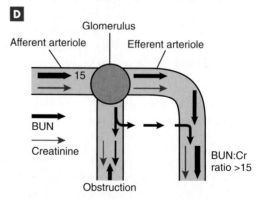

4-1: Blood urea nitrogen (BUN) and creatinine (Cr) ratios in normal persons (**A**) and in prerenal (**B**), renal (**C**), and postrenal azotemia (**D**). See text for discussion.

> BUN:Cr ratio that is <15. For example: serum BUN 80 mg/dL and serum creatinine 8 mg/dL has a ratio of 10. When creatinine and urea are filtered, both are lost in the urine because renal tubules are either dysfunctional or epithelium is sloughed off.

c. Postrenal azotemia
   (1) Azotemia is due to urinary tract obstruction below the level of the kidneys.
   (2) Examples
      (a) Prostate hyperplasia with obstruction of the urethra
      (b) Bladder or cervical cancer with obstruction of ureters
      (c) Blockage of ureters by stones

> In postrenal azotemia (Fig. 4-1D), obstruction to urine flow causes a decrease in GFR (back-up of urea and creatinine in blood) and back-diffusion of urea from the tubules into the blood causing the ratio to be >15. For example: serum BUN 60 mg/dL and serum creatinine 3 mg/dL produce a ratio of 20. If the obstruction is *not* relieved, tubular damage occurs and the ratio is <15.

Postrenal azotemia: BUN:creatinine ratio > 15

E. **Creatinine clearance (CCr)**
  1. Correlates with GFR
    • Annual decrease in CCr of 1 mL/minute beyond age 50
  2. CCr is useful in the following areas
    a. Detecting renal dysfunction
      • When comparing previous CCr values, a change >22 mL/minute in either direction is considered medically significant.
    b. Calculating dose intervals for nephrotoxic drugs

> Elderly patients normally have a decrease in CCr. Therefore, it is important to calculate the dose and dose interval for drugs that are nephrotoxic (e.g., aminoglycosides) in order to prevent acute renal failure due to nephrotoxic acute tubular necrosis.

    c. Evaluating the effectiveness of therapy of progressive renal diseases
      • Example—use of angiotensin-converting enzyme inhibitors in the treatment of diabetic glomerulopathy

Creatinine clearance: ↓ with age

  3. Creatinine clearance formula
    a. Measured CCr = UCr (mg/dL) × V (mL/min) ÷ PCr (mg/dL)
      • V = volume of a 24-hour urine collection in mL/minute, and UCr and PCr = the creatinine concentration of urine and plasma, respectively
    b. CCr is estimated with the following formula
      (1) CCr (adult male) = (140 − age) × weight in kg/PCr (mg/dL) × 72 (multiply the result by 0.85 to arrive at an estimated CCr for adult females)

**TABLE 4-3
Causes of
Increased and
Decreased CCr**

CCr Results	Discussion
Increased CCr	
Normal pregnancy	Range is 115–185 mL/min depending on the time of gestation; highest at the end of the first trimester
	Increase in plasma volume causes an increase in the GFR leading to an increase in CCr
Early diabetic glomerulopathy	Efferent arteriole becomes constricted due to hyaline arteriolosclerosis causing an increase in the GFR and CCr
	Increased GFR damages the glomerulus (hyperfiltration injury)
Decreased CCr	
Elderly people	GFR normally decreases with age causing a corresponding decrease in the CCr
Acute and chronic renal disease	Examples: ARF due to ATN, RPGN, drug hypersensitivity, postrenal obstruction; CRF due to diabetic glomerulopathy, hypertension, cystic disease

ARF, acute renal failure; ATN, acute tubular necrosis; CCr, creatinine clearance; CRF, chronic renal failure; GFR, glomerular filtration rate; RPGN, rapidly progressive glomerulonephritis.

(2) Estimated CCr is often more accurate than the measured CCr, because it does *not* require a urine collection.

c. Normal adult CCr range is 97 to 137 mL/minute.
  (1) In general, a CCr < 100 mL/minute is abnormal.
  (2) CCr < 10 mL/minute indicates renal failure.
  (3) CCr results are dependent on a correct 24-hour urine collection.
    • Undercollection or overcollection provides erroneous results.

4. Causes of increased and decreased CCr (Table 4-3)

F. **Urine osmolality (UOsm)**
  1. Useful in evaluating the concentrating ability of the kidney
    • Loss of urine concentration is the first laboratory sign of tubular dysfunction.
  2. UOsm > 500 mOsm/kg
    • Indicates good concentrating ability and normal tubular function
  3. UOsm < 350 mOsm/kg
    • Indicates poor concentrating ability and correlates with tubular dysfunction

G. **Fractional excretion of sodium (FENa$^+$)**
  1. Most sensitive and specific test for acute tubular necrosis (ATN)
  2. Calculation of the fractional excretion of sodium (FENa$^+$)
    a. FENa$^+$ is the amount of sodium excreted in the urine divided by the amount of sodium that is filtered.
    b. Calculation: FENa$^+$ = [(UNa$^+$ × PCr) ÷ (PNa$^+$ × UCr)] × 100
      (1) UNa$^+$ is a random urine sodium, PNa$^+$ serum sodium, UCr random urine creatinine, and PCr plasma creatinine.
      (2) Creatinine is used in the formula because the amount of sodium filtered is dependent on the GFR, which closely approximates the CCr.

↑ Creatinine clearance: pregnancy

FENa$^+$: most sensitive/ specific test for acute tubular necrosis

    c. $FENa^+ < 1\%$
- Indicates good tubular function and excludes ATN

    d. $FENa^+ > 2\%$
- Indicates tubular dysfunction and is highly predictive of ATN

    e. $FENa^+$ is falsely increased if a patient is losing sodium in the urine.
- Examples—diuretics, Addison's disease, 21-hydroxylase deficiency

III. **Urinalysis**
- Gold standard test in the initial workup of renal disease

  A. **Components of a basic urinalysis**
    1. General examination
      a. Color
      b. Clarity
      c. Specific gravity (usually part of the dipstick)
    2. Reagent strip (dipstick) examination
    3. Sediment examination

  B. **Urine color**
    1. Normal color is due to urobilin from oxidation of urobilinogen (UBG).
    2. Causes of urine color variations (Table 4-4)

> Urobilin: color of urine and stool; oxidation product of UBG

  C. **Urine clarity** (Table 4-4)

  D. **Urine specific gravity** (Table 4-4)
    1. Measure of the weight of solutes in water in the urine
      a. Solutes include urea, chloride, sulfate, and phosphate.
      b. Reagent strip specific gravity
- *Not* affected by excess glucose or radiocontrast material

      c. Specific gravity is a crude indicator of UOsm.
- UOsm is the most accurate measurement of solutes in urine.

TABLE 4-4
General Findings in Urinalysis

Components	Discussion
Color	Dark yellow: concentrated urine, bilirubinuria, ↑ UBG, vitamins Red or pink: hematuria, hemoglobinuria, myoglobinuria, drugs (e.g., phenazopyridine, urinary anesthetic), porphyria Smoky-colored urine: acid pH urine converts Hb to hematin; common finding in nephritic type of glomerulonephritis Black urine after exposure to light: alkaptonuria (AR disease with deficiency of homogentisate oxidase) with an increase in homogentisic acid in the urine
Clarity	Cloudy urine with alkaline pH: normal finding most often due to phosphates Cloudy urine with acid pH: normal finding most often due to uric acid Other: bacteria, WBCs, Hb, myoglobin also decrease clarity
Specific gravity	Evaluates urine concentration and dilution Specific gravity >1.023 indicates urine concentration and excludes intrinsic renal disease Fixed specific gravity (1.008–1.010): lack of concentration and dilution (e.g., chronic renal failure)

AR, autosomal recesssive; Hb, hemoglobin; UBG, urobilinogen.

2. Hypotonic urine
   - Specific gravity < 1.015 (~UOsm 220 mOsm/kg)
3. Concentrated urine
   a. Specific gravity > 1.023 (~UOsm 900 mOsm/kg)
   b. Urine specific gravity > 1.023 essentially excludes tubular dysfunction.
4. Fixed specific gravity (isosthenuria)
   a. Specific gravity is always between 1.008 and 1.010.
   b. Indicates complete loss of concentration and dilution
   c. Causes
      (1) Chronic renal failure
      (2) Sickle cell trait/disease
         - Microinfarcts in the renal medulla destroy tubular function
      (3) Chronic tubulointerstitial nephritis (e.g., analgesic abuse)

E. **Urine reagent strip reactions** (Table 4-5)
   1. pH
      a. Pure vegans have an alkaline pH
         - Citrate in fruits is converted to bicarbonate
      b. Diets including meat products produce an acid pH
         - Due to increased excretion of organic acids.

> Manipulation of urine pH is useful in certain clinical disorders. In patients with uric acid stone formation, alkalinizing the urine (e.g., use of a carbonic anhydrase inhibitor) causes uric acid to be soluble in urine and less likely to form uric acid crystals. Alkalinizing the urine is used in the treatment of salicylate intoxication, because it increases the rate of salicylate excretion in the urine. Acidifying the urine (e.g., ascorbic acid) is useful when treating a urinary tract infection, because urinary antiseptics have a greater bactericidal effect in an acid pH urine.

   c. Alkaline urine pH and an ammonia smell indicates a *Proteus* infection.
      - *Proteus* species are urease producers and convert urea to ammonia.
   2. Protein
      a. Proteinuria is often an early sign of renal dysfunction.
      b. Reagent strip detects albumin *not* globulins (e.g., light chains).
         - It detects concentrations of albumin as low as 30 mg/dL, which is equivalent to 150 mg/24 hours, the cutoff point for medically significant proteinuria.
      c. Positive reactions for protein are further evaluated with sulfosalicylic acid (SSA).
         (1) SSA detects *both* albumin and globulins (i.e., light chains, immunoglobulins).
         (2) If albuminuria alone is present
            - Reagent strip reaction and SSA reaction produce similar results (i.e., both have +1 results)
         (3) If albuminuria plus globulins are present
            - SSA reaction is greater than the reagent strip reaction (i.e., reagent strip is +1 and SSA is +4)

Margin notes:

Urine specific gravity >1.023: excludes tubular dysfunction

Fixed specific gravity: chronic renal failure

Alkaline urine + ammonia smell: urease producer (e.g., *Proteus*)

Reagent strip for protein: detects albumin

SSA: detects albumin + globulins; detects BJ protein (light chains)

TABLE 4-5
Urine Reagent
Strip Examination

Component	Description and Significance
pH	Determined by diet and acid-base status of the patient Alkaline pH + smell of ammonia: urease-producing pathogen (e.g., *Proteus*)
Protein	Detects albumin (not globulins) SSA: detects albumin and globulins (e.g., BJ protein) Albuminuria: reagent strip and SSA have the same results BJ protein: SSA greater than reagent strip result
Glucose	Specific for glucose ↑ Serum glucose + glucosuria: diabetes mellitus Normal serum glucose + glucosuria: normal pregnancy (low renal threshold for glucose), benign glucosuria (low renal threshold for glucose)
Ketones	Detects acetone, acetoacetic acid (not β-OHB) Ketonuria: DKA, starvation, ketogenic diets, pregnancy (normal finding), isopropyl alcohol poisoning
Bilirubin	Detects conjugated (water-soluble) bilirubin Bilirubinuria: viral hepatitis, obstructive jaundice
Urobilinogen	Normal to have trace amounts (normal urine color is due to urobilin) Absent urine UBG, ↑ urine bilirubin: obstructive jaundice ↑ Urine UBG, absent urine bilirubin: extravascular hemolytic anemia (e.g., hereditary spherocytosis) ↑ Urine UBG, ↑ urine bilirubin: hepatitis
Blood	Detects RBCs, Hb, and myoglobin Hematuria: e.g., renal stone Hemoglobinuria: e.g., intravascular hemolytic anemia Myoglobinuria: e.g., crush injuries, ↑ serum creatine kinase
Nitrites	Detects nitrites produced by nitrate reducing uropathogens (e.g., *E. coli*)
Leukocyte esterase	Detects esterase in neutrophils (pyuria) Infections: urethritis, cystitis, pyelonephritis Sterile pyuria (neutrophils present but negative standard urine culture): *Chlamydia trachomatis* urethritis, tuberculosis, drug-induced interstitial nephritis

BJ, Bence Jones; β-OHB, β-hydroxybutyric acid; DKA, diabetic ketoacidosis; Hb, hemoglobin; SSA, sulfosalicylic acid; UBG, urobilinogen.

In multiple myeloma, light chains are invariably present in the urine (i.e., Bence Jones proteinuria). SSA detects light chains, while the reagent strip does not.

  d. Microalbuminuria in diabetic glomerulopathy
    (1) Microalbuminuria (30–300 mg albumin/24 hours)
      • First sign of diabetic glomerulopathy
    (2) Detection requires special reagent test strips and quantitative immunoassays

Microalbuminuria: first sign of diabetic glomerulopathy

 3. Glucose
  a. Glucosuria is highly predictive of diabetes mellitus.
    (1) Normal renal threshold for glucose is 165 to 200 mg/dL.
    (2) Renal threshold often increases in diabetics.

Glucosuria: diabetes mellitus most common cause

    b. Reagent strip is specific for glucose.
- Does *not* detect other sugars (e.g., fructose, galactose)

    c. Causes of glucosuria (Table 4-5)

    d. Clinitest tablets
      (1) Detect reducing substances in urine
- Examples—glucose, galactose, fructose, lactose, pentoses (sucrose is *not* a reducing sugar)

      (2) Used as a screening test in newborns to exclude inborn errors of metabolism
- Examples—galactosemia, hereditary fructose intolerance

  4. Ketones

    a. Ketone body synthesis
      (1) Occurs in the liver when excess acetyl CoA is available from β-oxidation of fatty acids
      (2) Ketone bodies include acetone, acetoacetate (AcAc), β-hydroxybutyrate (β-OHB).

    b. Reagent strip detects AcAc and acetone.
- Does *not* detect β-hydroxybutyrate (β-OHB)

Reagent strip ketone bodies: does *not* detect β-OHB

> β-OHB is increased in alcoholics, because the increase in NADH derived from the metabolism of alcohol converts AcAc to β-OHB. A special test is required to detect β-OHB.

    c. Causes of ketonuria (Table 4-5)

  5. Bilirubin

    a. Bilirubinuria is *always* a pathologic finding.

    b. Only conjugated (CB; water-soluble) bilirubin is filtered in the urine.
- Unconjugated bilirubin (lipid soluble) is *not* filtered in the urine.

Bilirubinuria: conjugated bilirubin; hepatitis, obstructive jaundice

    c. Bilirubinuria
      (1) Hepatitis
- Examples—hepatitis A, alcoholic hepatitis

> Bilirubinuria is due to damage of intrahepatic bile ductules containing conjugated bilirubin. Conjugated bilirubin has access to blood in the hepatic sinusoids, which, in turn, has access to the systemic circulation.

      (2) Obstructive jaundice
- Examples—stone in common bile duct, blockage of intrahepatic bile ducts

↑ Bilirubin, ↑ UBG: hepatitis

> Bilirubinuria in obstructive jaundice is due to back-flow of bile containing CB into the bile ductules in hepatocytes. The bile ductules distend with bile and eventually rupture. CB has access to blood in the hepatic sinusoids, which empty into the central vein. The central vein becomes the hepatic vein, which empties into the vena cava.

6. Urobilinogen (UBG)
   a. CB in bile enters the small intestine via the common bile duct.
      (1) Colonic bacteria convert CB to UBG.
      (2) UBG is spontaneously oxidized to urobilin.
         • Color of stool is due to urobilin.
   b. Some UBG is reabsorbed from the colon into the blood.
      (1) Most UBG is taken up by the liver (enterohepatic circulation).
      (2) Remainder of UBG is directed to the kidneys.
         • Color of urine is due to urobilin.
   c. Increased urine UBG
      (1) Extravascular hemolytic anemia
         • Examples—hereditary spherocytosis, autoimmune hemolytic anemia

      > Most bilirubin in blood is unconjugated bilirubin (UCB) derived from macrophage destruction of senescent RBCs. In extravascular hemolytic anemias, more UCB is produced with a concomitant increase in CB, UBG (darker stools), and the amount of UBG recycled to the kidneys. The urine has a dark yellow color.

      Reagent strip negative for bilirubin, increased UBG: extravascular hemolytic anemia

      (2) Hepatitis
         • UBG recycled to the liver is redirected to the kidneys.

      Reagent strip positive for bilirubin, increased UBG: hepatitis

      (3) Porphyria

      > UBG is a porphyrin. Other porphyrins that are detected by the reagent strip include porphobilinogen (increased in acute intermittent porphyria) and uroporphyrin I (increased in porphyria cutanea tarda).

   d. Absence of urine UBG
      • Indicates obstructive jaundice (e.g., stone in common bile duct)

   Reagent strip positive for bilirubin, absent UBG: obstructive jaundice

7. Blood
   a. Reagent strip *cannot* distinguish Hb (within RBCs or free) from myoglobin.
   b. Causes of a positive reagent strip for blood
      (1) Hematuria
         • Examples—renal stone (most common), glomerulonephritis, renal cell carcinoma, ureteral stone, cystitis, transitional cell carcinoma of bladder, prostate hyperplasia
      (2) Hemoglobinuria
         • Examples—intravascular hemolysis (e.g., microangiopathic hemolytic anemia, glucose-6-phosphate dehydrogenase deficiency)
      (3) Myoglobinuria
         (a) Examples—rhabdomyolysis (rupture of striated muscle) from excessive exercise, muscle trauma
         (b) Serum creatine kinase is increased in myoglobinuria.

Reagent strip nitrite: detects nitrate reducers (e.g., *E. coli*)

8. Nitrite
    a. Most uropathogens (e.g., *Escherichia coli*) are nitrate reducers.
    b. Test sensitivity and specificity are 30% and 90%, respectively.

> Increased frequency of urination in urinary tract infections does *not* allow time for uropathogens to convert nitrate to nitrite; hence, the low test sensitivity.

9. Leukocyte esterase
    a. Neutrophils contain esterase in their lysosomes.
    b. Sensitivity and specificity of 80% for detecting neutrophils
    c. Causes of a positive reagent strip for leukocyte esterase
        (1) Urinary tract infection is the most common cause.
        (2) Sterile pyuria
            (a) Neutrophils present *without* identifiable organisms using standard urine cultures
            (b) Examples—*Chlamydia trachomatis* urethritis, renal tuberculosis, drug-induced interstitial nephritis

Sterile pyuria: neutrophils present but negative routine urine culture

F. **Cells in urine sediment** (Table 4-6)
    1. RBCs (hematuria)
        a. Greater than 2 RBCs/high-powered field (HPF) is significant.
        b. Upper urinary tract (kidneys, ureter) causes of hematuria

TABLE 4-6
Urine Sediment Examination

Component	Discussion
Cells	Bacteria: usually a sign of a urinary tract infection Red blood cells (hematuria): renal stone, cancer (bladder, renal), glomerulonephritis Dysmorphic RBCs: indicates hematuria of glomerular origin Neutrophils (pyuria): urinary tract infection, sterile pyuria Oval fat bodies: renal tubular cells with lipid (nephrotic syndrome)
Casts	Cylindrical structure (mold of tubule lumen) with entrapped cells, debris, and protein Hyaline cast: acellular, ghost-like cast containing protein; no significance in the absence of proteinuria RBC cast: nephritic type of glomerulonephritis (e.g., poststreptococcal glomerulonephritis) WBC cast: acute pyelonephritis, acute tubulointerstitial nephritis Renal tubular cell cast: acute tubular necrosis Fatty cast: contain lipid (e.g., cholesterol); sign of nephrotic syndrome (e.g., lipoid nephrosis) Waxy (broad) cast: refractile, acellular cast; sign of chronic renal failure
Crystals	Calcium oxalate: pure vegan diet, ethylene glycol poisoning, calcium oxalate stone Uric acid: hyperuricemia associated with gout or massive destruction of cells after chemotherapy Triple phosphate: may be a sign of urinary tract infection due to urease uropathogens (e.g., *Proteus* species) Cystine: hexagonal crystal seen in cystinuria

(1) Renal stone
- Most common cause (~40% of cases)

(2) Glomerulonephritis, medullary sponge kidney, renal papillary necrosis
- Account for ~ 20% of cases

(3) Renal cell carcinoma
- Hematuria is the most common initial finding.

(4) Sickle cell trait and disease
- Reduced oxygen tension causes sickling in peritubular capillaries leading to microinfarctions (microscopic hematuria) and the potential for renal papillary necrosis.

c. Lower urinary tract (bladder, urethra, prostate) causes of hematuria

(1) Infection
- Most common cause

(2) Transitional cell carcinoma of the bladder
- Most common cause of gross hematuria in the *absence* of infection

(3) Benign prostatic hyperplasia
- Most common cause of microscopic hematuria in adult males

d. Drugs associated with hematuria

(1) Anticoagulants (warfarin, heparin)
- Most common cause of hematuria due to drugs

(2) Cyclophosphamide
  (a) Produces hemorrhagic cystitis
  (b) Risk factor for transitional cell carcinoma of the bladder

(3) Drugs causing acute and chronic tubulointerstitial nephritis
  (a) Methicillin produces acute tubulointerstitial nephritis
  (b) Aspirin plus acetaminophen cause renal papillary necrosis

e. Dysmorphic RBCs
- RBCs that have protrusions from the surface

> Dysmorphic RBCs indicate a glomerular source of hematuria (e.g., glomerulonephritis). Phase contrast microscopy of the urinary sediment is very useful in identifying these RBCs (Fig. 4-2).

f. Initial steps in evaluating hematuria

(1) Complete urinalysis

(2) Urine culture

(3) Other tests that may be required pending the results of the foregoing studies
  (a) Kidney/ureter/bladder (KUB) radiograph to rule out renal stone
  (b) Intravenous pyelogram or renal ultrasound evaluates upper urinary tract causes of hematuria.
  (c) Cystoscopy evaluates causes of gross hematuria in the lower urinary tract.
  (d) Urine cytologic examination to rule out transitional cell carcinoma of the bladder

Cancers with hematuria: renal cell carcinoma, transitional cell carcinoma bladder

Elderly male with hematuria: benign prostatic hyperplasia

Most common drug-induced cause of hematuria: anticoagulants heparin and warfarin

Dysmorphic RBCs: sign of glomerulonephritis

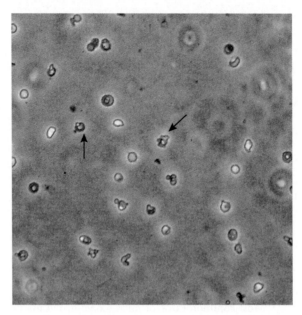

4-2: *This is a phase-contrast microscopy of urine sediment showing dysmorphic RBCs (arrows) with protrusions from the RBC membrane. They are a sign of hematuria of glomerular origin. (From Forbes C, Jackson W: Color Atlas and Text of Clinical Medicine, 2nd ed. St. Louis, Mosby, 2003, Fig. 6.10.)*

(e) Renal biopsy if hematuria is accompanied by dysmorphic RBCs and RBC casts indicating glomerulonephritis

2. Neutrophils
    a. Normal number of WBCs in urine is <2 WBCs per HPF.
    b. Causes of pyuria (WBCs in urine; Fig. 4-3)
        (1) Urinary tract infection
            • Most common cause
        (2) Sterile pyuria (see III.E)
    c. Eosinophils in urine (eosinophiluria)
        • Marker for acute drug-induced tubulointerstitial nephritis (see Section IV.E)
3. Oval fat bodies
    a. Epithelial cells or macrophages with lipid in the cytosol
        • Sign of nephrotic syndrome (see Section IV)
    b. Polarization shows Maltese crosses due to cholesterol (Fig. 4-4A, B)
    c. Fatty casts are usually present as well.
        • Epithelial cells are usually a sign of an improperly collected urine sample.

G. **Hemosiderinuria**
    • Hemosiderin in the urine
    1. Hemosiderin is storage iron that is normally located in bone marrow macrophages (see Chapter 5).
    2. Intravascular hemolysis produces hemosiderinuria (see Chapter 5).
        a. Destruction of RBCs in the vessels leads to the release of hemoglobin.

Most common cause of pyuria: urinary tract infection

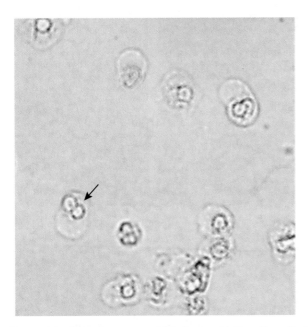

4-3: *Sediment with neutrophils. The arrow points to a bilobed neutrophil. (From Henry JB: Clinical Diagnosis and Management by Laboratory Methods, 20th ed. Philadelphia, WB Saunders, 2001, Plate 18-4.)*

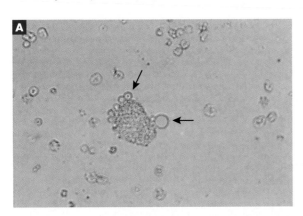 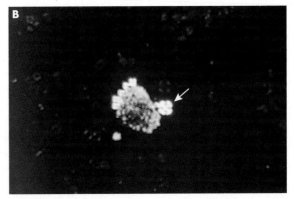

4-4: *Sediment with an oval fat body (**A**) and oval fat body after polarization (**B**). Oval fat bodies are renal tubular cells that have phagocytosed lipid, in this case, cholesterol. The arrows in A show fat droplets attached to the outer surface of a renal tubular cell. When polarized (**B**), the fat droplets have the appearance of a Maltese cross. Smaller fat droplets are present within the cytosol. (From Henry JB: Clinical Diagnosis and Management by Laboratory Methods, 20th ed. Philadelphia, WB Saunders, 2001, Plate 18-11 and Plate 18-12.)*

    b. Hemoglobin in the urine is metabolized by renal tubular cells with formation of hemosiderin granules.

    c. Hemosiderin granules stain blue with a Prussian blue stain.

    d. Examples of intravascular hemolysis

        (1) Microangiopathic hemolytic anemia (schistocytes in the peripheral blood)

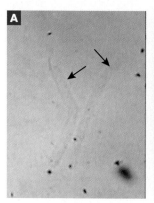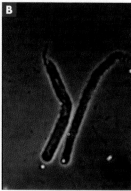

4-5: *Hyaline casts. The arrows in **A** show two hyaline casts (arrows) that are acellular and have smooth borders. Phase contrast microscopy of the casts (**B**) delineates the casts more clearly. (From Henry JB: Clinical Diagnosis and Management by Laboratory Methods, 20th ed. Philadelphia, WB Saunders, 2001, Plate 18-13AB.)*

        (2) Paroxysmal nocturnal hemoglobinuria, glucose-6-phosphate dehydrogenase deficiency, cold immune hemolytic anemias

H. **Urine casts**

1. Casts are formed in the tubules.
   - Protein matrix (Tamm-Horsfall protein) entraps cells, debris, or protein leaking through the glomeruli and forms casts in the tubule lumens.
2. Hyaline casts
   a. Most common cast
   b. Acellular ghost-like casts that are nonrefractile and have smooth rather than sharp borders (Fig. 4-5A, B)
   c. They have no clinical significance in the absence of proteinuria.
3. RBC casts
   a. Sign of the nephritic type of glomerulonephritis (e.g., poststreptococcal glomerulonephritis; Fig. 4-6)
   b. Usually accompanied by dysmorphic RBCs
4. WBC casts
   a. Cast contains bi- and trilobed neutrophils (Fig. 4-7).
   b. Causes
       (1) Acute pyelonephritis (most common cause)
       (2) Acute drug-induced tubulointerstitial nephritis
5. Renal tubular cell casts
   a. Sign of acute tubular necrosis (ischemic or nephrotoxic; Fig. 4-8)
   b. Often pigmented due to the presence of hemoglobin
6. Cellular cast degeneration
   a. Cellular cast progression
   - WBC cast or renal tubular cell cast → coarsely granular cast → finely granular cast → waxy (broad) cast (Fig. 4-9)
   b. Requires ~3 months to develop a waxy (broad) cast
       (1) Sign of chronic renal failure

Urine casts: renal tubule origin

RBC cast: sign of nephritic type of glomerulonephritis

WBC cast: sign of acute pyelonephritis or acute drug-induced tubulointerstitial nephritis

Renal tubular cell cast: sign of acute tubular necrosis

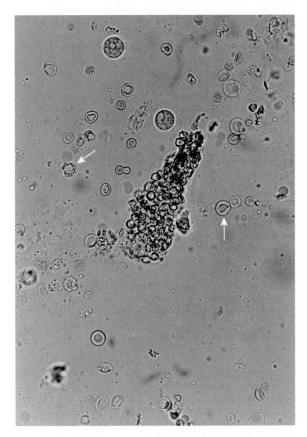

4-6: Red blood cell cast. The cast shows numerous red blood cells imparting a red color to the cast. The arrows show dysmorphic red blood cells. The patient has a nephritic type of acute glomerulonephritis. (From Forbes C, Jackson W: Color Atlas and Text of Clinical Medicine, 2nd ed. St. Louis, Mosby, 2003, Fig. 6.11.)

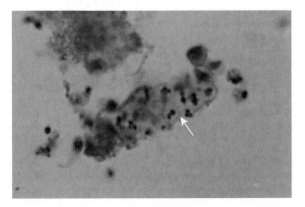

4-7: White blood cell cast. The cast is filled with multilobed cells (arrow) representing neutrophils. WBC casts are present in acute pyelonephritis and other types of acute tubulointerstitial nephritis. (From Henry JB: Clinical Diagnosis and Management by Laboratory Methods, 20th ed. Philadelphia, WB Saunders, 2001, Plate 18-17.)

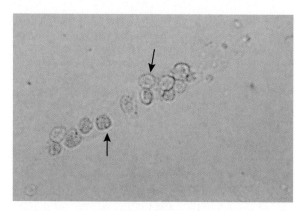

4-8: *Renal tubular cell cast. The cast has numerous renal tubular cells with round nuclei (arrows). These casts are a sign of acute tubular necrosis. (From Henry JB: Clinical Diagnosis and Management by Laboratory Methods, 20th ed. Philadelphia, WB Saunders, 2001, Plate 18-18.)*

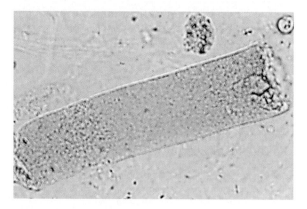

4-9: *Waxy (broad) cast. The cast is refractile and has sharp borders. Finely granular material is present at both ends of the cast. The diameter of the cast is increased indicating tubular atrophy. Waxy (broad) casts are a sign of chronic renal failure. (From Henry JB: Clinical Diagnosis and Management by Laboratory Methods, 20th ed. Philadelphia, WB Saunders, 2001, Plate 18-14.)*

Waxy (broad) cast: sign of chronic renal failure

(2) Tubular atrophy in chronic renal failure increases the diameter of a waxy cast producing a broad cast.
7. Fatty casts
   a. Sign of nephrotic syndrome
      • Hypoalbuminemia in nephrotic syndrome increases liver synthesis of cholesterol.

Fatty cast, oval fat bodies: sign of nephrotic syndrome

   b. Cholesterol enters the urine through damaged glomeruli.
   c. When polarized, cholesterol (*not* triglyceride) produces Maltese crosses similar to those seen in oval fat bodies (Fig. 4-4A, B).
I. **Urine crystals**
   1. Calcium oxalate
      a. Occur in an acid pH urine
      b. Look like a square with an X (Fig. 4-10)

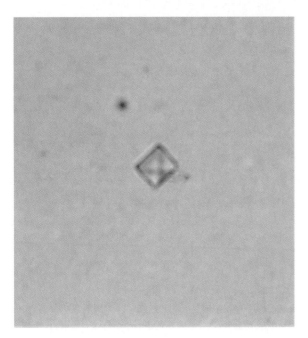

4-10: *Calcium oxalate crystal. The crystal has the appearance of a square box with an X connecting the corners. (From Henry JB: Clinical Diagnosis and Management by Laboratory Methods, 20th ed. Philadelphia, WB Saunders, 2001, Plate 18-31.)*

    c. Clinical associations
        (1) Renal stones (see Section IV)
        (2) Crohn's disease
           • Increased reabsorption of oxalate by the inflamed mucosa
        (3) Ethylene glycol poisoning
           • Ethylene glycol is converted to oxalic acid by alcohol dehydrogenase (see Chapter 2).

> Calcium oxalate crystals: ethylene glycol poisoning, Crohn's disease

2. Uric acid crystals
    a. Occur in an acid pH urine
    b. Clinical associations
        (1) Gout
        (2) Urate nephropathy

> Excess purines released from neoplastic cells during chemotherapy are converted to urate crystals causing urinary obstruction and acute renal failure.

> Urate nephropathy: prevent with allopurinol (xanthine oxidase inhibitor)

3. Triple phosphate
    a. Occur in an alkaline pH urine
    b. Occur in urine with urease-producing organisms (e.g., *Proteus* species)
        • Often associated with a magnesium ammonium phosphate stone (staghorn calculus)
4. Cystine

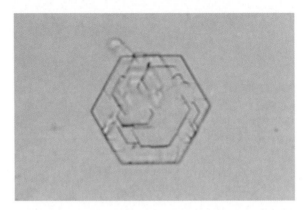

4-11: *The cystine crystal is hexagonal. It is present in cystinuria, a rare inborn error of metabolism. (From Henry JB: Clinical Diagnosis and Management by Laboratory Methods, 20th ed. Philadelphia, WB Saunders, 2001, Plate 18-37.)*

a. Hexagonal crystal (Fig. 4-11)
b. Indicates cystinuria

Hexagonal crystal: cystinuria

  • Autosomal recessive inborn error of metabolism
c. May be associated with cystine stones

IV. **Selected Renal Disorders**
   A. **Proteinuria**
      1. General

Proteinuria: >150 mg/24 hours

         a. Proteinuria is defined as protein >150 mg/24 hours or >30 mg/dL (reagent strip).
         b. Persistent proteinuria usually indicates renal disease.
         c. Qualitative tests include reagent strips and SSA.
         d. Quantitative test is a 24-hour urine collection.
            • Best screen to evaluate proteinuria
         e. Types of proteinuria
            (1) Functional
            (2) Overflow
            (3) Glomerular (selective and nonselective)
            (4) Tubular
      2. Functional proteinuria

Functional proteinuria: proteinuria *not* due to renal disease

         a. Proteinuria that is *not* associated with renal disease
            • Protein <2 g/24 hours
         b. Causes
            (1) Fever, strenuous exercise, stress, congestive heart failure, seizures
            (2) Idiopathic transient proteinuria
               • Common in children and young adults
            (3) Orthostatic proteinuria
               (a) Proteinuria occurs with standing and is absent in the recumbent state.
                  • Urine protein is absent in the first morning void.

      (b) Present in 15% to 20% of healthy young male adults

      (c) *No* progression into renal disease

3. Overflow proteinuria

  a. Low-molecular-weight proteinuria

    (1) Amount filtered exceeds the tubular capacity to reabsorb it

    (2) Protein loss is variable (0.2 to 10 g/24 hours)

  b. Causes

    (1) Multiple myeloma with Bence Jones proteinuria

    (2) Hemoglobinuria

      • Examples—intravascular hemolysis, hypophosphatemia (decreased ATP)

    (3) Myoglobinuria

      • Examples—hypophosphatemia (decreased ATP), crush injuries, McArdle's glycogenosis (deficient muscle phosphorylase), hyperthermia

    (4) Systemic inflammation (e.g., HIV, sepsis)

      • Urinary loss of acute phase reactants synthesized by the liver (e.g., transferrin)

    (5) Acute monocytic or myelomonocytic leukemia

      • Urinary loss of lysozyme (i.e., muramidase, a lysosomal enzyme)

4. Glomerular proteinuria

  a. Protein loss varies depending on the type of glomerular disease.

    (1) Nephritic syndrome has proteinuria >150 mg/24 hours but <3.5 g/24 hours.

    (2) Nephrotic syndrome has proteinuria >3.5 g/24 hours.

  b. Selective proteinuria

    (1) Loss of albumin *without* globulins

    (2) Due to loss of the negative charge in the glomerular basement membrane (GBM)

    (3) Negative charge of the GBM is due to heparan sulfate.

      • Example—nephrotic syndrome caused by minimal change disease (i.e., lipoid nephrosis)

  c. Nonselective proteinuria

    (1) Loss of plasma proteins (e.g., albumin and globulins) in the urine.

    (2) Due to damage of the GBM

  d. Causes of glomerular damage

    (1) Immunocomplexes (type III hypersensitivity)

      • Activate the complement system, which recruits neutrophils that damage the GBM (e.g., poststreptococcal glomerulonephritis).

    (2) Antibodies directed against GBM antigens (type II hypersensitivity)

      • Activate the complement system, which recruits neutrophils that damage the GBM (e.g., Goodpasture's syndrome).

    (3) Defects in T-cell–mediated immunity

      • Cause the release of cytokines that damage visceral epithelial cells.

    (4) Nonenzymatic glycosylation of GBM

Orthostatic proteinuria: proteinuria when standing, absent when reclining

Overflow proteinuria: amount filtered > amount reabsorbed

Selective proteinuria: albuminuria due to loss of negative charge of GBM

Nonselective proteinuria: loss of plasma proteins due to damage of GBM

- Glucose attaches to amino acids in the basement membrane; glycosylation end products render the GBM permeable to proteins (e.g., diabetic glomerulopathy).

5. Tubular proteinuria

a. Defect in the proximal tubule reabsorption of low-molecular-weight proteins (e.g., β_2-microglobulin, amino acids) at normal filtered loads

- Protein <2 g/24 hours

b. Causes

(1) Heavy metal poisoning (e.g., lead and mercury)
- Cause coagulation necrosis of the proximal tubules (i.e., nephrotoxic acute tubular necrosis)

(2) Fanconi syndrome
- Inability of the proximal tubule to reabsorb glucose, amino acids, uric acid, phosphate, bicarbonate, and uric acid

(3) Hartnup disease
(a) Autosomal recessive disease
(b) Defect in the reabsorption of neutral amino acids (e.g., tryptophan) in the gastrointestinal tract and kidneys.

(4) Galactosemia
(a) Autosomal recessive disease
(b) Deficiency of galactose 1-phosphate uridyl transferase
(c) Excess galactose 1-phosphate is toxic to the proximal tubules.

(5) Hereditary fructose intolerance
(a) Autosomal recessive disease
(b) Deficiency of aldolase B
(c) Excess fructose 1-phosphate is toxic to the proximal tubules.

(6) Tubulointerstitial nephritis (see Section IV.D)

(7) Acute renal failure
(a) Destruction of proximal renal tubule cells
(b) Due to ischemia (decreased renal blood flow) or nephrotoxic agents (e.g., aminoglycosides)

B. **Differentiation of the oliguric states**

1. Oliguria is defined as a urine output <400 mL/day or <20 mL/hour

2. Causes of oliguria (Table 4-7)

Tubular proteinuria: defect in proximal tubule reabsorption

TABLE 4-7 Differentiation of Oliguria

Disorder	FENa+%	BUN:Cr	UNa+	UOsm	Urinalysis
Prerenal azotemia	<1	>15	<20	>500	Normal sediment or hyaline casts
Acute glomerulonephritis	<1	>15	<20	>500	RBC casts, hematuria
Acute tubular necrosis	>2	<15	>40	<350	Renal tubular cell casts
Postrenal azotemia (prolonged obstruction)	>2	<15	>40	<350	Normal sediment

BUN, blood urea nitrogen; Cr, creatinine; FENa+, fractional excretion of sodium; RBC, red blood cell.

a. Prerenal azotemia (most common cause)

b. Acute glomerulonephritis (nephritic type)

c. Acute tubular necrosis (renal azotemia)

d. Postrenal azotemia

3. Laboratory tests used to evaluate tubular function

a. UOsm (see Section IIF)

(1) UOsm > 500 mOsm/kg indicates intact tubular function.

(2) UOsm < 350 mOsm/kg indicates tubular dysfunction.

b. $FENa^+$ (see Section IIG)

(1) $FeNa^+ < 1\%$ indicates good tubular function.

(2) $FeNa^+ > 2\%$ indicates tubular dysfunction.

c. Random UNa^+

(1) $UNa^+ < 20$ mEq/L indicates intact tubular function.

(2) $UNa^+ > 40$ mEq/L indicates tubular dysfunction.

d. Serum BUN:creatinine ratio (see Section IID)

(1) Ratio > 15 indicates intact tubular function.

(2) Ratio < 15 indicates tubular dysfunction.

4. Prerenal azotemia and acute glomerulonephritis (nephritic type)

a. Both have preservation of tubular function

b. UOsm > 500 mOsm/kg

c. $UNa^+ < 20$ mEq/L

d. $FENa^+ < 1\%$

e. Serum BUN:Cr ratio >15

f. Urine sediment

(1) Prerenal azotemia

• No abnormal findings or may have a few hyaline casts

(2) Acute glomerulonephritis (nephritic type)

• Hematuria (dysmorphic RBCs) and RBC casts

5. Acute tubular necrosis (ATN) and postrenal azotemia (long-standing obstruction)

a. Both disorders have tubular dysfunction

• Postrenal azotemia of short duration has normal tubular function and would have laboratory findings similar to prerenal azotemia.

b. UOsm < 350 mOsm/kg

c. $UNa^+ > 40$ mEq/L

d. $FENa^+ > 2\%$

e. Serum BUN:Cr ratio <15

f. Urine sediment

(1) ATN has renal tubular cell casts.

(2) Postrenal azotemia usually has a normal sediment.

C. **Glomerulopathy**

1. Subdivided into nephritic and nephrotic syndromes

2. Nephritic syndrome characteristics

a. Hypertension due to salt retention

• Also see periorbital puffiness due to looseness of the skin in that area

b. Oliguria due to decreased GFR from inflamed glomeruli

Sidebar notes:

Intact tubular function: UOsm > 500 mOsm/kg, $FENa^+ < 1\%$, random $UNa^+ < 20$ mEq/L, BUN:Cr ratio >15

Tubular dysfunction: UOsm < 350 mOsm/kg, $FENa^+ > 2\%$, random $UNa^+ > 40$ mEq/L, BUN:Cr ratio <15

Prerenal azotemia, acute glomerulonephritis: oliguria with intact tubular function

ATN, postrenal azotemia with long-standing obstruction: oliguria with tubular dysfunction

    c. Hematuria with dysmorphic RBCs

    d. Neutrophils in the sediment, particularly in the immunocomplex types

    e. RBC casts are a key finding.

    f. Proteinuria > 150 mg/24 hours but <3.5 g/24 hours.

    g. Azotemia with a BUN:Cr ratio >15

    h. UOsm > 500 mOsm/kg

    i. Random UNa^+ < 20 mEq/L

    j. $FENa^+$ < 1%

    k. Summary of glomerular diseases with a predominantly nephritic syndrome presentation (Table 4-8)

3. Nephrotic syndrome characteristics

    a. Proteinuria > 3.5 g/24 hours

    b. Generalized pitting edema and ascites

      • Due to hypoalbuminemia

    c. Hypercoagulable state

> Nephritic syndrome: proteinuria < 3.5 g/24 hours, RBC casts, dysmorphic RBCs

TABLE 4-8
Glomerular Diseases That Are Predominantly Nephritic

Type of Glomerulopathy	Discussion
IgA glomerulonephritis	Most common glomerulopathy May have a nephrotic presentation Affects children and adults Overlapping features with HSP Episodic microscopic or gross hematuria usually following a URI ↑ Serum IgA (50% of cases)
Poststreptococcal glomerulonephritis	Most common postinfectious glomerulonephritis Usually follows group A streptococcal infection of skin (e.g., scarlet fever) or pharynx Hematuria with smoky colored urine 1–3 wks following group A streptococcal infection CRF uncommon ↑ ASO titers in pharyngeal infections; ↑ anti-DNase B titers in skin infections
Diffuse proliferative glomerulonephritis (SLE)	Kidneys are major target organ in SLE (~90% of cases) Serum indirect IF ANA test: rim pattern indicating presence of anti-double-stranded DNA antibodies Commonly evolves into CRF
Rapidly progressive glomerulonephritis	Rapid loss of renal function progresses to ARF over days to weeks Clinical associations: Goodpasture's syndrome, microscopic polyarteritis (p-ANCA), Wegener's granulomatosis (c-ANCA) Goodpasture's syndrome: anti-BM antibodies against glomerular and pulmonary capillaries; young male dominant disease; usually begins with hemoptysis and ends with ARF

ANA, antinuclear antibody; ANCA, anti-neutrophil cytoplasmic antibody; ARF, acute renal failure; ASO, antistreptolysin O; BM, basement membrane; CRF, chronic renal failure; HSP, Henoch-Schönlein purpura; ICs, immunocomplexes; IF, immunofluorescence; SLE, systemic lupus erythematosus; URI, upper respiratory infection.

      (1) Due to loss of antithrombin III, which normally neutralizes many of the coagulation factors

      (2) Potential for renal vein thrombosis

    d. Hypercholesterolemia
* Hypoalbuminemia causes increased liver synthesis of cholesterol (unknown mechanism).

    e. Hypogammaglobulinemia
* Due to the loss of γ-globulins in the urine

    f. Fatty casts and oval fat bodies with Maltese crosses (key finding)

    g. Summary of glomerular diseases with a predominantly nephrotic syndrome presentation (Table 4-9)

> Nephrotic syndrome: proteinuria > 3.5 g/24 hours, pitting edema, fatty casts

TABLE 4-9 Glomerular Diseases That Are Predominantly Nephrotic

Type of Glomerulopathy	Discussion
Minimal change disease (lipoid nephrosis)	Most common cause of nephrotic syndrome in children Loss of negative charge of GBM; selective proteinuria (i.e., albuminuria) Often preceded by a respiratory infection or routine immunization
Focal segmental glomerulosclerosis	Most common glomerulopathy in AIDS and intravenous heroin abuse Nonselective proteinuria and hematuria most common initial presentations Progresses to CRF
Diffuse membranous glomerulopathy	Most common cause of nephrotic syndrome in adults Secondary causes: drugs (e.g., captopril), infections (e.g., HBV, *P. malariae,* syphilis), malignancy (e.g., malignant lymphoma)
Type I membranoproliferative glomerulonephritis	May have a nephritic presentation Secondary causes: HCV, cryoglobulinemia
Type II membranoproliferative glomerulonephritis	Associated with the C3 nephritic factor, an autoantibody that binds with C3 convertase (C3bBb) to stabilize it; very low C3 levels
Diabetic glomerulopathy	Occurs in type 1 and 2 diabetes mellitus Most common cause of CRF in United States GFR initially increased due to hyaline arteriolosclerosis of efferent arterioles Microalbuminuria initial laboratory manifestation. Usually begins after ~10 yr of poor glycemic control. ACE inhibitors slow progression of glomerular disease by inhibiting ATII and its vasoconstriction of efferent arterioles
Renal amyloidosis	Primary amyloidosis accounts for 15%–20% of cases of nephrotic syndrome in patients >60 yr old

ACE, angiotensin-converting enzyme; ATII, angiotensin II; CRF, chronic renal failure; GBM, glomerular basement membrane; GFR, glomerular filtration rate; HBV, hepatitis B virus; HCV, hepatitis C virus.

D. **Acute tubulointerstitial nephritis**
 1. Inflammation of the tubules and interstitium
 2. Causes
   a. Acute pyelonephritis
    • Most common cause
   b. Drugs
    • Examples—penicillin (particularly methicillin), sulfonamides, nonsteroidal anti-inflammatory drugs, diuretics
   c. Infections
    • Examples—legionnaires' disease, leptospirosis
   d. Lead poisoning, urate nephropathy, multiple myeloma
 3. Acute pyelonephritis
   a. Pathogenesis
    (1) Vesicoureteral reflux (VUR) with ascending infection
      (a) Intravesical portion of the ureter is horizontally oriented
      (b) Predisposes to reflux of urine from the bladder to the kidneys
      (c) Uropathogens (e.g., *E. coli*) ascend to the kidneys producing acute pyelonephritis.
    (2) Other risk factors
      • Urinary tract obstruction, diabetes mellitus, pregnancy, sickle cell trait and sickle cell disease
   b. Clinical findings
    (1) Spiking fever
      • Due to infection and sepsis
    (2) Flank pain
    (3) Lower urinary tract signs
      • Increased frequency of urination and painful urination (dysuria)
   c. Laboratory findings
    (1) WBC casts are a key finding
      • Fever, flank pain, WBC casts are *not* present in a lower urinary tract infection.
    (2) Pyuria, bacteriuria (usually *E. coli*), hematuria
 4. Acute drug-induced tubulointerstitial nephritis
   a. Combination of type I and type IV hypersensitivity reactions
   b. Clinical findings
    (1) Abrupt onset of oliguria and fever
    (2) Rash
    (3) Recovery after discontinuing the drug.
   c. Laboratory findings
    (1) BUN:creatinine ratio <15
    (2) Sterile pyuria and WBC casts
    (3) Tubular proteinuria (see Section IV.A)
    (4) Type IV renal tubular acidosis

Acute pyelonephritis: vesicoureteral reflux with ascending infection

Acute pyelonephritis: fever, flank pain, WBC casts

Type IV renal tubular acidosis is due to destruction of the juxtaglomerular apparatus resulting in hyporeninemia

> hypoaldosteronism. This causes sodium wasting, hyperkalemia, and a normal anion gap metabolic acidosis (see Chapter 2).

Acute drug-induced tubulointerstitial nephritis: rash, eosinophilia, eosinophiluria

    (5) Eosinophilia, eosinophiluria

E. **Chronic renal failure (CRF)**
  1. Definition
    a. Progressive irreversible azotemia that develops over months to years
    b. Culminates in end-stage renal disease
      • CCr < 10 mL/minute
  2. Primary causes (in descending order)
    a. Diabetic mellitus
    b. Hypertension
    c. Glomerulonephritis
      • Notably rapidly progressive glomerulonephritis and focal segmental glomerulosclerosis
    d. Adult polycystic kidney disease

Most common cause CRF: diabetes mellitus

  3. Laboratory findings
    a. Electrolyte abnormalities
      (1) Hyperkalemia
      (2) Increased anion gap metabolic acidosis
        • Produces osteoporosis (decreased bone mass) due to buffering of excess hydrogen ions by bone
      (3) Serum sodium changes
        • Usually normal unless there is salt wasting (produces hyponatremia)
    b. Hypocalcemia
      (1) Due to hypovitaminosis D from decreased synthesis of 1-α-hydroxylase
      (2) Hypocalcemia stimulates synthesis and release of parathyroid hormone (PTH, secondary hyperparathyroidism)
        • Secondary hyperparathyroidism produces excess lysis of bone (osteitis fibrosa cystica)
      (3) Hypovitaminosis D
        (a) Decreases bone mineralization causing osteomalacia (rickets in children).
        (b) Bone fractures and pain are common

Secondary hyperparathyroidism in CRF: ↓ vitamin D → ↓ serum calcium → ↑ serum PTH

    c. Hyperphosphatemia
      (1) Due to decreased excretion of phosphate
      (2) Drives calcium into bone and other tissues (metastatic calcification)
        • Further contributes to hypocalcemia
    d. Urinalysis abnormalities
      • Fixed specific gravity, tubular proteinuria, and waxy (broad) casts
    e. Normocytic anemia
      • Due to decreased synthesis of erythropoietin
    f. Qualitative platelet defects
      • Due to toxic metabolites that interfere with platelet aggregation

Causes of hypocalcemia in CRF: hypovitaminosis D, hyperphosphatemia

F. **Renal stones (urolithiasis)**
  1. Risk factors

Hypercalciuria: most common metabolic abnormality in calcium stone formation

  a. Hypercalciuria in the absence of hypercalcemia
    (1) Most common metabolic abnormality
    (2) Due to increased gastrointestinal reabsorption of calcium
  b. Decreased urine volume
    (1) Most often due to decreased intake of water
    (2) Concentrates the urine
  c. Reduced urine citrate
    • Citrate normally chelates calcium
  d. Primary hyperparathyroidism
    • Hypercalciuria due to hypercalcemia
  e. Diets high in dairy products (contain phosphate) or oxalates
  f. Urease-producing uropathogens (e.g., *Proteus*)
  2. Types of renal stones

Renal stones adults/ children: calcium oxalate/calcium phosphate, respectively

  a. Calcium stones
    (1) Calcium oxalate is the most common type in adults.
      • Increased incidence in pure vegans and Crohn's disease
    (2) Calcium phosphate is the most common type in children.
      • Associated with excess ingestion of dairy products and distal type of renal tubular acidosis
  b. Magnesium ammonium phosphate
    (1) "Staghorn calculus" or struvite stone
    (2) Associated with urease producers (e.g., *Proteus*)
    (3) Urine is alkaline and smells like ammonia.
  c. Uric acid, cystine
  3. Clinical and laboratory findings
  a. Sudden onset of ipsilateral colicky pain in the flank with radiation into the groin
  b. Gross and microscopic hematuria
  4. Majority of stones contain calcium (~80%).
  a. Often visualized on a routine radiograph
  b. Renal ultrasound and intravenous pyelogram detect stones that do *not* visualize.

G. **Renal cell carcinoma**
  1. Epidemiology
  a. Occurs in the sixth to seventh decades of life; seen in men more often than women
  b. Smoking is the greatest risk factor.
  2. Clinical and laboratory findings
  a. Triad of hematuria, flank mass, and costovertebral angle pain

Renal cell carcinoma: microscopic hematuria, secondary polycythemia, hypercalcemia

  b. Ectopic secretion of hormones
    (1) Erythropoietin produces secondary polycythemia
    (2) Parathyroid hormone-related protein produces hypercalcemia

Questions

Each numbered item is followed by options arranged in alphabetical or logical order. Select the best answer to each question. Some options may be partially correct, but there is only *one best* answer.

1. A 35-year-old woman diagnosed with chronic hepatitis B has dependent pitting edema in the lower extremities. A urine reagent strip for protein is strongly positive and urinalysis shows numerous refractile appearing casts that when polarized show Maltese crosses. Which of the following renal disorders is most likely present?
A. Focal segmental glomerulosclerosis
B. Goodpasture's syndrome
C. IgA glomerulonephritis
D. Membranous glomerulopathy
E. Minimal change disease

2. A 25-year-old man develops hemoptysis. A few weeks later, he experiences sudden onset of acute renal failure and dies. Prior to his death, urinalysis showed mild proteinuria, hematuria, and RBC casts. Which of the following is the most likely diagnosis?
A. Focal segmental glomerulosclerosis
B. Goodpasture's syndrome
C. IgA glomerulonephritis
D. Membranous glomerulopathy
E. Minimal change disease

3. A 10-year-old boy who recently recovered from scarlet fever develops hypertension, oliguria, and periorbital edema. His urine is smoke-colored and there is a positive urine reagent strip test for blood and protein. Which of the following casts are most likely present?
A. Fatty casts
B. Hyaline casts
C. RBC casts
D. Renal tubular cell casts
E. Waxy casts

4. A 50-year-old man with long-standing type 1 diabetes mellitus and poor glycemic control has oliguria. Examination of urinary sediment reveals waxy (broad) casts, some of which have a increased diameter. Which of the following additional laboratory test findings is most likely present?

A. Decreased serum parathyroid hormone
B. Decreased serum phosphorus
C. Increased serum calcium
D. Serum blood urea nitrogen (BUN):creatinine (Cr) ratio <15
E. Urine specific gravity >1.023

5. A 30-year-old man is found unconscious under a bridge and is brought to the emergency department. Initial laboratory studies show the following:

Serum
    Bicarbonate 14 mEq/L
    Blood urea nitrogen (BUN) 40 mg/dL
    Chloride 90 mEq/L
    Creatinine 4 mg/dL
    Potassium 5.0 mEq/L
    Sodium 136 mEq/L
Urine reagent strip test: negative for ketone bodies and glucose
Sediment examination: numerous calcium oxalate crystals

Which of the following is the most likely diagnosis?
A. Diabetic ketoacidosis
B. Ethylene glycol poisoning
C. Isopropyl alcohol poisoning
D. Methyl alcohol poisoning

6. A 10-year-old boy has an episodic history of developing pink-staining urine shortly after an upper respiratory infection. The patient is normotensive and afebrile. The urine reagent strip test is positive for blood and shows mild to moderate amounts of protein. The antistreptolysin O titer, anti-DNase B titer, and serum antinuclear antibody (ANA) test are all negative. Urinalysis shows RBCs and RBC casts. Which of the following is the most likely diagnosis?
A. Diffuse membranous glomerulopathy
B. Glomerulonephritis in systemic lupus erythematosus (SLE)
C. IgA glomerulonephritis
D. Minimal change disease
E. Poststreptococcal glomerulonephritis

7. A routine physical examination of an asymptomatic 21-year-old black American woman is normal. Urinalysis shows RBCs; however, casts are not present. Phase contrast microscopy of the RBCs in the urine shows uniformly normal appearing RBCs. A urine culture is negative, a peripheral smear is normal, and renal ultrasonography is normal. Laboratory studies show a normal serum blood urea nitrogen, serum creatinine, and hemoglobin. Which of the following tests should be ordered?
A. Bone marrow examination
B. Cystoscopy
C. Renal biopsy
D. Serum ferritin
E. Sickle cell screen

8. A febrile 25-year-old woman develops an acute onset of right flank pain, suprapubic discomfort, dysuria, and urinary frequency. She states that she has had recurrent urinary tract infections since early childhood. The urinary sediment examination shows clumps of WBCs, WBC casts, occasional RBCs, and numerous motile bacteria. What is the most likely diagnosis?
A. Cystitis
B. Glomerulonephritis
C. Pyelonephritis
D. Tubular necrosis
E. Urethritis

9. A 55-year-old woman with hypertension and a recurrent history of peptic ulcer disease and pancreatitis suddenly develops right flank pain that radiates to the right groin. Urinalysis shows a positive reagent strip for blood and a negative reagent strip for nitrite and leukocyte esterase. Urine sediment contains numerous RBCs and calcium oxalate crystals. Which of the following parathyroid hormone (PTH) and calcium findings is most likely present?

	Serum PTH	Serum Calcium
A.	Decreased	Decreased
B.	Decreased	Increased
C.	Increased	Decreased
D.	Increased	Increased

10. A 50-year-old man has chronic myelogenous leukemia that has progressed into an acute blast crisis. He is currently being treated with multiple antileukemic agents. One week into therapy, he develops oliguric renal failure. A urinalysis demonstrates an acid pH and numerous uric acid crystals. Which of the following best explains the mechanism for the renal failure?
A. Drug nephrotoxicity
B. Increased degradation of purine nucleotides
C. Increased degradation of pyrimidine nucleotides
D. Leukemic infiltration of the kidneys

11. A 70-year-old man with a 60-year history of smoking cigarettes develops weight loss, jaundice, and light-colored stools. Physical examination reveals a palpable gallbladder. The total bilirubin is 10 mg/dL (normal range, 0.1–1.0 mg/dL) and conjugated bilirubin is 8 mg/dL (normal range, 0.0–0.3 mg/dL). Computerized tomography shows a mass in the head of the pancreas and dilation of the common bile duct. Which of the following sets of laboratory data is most likely present?

	Urine Bilirubin	Urine Urobilinogen
A	0	+1
B.	0	+2
C.	+2	0
D.	+2	+2

12. A 62-year-old woman with chronic ischemic heart disease has dyspnea and decreased urine output. Physical examination reveals bibasilar crackles in the lungs. There is no neck vein distention or dependent pitting edema. A serum BUN is 60 mg/dL and serum creatinine is 2 mg/dL. The patient is not taking diuretics. Which of the following laboratory findings is most likely present?
A. $FENa^+ < 1\%$
B. Random urine sodium >40 mEq/L
C. UOsm < 350 mOsm/kg
D. Urine sediment with renal tubular cell casts

13. An afebrile, non–sexually active 20-year-old woman complains of burning urine and increased frequency of urination. Which of the following urine laboratory findings is most likely present?
A. Dysmorphic RBCs
B. Negative reagent strip for nitrites
C. Negative routine urine culture
D. Positive reagent strip for leukocyte esterase
E. Urine sediment with WBC casts

14. A professional body builder has a serum creatinine of 6.0 mg/dL (normal range, 0.6–1.2 mg/dL) and a normal serum blood urea nitrogen. A complete urinalysis is reported as normal. Which of the following best explains the increased serum creatinine?
A. Acute renal failure
B. Creatine supplementation
C. Excess protein intake
D. Excess vitamin intake

15. A 28-year-old man who delivers mail for a living is applying for health insurance. A urine sample has a positive reagent strip and sulfosalicylic acid test for protein. All the other urinalysis reagent strip tests are negative and the sediment examination is normal. A repeat test is requested. The patient is specifically asked to submit the first morning urine specimen for repeat analysis. On the repeat test, the reagent strip is negative for protein. Which of the following types of proteinuria is present in this patient?
A. Functional
B. Glomerular
C. Overflow
D. Tubular

16. An afebrile, sexually active 26-year-old man complains of increased frequency of urination, dysuria, and penile drainage. His last sexual encounter was 10 days ago. The urine reagent strip is positive for leukocyte esterase and negative for nitrite and blood. Sediment examination shows neutrophils in clumps; however, bacteria are not present. A standard urine culture is negative for organisms. What is the most likely diagnosis?

A. *Escherichia coli* urethritis or cystitis
B. *Chlamydia trachomatis* urethritis
C. Renal tuberculosis
D. Renal stone

17. A 70-year-old man complains of generalized bone pain and fatigue. The CBC exhibits a normocytic anemia with prominent rouleaux. The serum BUN is 60 mg/dL (normal range, 7–18 mg/dL) and serum creatinine is 6 mg/dL (normal range, 0.6–1.2 mg/dL). A urinalysis reveals a +1 reagent strip reaction for protein and a +4 sulfosalicylic acid reaction. The results of a bone marrow aspirate are pending. What type of proteinuria is most likely present?
A. Functional
B. Glomerular
C. Overflow
D. Tubular

18. A 48-year-old man with chronic urinary tract infections and poorly controlled type 2 diabetes mellitus has ultrasound evidence of a large stone in the left renal pelvis producing hydronephrosis. The urine has an ammonia smell. A CBC is normal. Which of the following additional urine laboratory findings is expected?
A. Alkaline urine pH
B. Calcium oxalate crystals
C. Hemoglobinuria
D. Ketonuria
E. RBC casts

19. An obese 45-year-old man decides to undertake a strenuous training program to lose weight. On the morning after his first 2-hour workout, he has generalized muscle aches and pains and pink urine. A urine reagent strip is positive for blood and protein. The serum blood urea nitrogen and creatinine are normal. A CBC is normal. What is the most likely diagnosis?
A. Acute glomerulonephritis
B. Acute renal failure
C. Hemoglobinuria
D. Myoglobinuria

20. A 45-year-old man who is under treatment for acute sinusitis develops a sudden onset of fever, a diffuse erythematous rash, and oliguria. The serum BUN is 50 mg/dL and creatinine is 5 mg/dL. A CBC reveals a mild normocytic anemia and eosinophilia. A urinalysis shows mild proteinuria, hematuria, and presence of WBCs and WBC casts. Some of the WBCs in the urine have refractile granules consistent with eosinophils. What is the most likely diagnosis?
A. Acute drug-induced tubulointerstitial nephritis
B. Acute glomerulonephritis
C. Acute pyelonephritis
D. Prerenal azotemia

21. A 22-year-old woman is currently in her third trimester of pregnancy. Which of the following laboratory test findings is expected?
 A. Increased creatinine clearance
 B. Increased serum and urine glucose
 C. Increased serum blood urea nitrogen
 D. Increased serum creatinine

22. A 75-year-old man has acute urinary retention. A serum blood urea nitrogen is 40 mg/dL and serum creatinine is 2 mg/dL. Which of the following additional laboratory test findings is most likely present?
 A. FENa$^+$ < 1%
 B. Random urine sodium >40 mEq/L
 C. UOsm < 350 mOsm/kg
 D. Urine sediment with renal tubular cell casts

Answers

1. **D** (membranous glomerulopathy) is correct. A chronic hepatitis B infection, dependent pitting edema, heavy proteinuria, and fatty casts with Maltese crosses suggest a diagnosis of a nephrotic syndrome. Chronic hepatitis B may be associated with diffuse membranous glomerulopathy, the most common cause of the nephrotic syndrome in adults.

A (focal segmental glomerulosclerosis) is incorrect. Focal segmental glomerulosclerosis is most often associated with AIDS and with intravenous heroin addiction. It causes the nephrotic syndrome and is associated with hypertension. There is no association with hepatitis B.

B (Goodpasture's syndrome) is incorrect. Goodpasture's syndrome has anti–basement membrane antibodies directed against pulmonary capillary and glomerular capillary basement membranes. It is more common in men than women and usually presents with hemoptysis followed by acute renal failure due to rapidly progressive glomerulonephritis. This type of glomerulonephritis most often presents with a nephritic syndrome with RBC casts rather than a nephrotic syndrome.

C (IgA glomerulonephritis) is incorrect. IgA glomerulonephritis is an immunocomplex type of glomerulonephritis associated with episodic bouts of microscopic or macroscopic hematuria. This type of glomerulonephritis most often presents with a nephritic syndrome with RBC casts rather than a nephrotic syndrome.

E (minimal change disease) is incorrect. Minimal change disease (lipid nephrosis) is the most common cause of the nephrotic syndrome in children. Cytokine damage to the basement membrane causes a loss of the negative charge, resulting in a selective loss of albumin in the urine. There is no association with hepatitis B.

2. **B** (Goodpasture's syndrome) is correct. Goodpasture's syndrome is more common in men than women. It is associated with IgG anti–basement membrane antibodies that are directed against pulmonary capillary basement membranes causing hemoptysis and glomerular capillary basement membranes producing acute renal failure due to rapidly progressive glomerulonephritis. This type of acute glomerulonephritis is associated with a nephritic syndrome presentation (hematuria, RBC casts, mild proteinuria), as in this case.

A (focal segmental glomerulosclerosis) is incorrect. Focal segmental glomerulosclerosis is most often associated with AIDS and with intravenous heroin addiction. It causes the nephrotic syndrome and is not associated with pulmonary disease.

C (IgA glomerulonephritis) is incorrect. IgA glomerulonephritis is an immunocomplex type of glomerulonephritis associated with episodic bouts of microscopic or macroscopic hematuria. Although it usually presents as a nephritic syndrome, pulmonary disease is not a feature of the disease.

D (membranous glomerulopathy) is incorrect. Membranous glomerulopathy is the most common cause of the nephrotic syndrome in adults (pitting edema, fatty casts). It is not associated with pulmonary disease.

E (minimal change disease) is incorrect. Minimal change disease is the most common cause of the nephrotic syndrome in children. Cytokine damage to the basement membrane causes a loss of the negative charge, resulting in a selective loss of albumin in the urine. It does not present with pulmonary disease.

3. **C** (RBC casts) is correct. The patient has poststreptococcal glomerulonephritis secondary to scarlet fever, which is caused by an erythrogenic strain of group A streptococcus. Poststreptococcal glomerulonephritis presents as a nephritic syndrome with mild to moderate proteinuria, hematuria, and RBC casts.

A (fatty casts) is incorrect. Fatty casts are present in the nephrotic syndrome, which is characterized by heavy proteinuria and pitting edema. These findings are not present in this patient.

B (hyaline casts) is incorrect. Hyaline casts are acellular casts that occur in any proteinuric state. In the absence of proteinuria, they have no clinical significance. Although occasional hyaline casts may occur in poststreptococcal glomerulonephritis, they are not the predominant cast that is present.

D (renal tubular cell casts) is incorrect. Renal tubular cell casts are present in acute tubular necrosis, the most common cause of acute renal failure. Renal failure rarely occurs in poststreptococcal glomerulonephritis.

E (waxy casts) is incorrect. Waxy (broad) casts are present in chronic renal failure, which rarely occurs in poststreptococcal glomerulonephritis.

4. **D** (serum blood urea nitrogen:creatinine ratio <15) is correct. Waxy (broad) casts are a sign of chronic renal failure (CRF). Diabetes mellitus is the most common cause of CRF in the United States. The glomerular filtration rate is decreased in CRF, resulting in decreased clearance of creatinine and urea by the kidneys. In addition, some of the urea is excreted in the skin and gastrointestinal tract causing a disproportionate increase in creatinine leading to a serum BUN:creatinine ratio <15. Because CRF is characterized by tubular dysfunction, filtered urea and creatinine are both lost in the urine.

A (decreased serum parathyroid hormone) and **C** (increased serum calcium) are incorrect. In CRF, the second hydroxylation of vitamin D is impaired due to the loss of 1-α-hydroxylase in the proximal renal tubules. Hypovitaminosis D occurs, which causes hypocalcemia due to decreased reabsorption of calcium from the gastrointestinal tract and the kidneys. Hypocalcemia, in turn, is a stimulus for the synthesis and release of parathyroid hormone (secondary hyperparathyroidism).

B (decreased serum phosphorus) is incorrect. Phosphorus is normally reabsorbed in the proximal tubules of the kidneys. In CRF, the decrease in the glomerular filtration rate along with tubular dysfunction causes an accumulation of phosphorus in the blood, leading to hyperphosphatemia. Hyperphosphatemia drives calcium into tissue and contributes to the development of hypocalcemia.

E (urine specific gravity >1.023) is incorrect. An increase in urine specific gravity corresponds with an increase in urine osmolality. Both measurements reflect the ability of the renal tubules to concentrate and dilute urine. A specific gravity >1.023 indicates excellent concentrating ability and essentially excludes intrinsic renal disease. In CRF, there is tubular dysfunction and neither concentration nor dilution occurs. Therefore, the urine specific gravity is essentially the same as the glomerular filtrate, which is ~1.010. This decreased specific gravity remains unchanged regardless of time of day and fluid intake (fixed specific gravity).

5. **B** (ethylene glycol poisoning) is correct. The patient most likely has ethylene glycol poisoning from drinking antifreeze. Ethylene glycol is converted to oxalic acid by alcohol dehydrogenase. Oxalic acid combines with calcium to form calcium oxalate crystals, which obstruct the kidney tubules and cause acute renal failure. Laboratory findings in this patient show an increased serum BUN and creatinine with a BUN:creatinine ratio of 10 (40/4), which indicates renal azotemia (uremia). Electrolytes in ethylene glycol poisoning show an increased anion gap metabolic acidosis due to an increase in oxalic acid. In this case, the anion gap is calculated as follows: Anion gap = serum sodium − (serum chloride + serum bicarbonate); 136 − (90 + 14) = 32 (normal, 12 ± 2).

A (diabetic ketoacidosis) is incorrect. The urine reagent strip test is negative for ketone bodies and glucose; therefore, diabetic ketoacidosis is excluded.

C (isopropyl alcohol poisoning) is incorrect. Isopropyl alcohol is rubbing alcohol. When ingested, it is converted to acetone; however, no acid is produced. Because the urine reagent strip for ketone bodies is negative and the patient has metabolic acidosis, this diagnosis is excluded.

D (methyl alcohol poisoning) is incorrect. Methyl alcohol is present in solvents such as window washing fluid. When ingested, it is converted to formic acid by alcohol dehydrogenase, and produces an increased anion gap metabolic acidosis. Formic acid damages the optic nerve, resulting in optic neuritis, which is not present in this patient.

6. **C** (IgA glomerulonephritis) is correct. RBC casts, hematuria, and proteinuria are characteristic of a nephritic type of glomerulonephritis. The episodic history of hematuria following upper respiratory infections and the absence of hypertension are characteristic of IgA glomerulonephritis, which is the most common type of acute glomerulonephritis.

A (diffuse membranous glomerulopathy) and **D** (minimal change disease) are incorrect. Diffuse membranous glomerulopathy and minimal change disease are associated with a nephrotic type of glomerular disease, which is characterized by massive proteinuria (>3.5 g/24 h), pitting edema, and fatty casts. These findings are not present in this patient.

B (glomerulonephritis in systemic lupus erythematosus, SLE) is incorrect. A negative serum ANA test excludes SLE as a diagnosis.

E (poststreptococcal glomerulonephritis) is incorrect. Poststreptococcal glomerulonephritis is caused by an erythrogenic strain of group A streptococcus. Negative antistreptolysin O and DNase B titers and the absence of hypertension exclude the diagnosis of poststreptococcal glomerulonephritis.

7. **E** (sickle cell screen) is correct. The patient most likely has sickle cell trait, which causes recurrent microscopic hematuria. In sickle cell trait, the percentage of sickle hemoglobin is 40% to 45%, and the remainder of the hemoglobin is hemoglobin A. There are no sickle cells in the peripheral smear in sickle cell trait; therefore, a sickle cell screen is required to induce sickling of RBCs containing sickle hemoglobin. The oxygen tension in the renal medulla is low enough to induce sickling of RBCs in the peritubular capillaries. This causes microinfarctions in the renal medulla causing microscopic hematuria. Repeated infarctions in the renal medulla may cause renal papillary necrosis.

A (bone marrow examination) is incorrect. A bone marrow examination is not warranted, because the patient does not have anemia or evidence of intrinsic bone marrow disease.

B (cystoscopy) is incorrect. If the sickle cell screen is negative, a cystoscopy may be necessary to determine the cause of the hematuria.

C (renal biopsy) is incorrect. If the sickle cell screen is negative, a renal biopsy may be necessary to rule out primary renal disease, particularly IgA glomerulonephritis, which is commonly associated with episodic hematuria. However, because the phase contrast microscopy of urine does not demonstrate dysmorphic RBCs (RBCs with protrusions from the membrane), a glomerular origin for the hematuria is unlikely.

D (serum ferritin) is incorrect. Although serum ferritin is decreased in the early stages of iron deficiency when anemia is not present, hematuria is rarely a cause of iron deficiency.

8. **C** (pyelonephritis) is correct. The patient has acute pyelonephritis, which is a bacterial infection (usually caused by *Escherichia coli*) that produces abscesses in the tubules and interstitium of the kidney. Classic signs include fever, flank pain, and WBC casts accompanied by signs of a lower urinary tract infection (e.g., suprapubic discomfort, dysuria, and urinary frequency). The majority of cases occur in women who have recurrent lower urinary tract infections complicated by vesicoureteral reflux, which allows the infected urine access to the kidneys where it produces acute pyelonephritis.

A (cystitis) and **E** (urethritis) are incorrect. Acute cystitis and urethritis are lower urinary tract infections. They are not associated with fever, flank pain, and WBC casts in the urine.

B (glomerulonephritis) is incorrect. Acute glomerulonephritis is characterized by oliguria (decreased glomerular filtration rate), proteinuria, hematuria, and urine casts (RBC, WBC, or fatty casts), depending on the type of glomerulonephritis. Most cases are immune-mediated and are not accompanied by lower urinary tract signs of dysuria and increased frequency.

D (tubular necrosis) is incorrect. Acute tubular necrosis is caused by ischemia (e.g., decreased cardiac output) or nephrotoxic drugs (e.g., aminoglycosides). Acute tubular necrosis is characterized by oliguria and is associated with renal tubular cell casts rather than WBC casts.

9. **D** (increased serum PTH, increased serum calcium) is correct. Renal stone formation is the most common presentation for primary hyperparathyroidism, which is the most common cause of hypercalcemia in ambulatory individuals. The majority of cases are due to a parathyroid adenoma, which increases production of PTH causing increased lysis of bone leading to hypercalcemia. In this patient, primary hyperparathyroidism is complicated by hypertension, peptic ulcer disease, pancreatitis, and a renal stone composed of calcium oxalate. Hypertension is due to calcium increasing contraction of the smooth muscle cells of the peripheral resistance arterioles. Hypercalcemia stimulates gastrin release and activates pancreatic phospholipase causing peptic ulcer disease and acute pancreatitis, respectively. Excess calcium in the urine predisposes to formation of calcium-containing stones.

A (decreased serum PTH, decreased serum calcium) is incorrect. A decrease in serum PTH and serum calcium defines primary hypoparathyroidism, which is most often due to previous thyroid surgery or autoimmune disease. Primary hypoparathyroidism is not associated with hypertension, peptic ulcers, pancreatitis, or renal stones.

B (decreased serum PTH, increased serum calcium) is incorrect. A decrease in serum PTH and an increase in serum calcium defines hypercalcemia due to malignancy (most common cause) or other non–parathyroid gland-related disorders (e.g., sarcoidosis, hypervitaminosis D). Hypercalcemia suppresses the release of PTH by the parathyroid gland. Primary hyperparathyroidism is the most common cause of hypercalcemia in the ambulatory population, and is a more likely cause of the findings in this patient.

C (increased serum PTH, decreased serum calcium) is incorrect. An increase in serum PTH and a decrease in serum calcium defines secondary hyperparathyroidism. Hypocalcemia that is not due to primary hypoparathyroidism stimulates the parathyroid glands to synthesize and release PTH. Hypovitaminosis D is the most common pathologic cause of hypocalcemia. Secondary hyperparathyroidism does not cause hypertension, peptic ulcer disease, pancreatitis, or renal stones.

10.   **B** (increased degradation of purine nucleotides) is correct. Treatment of disseminated malignancies with chemotherapy drugs results in the release of purine nucleotides from the nuclei of the killed cancer cells. Uric acid is the end product of degradation of purine nucleotides. An acid urine pH crystallizes the uric acid within the renal tubules leading to urate nephropathy and acute renal failure. This complication is prevented by allopurinol, which blocks xanthine oxidase and prevents conversion of xanthine to uric acid.

A (drug nephrotoxicity) is incorrect. Although many chemotherapy drugs are directly nephrotoxic, this patient has uric acid crystals reported in his urine, hence negating drug nephrotoxicity as the cause of the renal failure.

C (increased degradation of pyrimidine nucleotides) is incorrect. Although pyrimidine nucleotide degradation also occurs in patients being treated with chemotherapy drugs, pyrimidines are degraded to CO_2, ammonia, and amino acids. Ammonia is metabolized in the urea cycle and urea is excreted in the kidneys. Urea does not produce crystals in the urine.

D (leukemic infiltration of the kidneys) is incorrect. Although leukemic cells metastasize to all organ systems, the report of uric acid crystals in the urine negates leukemic infiltration as the primary cause of renal failure.

11.   **C** (urine bilirubin: +2, urine urobilinogen: 0) is correct. The patient has carcinoma of the head of pancreas, which is most commonly due to carcinogens that are present in cigarette smoke. Because the common bile duct (CBD) passes through the head of pancreas, there is complete obstruction of the CBD leading to distention of the CBD and gallbladder. The bile containing conjugated bilirubin refluxes back into the hepatocytes and out into the sinusoids. Conjugated bilirubin (CB) is water soluble, so bilirubin is filtered and excreted in the urine. Urobilinogen (UBG) in the stool derives from degradation of CB by colonic bacteria. Urobilin, its oxidation product, is responsible for the color of stool. A small fraction of UBG is recycled back into the blood where it is taken up by the liver (90%) and filtered in the kidneys (10%). The normal yellow color of urine is due to urobilin. Therefore, obstruction to bile flow causes light-colored stools, owing to the absence of UBG in stool, and absence of UBG in the urine.

A (urine bilirubin: 0, urine urobilinogen: +1) is incorrect. A slight increase in urobilinogen is normal in the urine. Urobilinogen is spontaneously oxidized to urobilin, which gives the normal color of urine.

B (urine bilirubin: 0, urine urobilinogen: +2) is incorrect. Absence of bilirubin in the urine and an increase in UBG occurs whenever there is an increase in unconjugated bilirubin presented to the liver for conjugation. This occurs in extravascular hemolytic anemias where there is macrophage destruction of RBCs leading to an increase in unconjugated bilirubin. Examples include hereditary spherocytosis, sickle cell anemia, ABO and Rh hemolytic disease of the newborn, and warm autoimmune hemolytic anemia. More unconjugated bilirubin is converted to CB, more CB is converted to UBG in the colon, and proportionately more UBG is recycled to the kidneys. Unconjugated bilirubin is lipid soluble and bound to albumin; therefore, it is not filtered by the kidneys.

D (urine bilirubin: +2, urine urobilinogen: +2) is incorrect. The presence of bilirubin in the urine and an increase in UBG occurs in hepatitis. In hepatitis, there is disruption of bile ductules in the liver, which allows CB to enter the sinusoids of the liver and gain access to the circulation. Furthermore, the UBG that is normally recycled to the liver is redirected to the kidneys causing an increase in urine UBG.

12. **A** ($FENa^+ < 1\%$) is correct. The patient has left-sided heart failure (dyspnea, pulmonary edema with inspiratory crackles) causing a decrease in cardiac output leading to a decrease in renal blood flow, glomerular filtration rate, and oliguria. The serum BUN:creatinine ratio is 30 (60/2), which is consistent with a prerenal azotemia. The $FENa^+$ is a sensitive indicator of tubular function. Values <1% indicate intact tubular function, while those >2% indicate tubular dysfunction. In prerenal azotemia, tubular function is intact; therefore, the $FENa^+$ is <1%.

B (random urine sodium >40 mEq/L) is incorrect. The patient has prerenal azotemia secondary to left-sided heart failure. Because tubular function is intact, reabsorption of sodium in the proximal and distal tubules is normal and the random urine sodium is <20 mEq/L. A random urine sodium >40 mEq/L indicates tubular dysfunction.

C (UOsm < 350 mOsm/kg) is incorrect. The patient has prerenal azotemia secondary to left-sided heart failure. Because tubular function is intact, renal concentration is normal and the UOsm is >500 mOsm/kg. A UOsm < 350 mOsm/kg indicates a loss of urine concentration, which is the first sign of tubular dysfunction.

D (urine sediment with renal tubular cell casts) is incorrect. The patient has prerenal azotemia secondary to left-sided heart failure. Because tubular function is intact, there should be no casts in the urine. Renal tubular cell casts are present in acute tubular necrosis.

13. **D** (positive reagent strip for leukocyte esterase) is correct. The patient has a lower urinary tract infection (dysuria, increased urine frequency) most likely due to *Escherichia coli*. Neutrophils are invariably present in the urine with bacterial infections; therefore, the reagent strip test for leukocyte esterase is positive.

   A (dysmorphic RBCs) is incorrect. Dysmorphic RBCs are RBCs that have protrusions from the cell membrane. They are best identified with phase contrast microscopy. Their presence indicates hematuria of glomerular origin (e.g., glomerulonephritis) and essentially excludes any lower urinary tract cause of hematuria, including a urinary tract infection.

   B (negative reagent strip for nitrites) is incorrect. The majority of uropathogens are bacteria that are nitrate reducers; therefore, the reagent strip is usually positive for nitrites.

   C (negative routine urine culture) is incorrect. The majority of lower urinary tract infections are due to *E. coli*, which is easily identified with routine urine cultures.

   E (urine sediment with WBC casts) is incorrect. The presence of WBC casts accompanied by lower urinary tract signs of infection indicates acute pyelonephritis, which is the most common upper urinary tract infection.

14. **B** (creatine supplementation) is correct. Creatinine is the metabolic end product of creatine in muscle. Creatine phosphate is the main storage depot for energy in muscle in that it is a ready source of phosphate for ATP synthesis. Creatine supplementation provides increased energy for body builders and causes an increase in the serum creatinine.

   A (acute renal failure, ARF) is incorrect. ARF is associated with an increase in serum creatinine and serum BUN and the urine sediment shows renal tubular cell casts. The patient has a normal serum BUN and the urinalysis is normal, hence excluding ARF as a diagnosis.

   C (excess protein intake) is incorrect. Body builders commonly increase protein intake to supply amino acids for muscle growth. However, the end product of amino acid metabolism is urea and not creatinine.

   D (excess vitamin intake) is incorrect. Body builders commonly take numerous vitamins to increase energy; however, vitamins have no effect on increasing serum creatinine.

15. **A** (functional) is correct. The patient has orthostatic proteinuria, which is a type of functional proteinuria that is not associated with an underlying renal disease. In orthostatic proteinuria, proteinuria occurs with standing and is absent in the recumbent state (e.g., first morning void). It occurs in 15% to 20% of healthy young male adults.

   B (glomerular) is incorrect. Glomerular proteinuria is associated with a loss of protein ranging from 150 mg/24 hours to >3 g/24 hours. It is subdivided into selective and nonselective proteinuria. Selective proteinuria refers to a loss of albumin and not globulins. It is due to loss of the negative charge in the glomerular basement membrane (e.g., nephrotic syndrome caused by minimal change disease). Nonselective proteinuria refers to the loss of plasma proteins (e.g., albumin and globulins) in urine. It is due to damage of the glomerular basement membrane (e.g., poststreptococcal glomerulonephritis). Glomerular proteinuria is unlikely in this patient, because proteinuria disappeared after reclining and no abnormal casts were present in the urine (e.g., RBC or fatty casts).

C (overflow) is incorrect. In overflow proteinuria, the protein loss is variable (0.2–10 g/24 hours). It is a low-molecular-weight proteinuria in which the amount filtered exceeds the tubular capacity to reabsorb it (e.g., Bence Jones proteinuria, hemoglobinuria, myoglobinuria). Overflow proteinuria is unlikely in this patient, because the proteinuria disappeared after reclining.

D (tubular) is incorrect. Tubular proteinuria is associated with a protein loss <2 g/24 hours. It is due to a defect in proximal tubule reabsorption of low-molecular-weight proteins (e.g., β_2-microglobulin, amino acids) at normal filtered loads (e.g., heavy metal poisoning, Hartnup disease). Tubular proteinuria is unlikely in this patient, because proteinuria disappeared after reclining.

16. **B** (*Chlamydia trachomatis* urethritis) is correct. The patient has a sterile pyuria, which refers to the presence of neutrophils in the urine (positive reagent strip for leukocyte esterase), a negative reagent strip for nitrites, and no growth of organisms with a standard urine culture. Owing to the close proximity of the patient's urinary findings with a previous sexual encounter, the patient most likely has urethritis due to *Chlamydia trachomatis.*

A (*Escherichia coli* urethritis or cystitis) is incorrect. In lower urinary tract infections due to *E. coli,* the reagent strip is positive for nitrites and leukocyte esterase and routine cultures isolate the organism.

C (renal tuberculosis) is incorrect. Renal tuberculosis produces a sterile pyuria; however, the history of symptoms within 10 days of a sexual encounter is more likely to represent urethritis due to *C. trachomatis* than renal tuberculosis.

D (renal stone) is incorrect. A renal stone presents with a sudden onset of flank pain with radiation of pain into the ipsilateral groin. Hematuria is invariably present. None of these findings are present in the patient.

17. **C** (overflow) is correct. In overflow proteinuria, the protein loss is variable (0.2–10 g/24 hours). It is a low-molecular-weight proteinuria in which the amount filtered exceeds the tubular capacity to reabsorb it. The patient most likely has multiple myeloma, a malignant plasma cell disorder associated with Bence Jones proteinuria (light chains in the urine). He has anemia and renal failure (BUN:creatinine ratio is 10). There is a disparity in the protein readings for the reagent strip and sulfosalicylic acid (SSA). This occurs in multiple myeloma with Bence Jones proteinuria, because the reagent strip for protein detects albumin and not globulins (e.g., light chains), and the SSA reaction detects albumin and globulins. A bone marrow aspirate confirms the presence of malignant plasma cells, while a serum and urine immunoelectrophoresis determine the immunoglobulin and light chain that is involved.

A (functional) is incorrect. A functional proteinuria is a proteinuria that is not associated with an underlying renal disease. Causes include fever, stress, sepsis, and orthostatic proteinuria. The patient has renal failure and proteinuria due to the presence of Bence Jones protein, which damages the tubular epithelium and blocks tubular lumens with proteinaceous material.

B (glomerular) is incorrect. Glomerular proteinuria is associated with a loss of protein ranging between 150 mg/24 hours to > 3.5 g/24 hours. It is subdivided into selective and nonselective proteinuria. Selective proteinuria refers to a loss of albumin and not globulins. It is due to loss of the negative charge in the glomerular basement membrane (e.g., nephrotic syndrome caused by minimal change disease). Nonselective proteinuria refers to the loss of plasma proteins (e.g., albumin and globulins) in urine. It is due to damage of the glomerular basement membrane (e.g., poststreptococcal glomerulonephritis). Glomerular proteinuria is unlikely in this patient, because no abnormal casts are present in the urine (e.g., RBC or fatty casts).

D (tubular) is incorrect. Tubular proteinuria is associated with a protein loss <2 g/24 hours. It is due to a defect in proximal tubule reabsorption of low-molecular-weight proteins (e.g., β_2-microglobulin, amino acids) at normal filtered loads (e.g., heavy metal poisoning). Tubular proteinuria is unlikely in this patient because Bence Jones protein damages the collecting tubules rather than the proximal renal tubules.

18. **A** (alkaline urine pH) is correct. The patient has an ammonia smell to urine, which is consistent with a urinary tract infection due to urease producers (e.g., *Proteus* species). Ammonia produces a urine with an alkaline pH. The renal stone is most likely a struvite stone composed of magnesium, ammonia, and phosphate ("staghorn" calculus).

B (calcium oxalate crystals) is incorrect. Calcium oxalate crystals and stones develop in an acid pH urine.

C (hemoglobinuria) is incorrect. Hemoglobinuria is most commonly due to an intravascular type of hemolytic anemia (e.g., glucose-6-phosphate dehydrogenase deficiency). Hemoglobinuria does not produce an alkaline urine or an ammonia smell. Furthermore, the patient does not have anemia.

D (ketonuria) is incorrect. Ketonuria occurs in type 1 diabetes mellitus and not type 2 diabetes mellitus. Furthermore, ketone bodies do not alkalinize the urine or produce an ammonia smell.

E (RBC casts) is incorrect. Casts of any type develop within renal tubules and imply intrinsic renal disease. A renal stone is likely to produce hematuria; however, RBC casts are not present.

19. **D** (myoglobinuria) is correct. The patient, who is most likely in poor physical condition, has damaged striated muscle (generalized muscle pain) causing the release of myoglobin, which produces a pink urine and a positive urine reagent strip for blood and protein. The reagent strip for blood does not distinguish hemoglobin from myoglobin. A serum creatine kinase would be markedly elevated in this patient.

A (acute glomerulonephritis) is incorrect. The nephritic type of acute glomerulonephritis produces hematuria and proteinuria; however, it is not associated with generalized muscle pain. Furthermore, acute glomerulonephritis is associated with an increase in serum BUN and creatinine (normal in this patient) due to a decrease in the glomerular filtration rate.

B (acute renal failure, ARF) is incorrect. Myoglobinuria is a potential cause of ARF; however, the serum blood urea nitrogen and creatinine are normal in this patient and it is increased in ARF.

C (hemoglobinuria) is incorrect. Hemoglobinuria is most commonly due to an intravascular hemolytic anemia (e.g., glucose-6-phosphate dehydrogenase deficiency). The urine reagent strip is positive for blood and protein. However, since the patient does not have anemia, this diagnosis is excluded.

20. **A** (acute drug-induced tubulointerstitial nephritis) is correct. The patient has acute sinusitis and is likely taking an antibiotic (e.g., amoxicillin) that has produced acute drug-induced tubulointerstitial disease. Key clinical features of the disease are an abrupt onset of fever, oliguria, and a rash. Laboratory findings include a serum BUN:creatinine ratio <15 (renal azotemia), WBCs and WBC casts, proteinuria, eosinophiluria and the presence of eosinophilia in the peripheral blood. Cessation of the drug causes reversal of the renal failure.

B (acute glomerulonephritis) is incorrect. Acute glomerulonephritis does not present with an abrupt onset of acute renal failure, fever, and rash, as in this patient. Furthermore, the type of urine cast is different, mainly RBC casts in the nephritic syndrome or fatty casts in the nephrotic syndrome.

C (acute pyelonephritis) is incorrect. Acute pyelonephritis is an example of an acute tubulointerstitial nephritis and is associated with WBC casts; however, it does not present with acute renal failure and is not associated with rash, eosinophilia, and eosinophiluria.

D (prerenal azotemia) is incorrect. Prerenal azotemia refers to oliguria that is due to hypoperfusion of the kidneys from a decrease in cardiac output. The serum BUN:creatinine ratio is >15 and the urine sediment is normal. The patient has renal azotemia with a serum BUN:creatinine ratio of 10.

21. **A** (increased creatinine clearance) is correct. In pregnancy, the plasma volume increases, which causes an increase in the glomerular filtration rate and a corresponding increase in the creatinine clearance.

B (increased serum and urine glucose) is incorrect. In pregnancy, the serum glucose is usually normal; however, glucosuria may be present because of a decrease in the renal threshold for reabsorbing glucose. An increase in serum and urine glucose in pregnancy is most often due to gestational diabetes.

C (increased serum blood urea nitrogen, BUN) is incorrect. In pregnancy, the plasma volume increases, which causes an increase in the glomerular filtration rate and increased clearance of urea causing a decrease in the serum BUN.

D (increased serum creatinine) is incorrect. In pregnancy, the plasma volume increases, which causes an increase in the glomerular filtration rate and increased clearance of creatinine causing a decrease in the serum creatinine.

22. **A** ($FENa^+ < 1\%$) is correct. The patient has acute urinary retention most likely due to benign prostate hyperplasia causing obstruction of urine outflow through the urethra. The serum BUN:creatinine ratio is 20 (40/2), which is consistent with a postrenal azotemia. Postrenal azotemia is most often due to urinary tract obstruction, which, in this case, is prostate hyperplasia. In the initial stages of urinary tract obstruction, tubular function is intact and there is a decrease in the glomerular filtration rate and back-diffusion of urea into the blood causing the BUN:creatinine ratio to be >15. The $FENa^+$ is a sensitive indicator of tubular function. An $FENa^+ < 1\%$ is compatible with intact tubular function. If urinary retention is not relieved, the patient will progress into acute renal failure, where the $FENa^+$ is >2% and the serum BUN:creatinine ratio <15.

B (random urine sodium >40 mEq/L) is incorrect. The patient has postrenal azotemia secondary to prostate hyperplasia. Because the serum BUN:creatinine ratio is 20 indicating intact tubular function, reabsorption of sodium in the proximal and distal tubules is normal and the random urine sodium should be <20 mEq/L. A random urine sodium >40 mEq/L indicates tubular dysfunction.

C (UOsm < 350 mOsm/kg) is incorrect. The patient has postrenal azotemia secondary to prostate hyperplasia. Because the serum BUN:creatinine ratio is 20 indicating intact tubular function, renal concentration is normal and the UOsm should be >500 mOsm/kg. A UOsm < 350 mOsm/kg indicates a loss of urine concentration, which is the first sign of tubular dysfunction.

D (urine sediment with renal tubular cell casts) is incorrect. The patient has postrenal azotemia secondary to prostate hyperplasia. Because the serum BUN:creatinine ratio is 20 indicating intact tubular function, there should be no casts in the urine. Renal tubular cell casts are present in renal azotemia.

Red Blood Cell Disorders

I. **Hematopoiesis**

   A. **Erythropoiesis and erythropoietin**

      1. Erythropoiesis
         a. Production of red blood cells (RBCs) in the bone marrow
            • Due to the release of erythropoietin (EPO) from the kidneys
         b. EPO stimulates erythroid stem cells in the bone marrow to divide.
      2. Stimuli for EPO release
         a. Decreased Pao_2 (hypoxemia)
         b. Severe anemia, left-shifted O_2-binding curve (OBC)

> Increased hemoglobin (Hb) in newborns is due to increased HbF (fetal Hb), which left-shifts the OBC causing the release of EPO.

↑ Hb newborn: ↑ HbF

   c. Increased O_2 content suppresses EPO release.
      (1) O_2 content $= 1.34$ (Hb) $\times O_2$ saturation $+ 0.003$ (Pao_2)
      (2) Example—in polycythemia vera, the serum EPO is decreased.

↑ O_2 content: ↓ EPO

   d. Other sources of EPO
      (1) Ectopic production by tumors
         • Examples—renal cell carcinoma, hepatocellular carcinoma
      (2) Ectopic production by benign renal lesions
         • Example—polycystic kidneys
      3. Peripheral blood reticulocytes
         a. Young RBCs that require 24 hours to become mature RBCs
            • Splenic macrophages are responsible for their maturation.
         b. Identified with supravital stains
            • Contain thread-like RNA filaments in the cytoplasm (Fig. 5-1)
         c. Polychromasia
            (1) RBCs with a blue discoloration
               • Routine Wright-Giemsa stain of peripheral blood (Fig. 5-2)
            (2) Bone marrow reticulocytes that require 2 to 3 days to become mature RBCs
      4. Reticulocyte count
         a. Best marker of effective erythropoiesis
            • Indicates that the bone marrow is responding appropriately to an anemia

Reticulocyte count: marker of effective erythropoiesis

         b. Reported as a percentage (normal is 0.5–1.5%)
         c. Initial percentage must be corrected for the degree of anemia (Fig. 5-3).

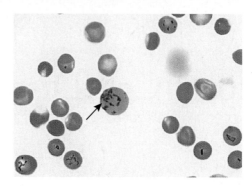

5-1: *Peripheral blood reticulocytes with supravital stain (methylene blue). The arrow shows a reticulocyte with thread-like material in the cytosol representing residual RNA filaments and protein. (From Naeim F: Atlas of Bone Marrow and Blood Pathology. Philadelphia, WB Saunders, 2001, Fig. 1-15B.)*

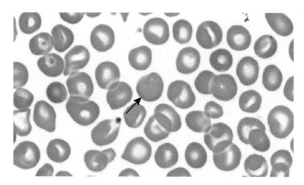

5-2: *Polychromasia. The arrow depicts a blue-discolored RBC without a central area of pallor. These types of reticulocytes appear when there is a very brisk type of hemolytic anemia (e.g., autoimmune hemolytic anemia). (From Naeim F: Atlas of Bone Marrow and Blood Pathology. Philadelphia, WB Saunders, 2001, Fig. 1-15A.)*

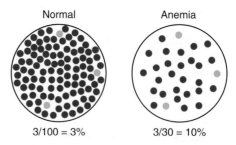

5-3: *Correction of the reticulocyte count for the degree of anemia. Note that the normal reticulocyte count is 3% when 3 reticulocytes (pale RBCs) are expressed as a percentage of 100 RBCs in the microscopic field. However, the same 3 reticulocytes account for 30% of the RBCs in the patient with anemia, who has only 30 RBCs in the microscopic field.*

(1) Corrected reticulocyte count = (patient Hct/45) × reticulocyte count
  - 45 represents the normal hematocrit (Hct).

(2) Example—Hct 15%, reticulocyte percentage 9%; corrected reticulocyte count is 3% (15/45 × 9% = 3%).

d. Presence of polychromasia requires an additional correction.
  (1) Falsely increases the percentage of reticulocytes entering peripheral blood in the last 24 hours
  (2) Correction for polychromasia
    - Divide the initial correction for anemia by 2 (called reticulocyte index)
  (3) Example—if polychromasia is present in the above example, the reticulocyte index is 3/2 = 1.5%.

e. Corrected reticulocyte count or reticulocyte index ≥3%.
  - Good bone marrow response to anemia (i.e., effective erythropoiesis)

> In hemolytic anemias (e.g., autoimmune), blood loss, and treatment of iron, folate, and vitamin B_{12} deficiency, the bone marrow responds to EPO stimulation by producing increased numbers of reticulocytes. The corrected reticulocyte count or reticulocyte index is ≥3%.

f. Corrected reticulocyte count or reticulocyte index is <3%.
  - Poor bone marrow response to anemia (i.e., ineffective erythropoiesis)

> In aplastic anemia, the bone marrow stem cells for producing RBCs are absent; therefore, there is ineffective erythropoiesis. The corrected reticulocyte count is <3%.

B. **Extramedullary hematopoiesis (EMH)**
  1. Hematopoiesis (RBC, white blood cell, and platelet production) occurs outside the bone marrow.
  2. Common sites for EMH
    (1) Liver and spleen
    (2) Become markedly enlarged (i.e., hepatosplenomegaly)

> In the fetus, hematopoiesis (blood cell formation) begins in the yolk sac and subsequently moves to the liver and finally the bone marrow by the fifth to sixth month of gestation.

  3. Causes of EMH
    a. Intrinsic bone marrow disease
      - Example—myelofibrosis, where the bone marrow is replaced by fibrous tissue
    b. Accelerated erythropoiesis
      - Example—severe hemolysis in sickle cell disease

Margin notes:

Corrected retic count: patient Hct/45 × % reticulocyte count

Corrected reticulocyte count ≥3%: effective erythropoiesis

Corrected reticulocyte count <3%: ineffective erythropoiesis

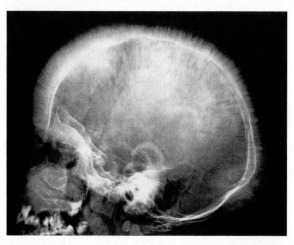

5-4: *Skull radiograph showing "hair-on-end" appearance. There is increased thickening of the parietal and frontal bones due to accelerated erythropoiesis in the marrow-containing diploic space. (From Wickramasinghe SE, McCullough J: Blood and Bone Marrow Pathology. Philadelphia, Churchill Livingstone, 2003, Fig. 6.6.)*

> Accelerated erythropoiesis often expands the bone marrow cavity, which produces frontal bossing of the skull and a "hair-on-end" appearance when viewing radiograph of the skull (Fig. 5-4).

II. **Complete Blood Count (CBC) and Other Tests**
   A. **Components of a CBC**
      1. Hb, Hct, RBC count
      2. RBC indices
      3. RBC distribution width (RDW)
      4. White blood cell (WBC) count with differential
      5. Platelet count
      6. Evaluation of peripheral blood morphology
   B. **Hb, Hct, RBC count**

$Hb \times 3 = Hct$

   1. Hb multiplied by 3 should approximate the Hct.
      • Example—Hb is 9 g/dL; therefore, the Hct is ~27%.
   2. Variables affecting reference intervals (see Chapter 1)
      • Age, sex, smoking, pregnancy
   3. Anemia
      a. Decrease in Hb, Hct, or RBC concentration
      b. Sign of an underlying disease rather than a specific diagnosis

Anemia: normal O_2 saturation and PaO_2

      c. Arterial O_2 saturation and PaO_2 are normal.
      d. Clinical findings
         (1) Fatigue
         (2) Dyspnea with exertion
            • Due to a lack of O_2
         (3) Anorexia, insomnia, inability to concentrate, dizziness

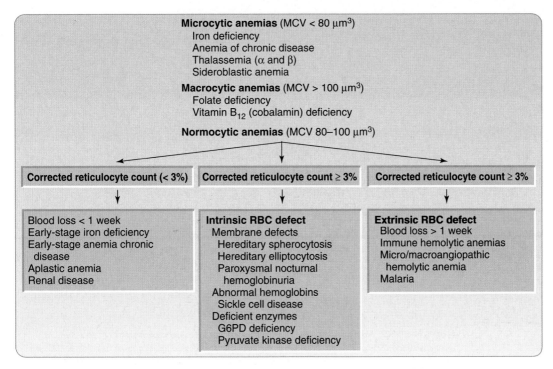

Microcytic anemias (MCV < 80 μm³)
Iron deficiency
Anemia of chronic disease
Thalassemia (α and β)
Sideroblastic anemia

Macrocytic anemias (MCV > 100 μm³)
Folate deficiency
Vitamin B₁₂ (cobalamin) deficiency

Normocytic anemias (MCV 80–100 μm³)

Corrected reticulocyte count (< 3%)	Corrected reticulocyte count ≥ 3%	Corrected reticulocyte count ≥ 3%

Blood loss < 1 week
Early-stage iron deficiency
Early-stage anemia chronic
 disease
Aplastic anemia
Renal disease
	Intrinsic RBC defect
	  Membrane defects
	    Hereditary spherocytosis
	    Hereditary elliptocytosis
	    Paroxysmal nocturnal
	      hemoglobinuria
	  Abnormal hemoglobins
	    Sickle cell disease
	  Deficient enzymes
	    G6PD deficiency
	    Pyruvate kinase deficiency
		Extrinsic RBC defect
		  Blood loss > 1 week
		  Immune hemolytic anemias
		  Micro/macroangiopathic
		    hemolytic anemia
		  Malaria

5-5: *Classification scheme for anemia. See text for discussion. (From Goljan EF: Rapid Review Pathology, 2nd ed. St. Louis, Mosby, 2007, Fig. 11-2.)*

  e. Thalassemia
    (1) Genetic globin chain disorder
    (2) Hb and Hct are decreased.
    (3) RBC count is increased (unknown mechanism).

C. **RBC indices**
  1. Clinically useful indices
    a. Mean corpuscular volume (MCV)
    b. Mean corpuscular Hgb concentration (MCHC)
  2. MCV
    a. Average volume of RBCs
    b. Useful for a classification scheme for anemias (Fig. 5-5)
      • Example—microcytic (<80 μm³), normocytic (80–100 μm³),
        macrocytic (>100 μm³)
    c. Mixture of microcytic and macrocytic RBCs produces a normal MCV.
      • Called a dimorphic RBC population
  3. MCHC
    a. Average Hb concentration in RBCs
    b. Mature RBCs are biconcave disks (Fig. 5-6).
      (1) Hb concentrates in the thick peripheral rim of the RBC.
      (2) Less Hb concentrates in the center where the RBC diameter is
        thinnest.
        • Correlates with the central area of pallor in normal RBCs.

Thalassemia: ↑ RBC count

MCHC: correlates with central area of pallor

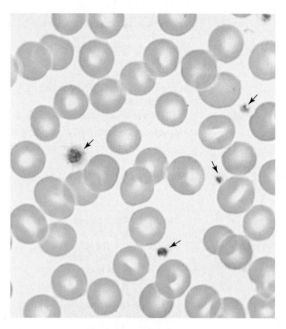

5-6: *Normal RBCs. Note the uniformity in the size of the RBCs and the central areas of pallor that are slightly less than 50% of the total diameter of the RBC. The four dark objects (arrows) outside the RBCs are platelets. (From Hoffbrand AV: Color Atlas: Clinical Hematology, 3rd ed. St. Louis, Mosby, 2000, Fig. 1.62.)*

      c. MCHC is decreased when there is a decrease in Hb synthesis.
         (1) Finding in all of the microcytic anemias
         (2) Increased central area of pallor in microcytic anemias

↑ MCHC: hereditary spherocytosis

      d. MCHC is increased when RBCs are spherical (i.e., spherocytes).
        • Spherocytes have no central area of pallor.
    D. **Red blood cell distribution width (RDW)**
      1. Measurement of size variation of RBCs in the peripheral blood
        • Called anisocytosis
      2. RDW is increased in dimorphic RBC populations.
      3. RDW is increased in iron deficiency anemia.

Iron deficiency: ↑ RDW

        • There is a mixture of normocytic and microcytic cells.
    E. **WBC count and differential**

> A 100 cell differential count divides leukocytes by percentage (neutrophils, lymphocytes, etc.) and further subdivides neutrophils into segmented and band neutrophils. Multiplication of the percentage times the total white blood cell count gives the absolute number of a particular leukocyte. Example: lymphocytes 30%, total WBC count 10,000/mm^3. Absolute lymphocyte count is $0.30 \times 10,000 = 3,000/mm^3$.

    F. **Platelet count**
      1. Anucleate cells
      2. Produced by cytoplasmic budding of megakaryocytes

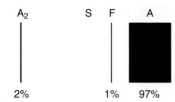

5-7: *Normal hemoglobin (Hb) electrophoresis. Hemoglobin A (2α/2β), hemoglobin A₂ (2α/2δ), and hemoglobin F (2α/2γ) separate out into three distinct bands on cellulose acetate. When these bands are stained, the density correlates with the concentration of the individual hemoglobins. When these densities are converted into a percentage by a densitometer, HbA accounts for 97%, HbA₂ 2%, and HbF 1% of the total.*

G. **Characteristics of mature RBCs**
   1. Anaerobic glycolysis is the main source of ATP.
      • Lactic acid is the end product of RBC metabolism.
   2. Pentose phosphate pathway
      • Synthesizes glutathione (GSH) to neutralize hydrogen peroxide
   3. Methemoglobin reductase pathway
      a. Reduces ferric (Fe^{3+}, methemoglobin) to ferrous (Fe^{2+}) in heme
      b. Heme group must be ferrous to carry O_2.
   4. Luebering-Rapaport pathway
      a. Synthesis of 2,3-bisphosphoglycerate
      b. Required to right-shift the OBC (i.e., release O_2 to tissue)
   5. No mitochondria or human leukocyte antigens (HLA)
   6. Senescent RBCs are removed by splenic macrophages.
      • End product of heme degradation in macrophages is unconjugated bilirubin.

H. **Hb electrophoresis**
   • Detects abnormalities in globin chain structure (e.g., sickle cell disease) and globin chain synthesis (e.g., thalassemia).

   > Different types of Hb migrate to different positions on cellulose acetate where they are stained, scanned with a densitometer, and reported as a percentage of total Hb. HbA is 2α/2β globin chains (97%), HbA₂ is 2α/2δ globin chains (2%), and HbF is 2α/2γ globin chains (1%; Fig. 5-7).

I. **Iron studies** (Fig. 5-8)
   1. Serum ferritin
      a. Primary soluble iron storage protein
         (1) Primary storage site is in the bone marrow macrophages
            • Shaded area in the small box in Figure 5-8A
         (2) Serum levels correlate with ferritin stores in the macrophages.
         (3) Synthesis of ferritin in macrophages increases in inflammation.
            • Due to release of interleukin 1 and tumor necrosis factor-α
      b. Decreased serum ferritin
         • Diagnostic of iron deficiency (Fig. 5-8B)
      c. Increased serum ferritin

Margin notes:

Methemoglobin: Fe^{3+}

Unconjugated bilirubin: end-product heme degradation in macrophage

HbA 2α/2β, HbA₂ 2α/2δ, HbF 2α/2γ

Serum ferritin: ↓ iron deficiency

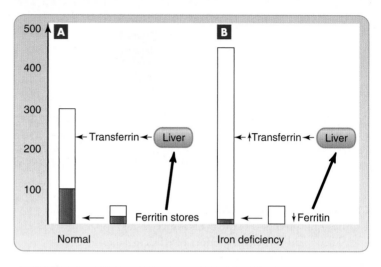

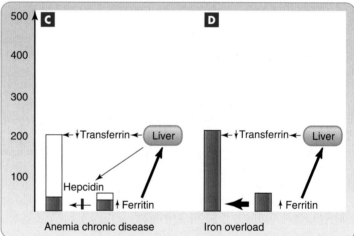

5-8: *Iron studies in normal people (**A**) and in iron deficiency (**B**), anemia of chronic disease (**C**), and iron-overload diseases (**D**). See text for discussion. (From Goljan EF: Rapid Review Pathology, 2nd ed. St. Louis, Mosby, 2007, Fig. 11-4.)*

↑ ACD, iron overload disease

      (1) Anemia of chronic disease (ACD; Fig. 5-8C)
      (2) Iron overload disease (Fig. 5-8D)
         • Examples—sideroblastic anemia, hemochromatosis
    d. Hemosiderin
      (1) Insoluble degradation product of ferritin
      (2) Levels directly correlate with changes in ferritin stores
  2. Serum iron
    a. Represents iron bound to transferrin, the binding protein of iron
      (1) Transferrin is synthesized in the liver.
      (2) Serum iron is the shaded area of the column in Figure 5-8A.
         • Note that the normal serum iron is 100 μg/dL.

b. Decreased serum iron
  (1) Iron deficiency (Fig. 5-8B)
  (2) ACD (Fig. 5-8C)
c. Increased serum iron
  • Iron overload diseases (Fig. 5-8D)

3. Serum total iron-binding capacity (TIBC)
  a. Serum TIBC correlates with the concentration of transferrin.
    (1) Height of the column correlates with serum transferrin and TIBC in Figure 5-8A.
    (2) Note that the normal TIBC is 300 µg/dL.
  b. Inverse relationship of transferrin synthesis with ferritin stores in macrophages
    (1) Decreased ferritin stores causes increased synthesis of transferrin (Fig. 5-8B).
      • Increase in transferrin and TIBC is present in iron deficiency.
    (2) Increased ferritin stores causes decreased synthesis of transferrin (Fig. 5-8C and D).
      • Decrease in transferrin and TIBC occurs in ACD (Fig. 5-8C) and iron overload disease (Fig. 5-8D).

4. Iron saturation (%)
  a. Represents the percentage of binding sites on transferrin occupied by iron
    (1) Iron saturation = serum iron/TIBC × 100
    (2) Normal saturation is 100/300 × 100, or 33% (Fig. 5-8A).
  b. Decreased iron saturation
    (1) Iron deficiency (Fig. 5-8B)
    (2) ACD (Fig. 5-8C)
  c. Increased iron saturation
    • Iron overload diseases (Fig. 5-8D)

III. Microcytic Anemias
A. Microcytic anemia classification
  1. Iron deficiency (most common)
  2. Anemia of chronic disease (ACD)
  3. Thalassemias (α and β)
  4. Sideroblastic anemias (least common)
B. Pathogenesis
  1. All have defects in the synthesis of Hb (Fig. 5-9).
    a. Defects in synthesis of heme (i.e., iron + protoporphyrin)
      • Examples—iron deficiency, ACD, sideroblastic anemia
    b. Defects in synthesis of globin chains (i.e., α or β)
      • Example—α- and β-thalassemia (thal)
  2. Cause of microcytosis
    • Extra cell divisions due to decreased concentration of Hb in developing normoblasts in the marrow
C. Iron deficiency anemia
  1. Epidemiology

Serum iron: ↓ iron deficiency, ACD ↑ iron overload disease

↓ TIBC = ↓ transferrin ↑ TIBC = ↑ transferrin

↓ Ferritin stores = ↑ TIBC; iron deficiency

↑ Ferritin stores = ↓ TIBC; ACD, iron overload

↓ % saturation: iron deficiency, ACD

↑ % saturation: iron overload disease

Microcytic anemia: ↓ Hb synthesis

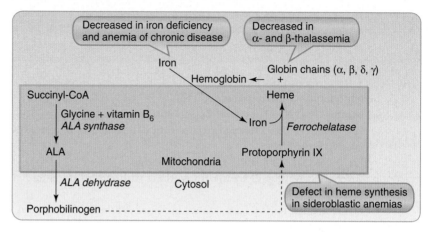

5-9: *Pathophysiology of microcytic anemias. Hemoglobin is produced when heme (iron + protoporphyrin IX) is combined with globin chains. Iron deficiency and anemia of chronic disease (ACD) are due to a lack of iron to produce heme. Sideroblastic anemias are produced when there is a defect in mitochondrial synthesis of heme. In thalassemia (α and β), there is a defect in globin chain synthesis. Note that heme synthesis begins in the mitochondria, moves into the cytosol, and then returns to the mitochondria for the final reactions. ALA, aminolevulinic acid. (From Goljan EF: Rapid Review Pathology, 2nd ed. St. Louis, Mosby, 2007, Fig. 11-5.)*

Iron deficiency: bleeding most common cause

    a. Most common overall anemia
    b. Bleeding is the most common cause of iron deficiency.
    c. Causes of iron deficiency (Table 5-1)
  2. Clinical findings
    a. Plummer-Vinson syndrome
      (1) Caused by chronic iron deficiency
      (2) Clinical findings
        (a) Esophageal web
          • Dysphagia for solids but not liquids
        (b) Achlorhydria
          • No acid in the stomach
        (c) Glossitis
          • Inflammation of the tongue
        (d) Spoon nails (koilonychia)
    b. Laboratory findings
      (1) Decreased MCV
      (2) Decreased Hb, Hct, RBC count
      (3) Decreased serum iron and iron saturation (%)
      (4) Decreased serum ferritin (<30 ng/mL)
        • Serum ferritin may be normal if there is coexisting ACD
      (5) Decreased MCHC
        • Decreased central area of pallor (Fig. 5-10)
      (6) Increased TIBC
      (7) Increased RDW
        • Microcytic and normocytic cells

TABLE 5-1
Causes of Iron Deficiency

Classification	Causes	Discussion
Blood loss	Gastrointestinal loss	Meckel's diverticulum (older children) PUD (most common cause adult men) Polyps/colorectal cancer (most common cause in adults >50 yr old) Hookworm; hereditary telangiectasia (AD, telangiectasia skin and GI tract); Crohn's disease; angiodysplasia (telangiectasia of vessels in cecum)
	Menorrhagia	Most common cause in women <50 yr old
	Genitourinary	Renal cell carcinoma, transitional cell carcinoma of bladder
Increased utilization	Pregnancy/lactation	Daily iron requirement in pregnancy is 3.4 mg and 2.5–3.0 mg in lactation
	Infants/children	Iron is required for tissue growth, development, and expansion of blood volume
Decreased intake	Infants/children	Most common cause of iron deficiency in young children; iron content is inadequate in milk (breast and other sources) and cereals
	Pure vegan/elderly	Non-heme iron (iron Fe^{3+}) is poorly absorbed in the duodenum
	Elderly	Restricted diets with little meat (lack of heme iron; Fe^{2+})
Decreased absorption	Celiac sprue	Absence of villous surface in the duodenum
	Achlorhydria (e.g., gastrectomy, pernicious anemia)	Hydrochloric acid chelates ferrous iron to stabilize iron in the soluble form for reabsorption
Intravascular hemolysis	Micro-, macroangiopathic hemolytic anemia, PNH	Chronic loss of Hb in urine leads to iron deficiency

AD, autosomal dominant; GI, gastrointestinal; Hb, hemoglobin; PNH, paroxysmal nocturnal hemoglobinuria; PUD, peptic ulcer disease.

(8) Increased serum free erythrocyte protoporphyrin (FEP)
- Less iron available to combine with protoporphyrin to form heme

> Stages of iron deficiency in sequence are as follows: absent iron stores; decreased serum ferritin; decreased serum iron, increased TIBC, decreased iron saturation; normocytic normochromic anemia; microcytic hypochromic anemia.

Iron deficiency: ↓ iron, % saturation, ferritin; ↑ TIBC, RDW, FEP

(9) Platelet count is variable.
- Thrombocytosis (increased platelet count) is a common finding in chronic iron deficiency due to blood loss.

(10) Leukocyte count is usually normal.
- Eosinophilia occurs in hookworm infestations.

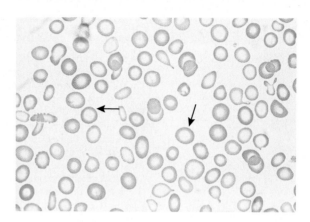

5-10: *Peripheral blood smear of iron deficiency anemia. Note the enlarged central areas of pallor in the majority of RBCs (arrows), which correlates with a decrease in the synthesis of hemoglobin (hypochromasia). A few of the RBCs are normocytic and normochromic. Other RBCs exhibit shape abnormalities (e.g., pencil-shaped, tear drops). The marked size variation in the RBCs is responsible for an increase in RBC distribution width in iron deficiency. (From Wickramasinghe SE, McCullough J: Blood and Bone Marrow Pathology. Philadelphia, Churchill Livingstone, 2003, Fig. 11.6.)*

3. Treat with ferrous sulfate
   a. Reticulocyte response
      • Begins about 3 days after therapy and peaks in 8 to 10 days
   b. Hct should increase ~0.5% to 1% per day after the initial lag period.
D. **Anemia of chronic disease**
   1. Epidemiology
      a. Causes
         (1) Chronic inflammation
            • Example—rheumatoid arthritis, tuberculosis
         (2) Alcoholism
            • Most common anemia
         (3) Malignancy
            • Most common anemia
      b. Most common anemia in hospitalized patients
   2. Pathogenesis
      a. Decreased production of EPO
         • Due to macrophage release of interleukin 1 (IL-1) and tumor necrosis factor (TNF)
      b. Hepcidin
         (1) Antimicrobial peptide synthesized in the liver
         (2) Released as an acute phase reactant in the liver in response to inflammation

> Acute phase reactants (APRs) are proteins that are synthesized and released by the liver in inflammation. APRs include coagulation factors (e.g., fibrinogen, factor V, factor VIII), complement, hepcidin, C-reactive protein, and serum

associated amyloid. IL-1 and TNF are the mediators that stimulate the liver to synthesize and release APRs.

(3) Prevents release of iron from marrow macrophages to transferrin for delivery to developing normoblasts (Fig. 5-8C)

(4) Inhibits iron uptake in the duodenum

c. Increased iron stores in marrow macrophages

(1) Normal input of iron into macrophages

(2) Output of iron is decreased due to hepcidin.

3. Laboratory findings

a. Decreased MCV (10–30% of cases)

b. Decreased Hb, Hct, RBC count

- Hb rarely <9 g/dL)

c. Decreased serum iron, TIBC, and iron saturation

d. Increased serum ferritin (>100 ng/mL)

e. Increased serum FEP

- Less iron available to combine with protoporphyrin to form heme

f. Platelet and leukocyte counts are variable.

E. **Thalassemias (α and β)**

1. Epidemiology

a. Autosomal recessive disorders

b. α-Thalassemia is common in Southeast Asia and in the black population.

c. β-Thalassemia is common in the black population, Greeks, and Italians.

2. Pathogenesis of α-thalassemia

a. Decrease in α-globin chain synthesis on chromosome 16

- Due to gene deletions

b. One gene deletion produces a silent carrier.

- It is *not* associated with anemia.

c. Two gene deletions is called α-thalassemia trait.

(1) Mild microcytic anemia

(2) Black population type has a loss of one gene on each chromosome (α/- α/-; Fig. 5-11A).

(3) Asian type has a loss of both genes on the same chromosome (-/- α/α, Fig. 5-11B).

- Increased risk for developing more severe types of α-thalassemia

(4) Laboratory findings

(a) Decreased MCV

(b) Decreased Hb, Hct

(c) Increased RBC count

(d) Decreased MCHC

(e) Normal RDW

(f) Normal serum ferritin

(g) Normal serum FEP

Hepcidin: "reticuloendothelial cell block"

ACD: ↓ iron, TIBC, % saturation; ↑ ferritin, FEP

α-Thal: gene deletions

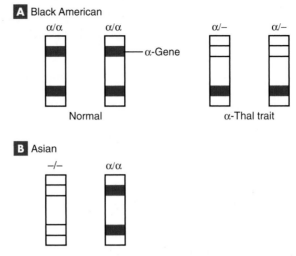

5-11: *Gene deletions in α-thalassemia in the black population (**A**) and Asian population (**B**). Four α-genes are involved in α-globin chain synthesis. The black population type is associated with a loss of one gene on each chromosome (trans configuration: α/- α/-; schematic A). This eliminates the possibility of developing severe types of α-thalassemia between members of the same race. In the Asian type, there is a loss of both genes on the same chromosome (cis configuration: -/- α/α, B). This poses an increased risk for developing more severe types of α-thalassemia (e.g., Hb H and Hb Barts disease) between members of the same race.*

(h) Normal Hb electrophoresis

> Hb electrophoresis is normal in α-thalassemia trait, because all Hb types require α-globin chains. All the Hb types are decreased; however, the relative proportions of the normal Hb types remain the same (Fig. 5-12B).

α-Thal trait: ↓ HbA, HbA$_2$, HbF (normal electrophoresis); ↑ RBC count

(5) There is no treatment.
  • Treatment with iron is *not* indicated because of the danger of developing iron overload.

d. Three gene deletions is called HbH (four β-chains) disease.
  (1) Severe hemolytic anemia
    (a) Due to the presence of excess β-chain inclusions
    (b) Macrophage destruction of RBCs with inclusions
    (c) Signal for apoptosis of the RBC

HbH: 4 β-chains

  (2) Hb electrophoresis detects HbH.

Hb Bart: 4 γ-chains

e. Four gene deletions is called Hb Bart (four γ-chains) disease.
  (1) Incompatible with life unless intrauterine transfusions are utilized
  (2) Increased incidence of spontaneous abortions
    • Predisposes to an increase in molar pregnancies
  (3) Hb electrophoresis shows an increase in Hb Bart.

3. Pathogenesis of β-thalassemia
  a. Decrease in β-globin chain synthesis on chromosome 11
    (1) Mild anemia
      • Most often due to DNA splicing defects

	Pattern				Type of anemia	Interpretation and discussion
A.	A_2 2%	S	F 1%	A 97%	None	Normal Hb electrophoresis
B.	A_2 2%	S	F 1%	A 97%	Microcytic	α - Thal trait. Note that the proportion of the Hb types remains the same; however, the patient has a microcytic anemia.
C.	A_2 5%	S	F 2%	A 93%	Microcytic	β - Thal minor. Note that HbA is decreased, because β-globin chain synthesis is decreased. There is a corresponding increase in HbA_2 and HbF.
D.	A_2 10%	S	F 90%	A	Microcytic	β - Thal major. Note that there is no synthesis of HbA.
E.	A_2 2%	S 45%	F 1%	A 52%	No anemia	Sickle cell trait. Note that there is not enough HbS to cause spontaneous sickling in the peripheral blood.
F.	A_2 2%	S 90%	F 8%	A	Normocytic	Sickle cell disease. Note that there is no HbA. There is enough HbS to cause spontaneous sickling.

5-12: Hemoglobin electrophoresis patterns in thalassemia and sickle cell disorders. Refer to text for discussion.

β-Thal: mild—DNA splicing defect; severe— stop codon

      (2) Severe anemia

         (a) Nonsense mutation with formation of a stop codon

         (b) Premature termination of β-globin chain synthesis or absent β-globin chain synthesis

  b. Normal synthesis of α-, δ-, γ-globin chains

> Normal β-globin chain synthesis is designated β; some β-globin chain synthesis is designated $β^+$; no β-globin chain synthesis is designated $β^0$.

  c. β-Thalassemia minor ($β/β^+$)

      (1) Mild microcytic hypochromic anemia

      (2) Mild protective effect against falciparum malaria infection

        • RBC life span is shorter than normal.

      (3) Peripheral blood RBCs

         (a) Tear drop cells (shape of a tear)

         (b) Target cells (RBCs with a bull's-eye appearance)

      (4) Decreased Hb, Hct, and MCHC

      (5) Increased RBC count

      (6) Normal RDW

      (7) Normal serum ferritin

      (8) Normal serum FEP

      (9) Hb electrophoresis (Fig. 5-12C)

β-Thal minor: ↓ HbA; ↑ RBC count, HbA_2, HbF

        • Decreased HbA ($2α/2β$); increased HbA_2 ($2α/2δ$) and HbF ($2α/2γ$)

     (10) There is no treatment.

        • Treatment with iron is *not* recommended because of the danger of developing iron overload.

  d. β-Thalassemia major (Cooley's anemia; $β^0/β^0$)

      (1) Severe hemolytic anemia with massive ineffective erythropoiesis

         (a) Excess α-chain inclusions in normoblasts initiates apoptosis

         (b) RBCs with inclusions in peripheral blood are phagocytosed and destroyed by splenic macrophages.

        • Produces an increase in serum unconjugated bilirubin

      (2) Extramedullary hematopoiesis

      (3) Peripheral blood RBCs

         (a) Target cells and tear drop cells

         (b) Basophilic stippling

        • RBCs with persistent ribosomes

         (c) Nucleated RBCs

      (4) Increased RDW

      (5) Reticulocytosis

        • Usually <10% due to high degree of ineffective erythropoiesis

      (6) Hb electrophoresis (Fig. 5-12D)

        • No synthesis of HbA; increase in HbA_2 and HbF

β-Thal major: no HbA; ↑ HbA_2, HbF

      (7) Unconjugated hyperbilirubinemia

        • Extravascular hemolysis by splenic macrophages

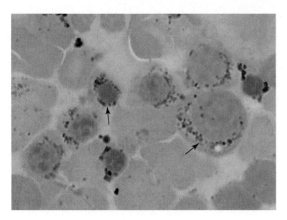

5-13: *Ringed sideroblasts in a bone marrow aspirate. Note the rim of dark, blue iron granules around the nucleus of developing normoblasts. These granules represent iron trapped within mitochondria and indicate a defect in heme synthesis within the mitochondria. (From Forbes C, Jackson W: Color Atlas and Text of Clinical Medicine, 2nd ed. St. Louis, Mosby, 2003, Fig. 10.27.)*

       (8) Transfusion is required together with chelation of iron to prevent iron overload.
         • Bone marrow transplantation is the only effective cure.

F. **Sideroblastic anemia**
  1. Epidemiology: causes
    a. Chronic alcoholism (most common cause)
    b. Pyridoxine (vitamin B_6) deficiency
    c. Lead (Pb) poisoning
    d. Refractory anemia with ringed sideroblasts (RARS; see Chapter 6)
  2. Pathogenesis
    a. Defect in heme synthesis within the mitochondria (see Fig. 5-9)
    b. Iron accumulates in mitochondria forming ringed sideroblasts (Fig. 5-13).
    c. Iron-overload types of anemia
      • Increase in iron stores in the bone marrow
  3. Chronic alcoholism
    a. Sideroblastic anemia occurs in ~30% of hospitalized chronic alcoholics.
    b. Alcohol is a mitochondrial poison.
      • Damages heme biosynthetic pathways in the mitochondria
  4. Pyridoxine deficiency
    a. Vitamin B_6 is a cofactor for δ-aminolevulinic acid synthase.
      • Rate-limiting reaction of heme synthesis (Fig. 5-9)
    b. Most common cause of deficiency is isoniazid (INH) therapy.
      • INH is used in the treatment of tuberculosis.
  5. Lead poisoning
    a. Epidemiology
      (1) Pica (abnormal craving) for eating lead-based paint
        • Common childhood cause in inner cities

Sideroblastic anemia: defect in mitochondrial heme synthesis; ringed sideroblasts

Sideroblastic anemia: alcohol most common cause

Pyridoxine deficiency: INH most common cause

(2) Pottery painter
  • Lead-based paints are commonly used for decoration.
(3) Working in a battery or ammunition factory
(4) Radiator repair

Pb poisoning: paint, batteries, radiators

b. Lead denatures (irreversibly inhibits) the following enzymes (Fig. 5-9)
  (1) Ferrochelatase (i.e., heme synthase)
    • Iron cannot bind with protoporphyrin to form heme causing an increase in FEP (proximal to enzyme block).
  (2) Aminolevulinic acid (ALA) dehydrase
    • δ-ALA is *not* converted to porphobilinogen causing an increase in δ- ALA (proximal to enzyme block).

Pb poisoning: ↑ FEP, δ-ALA

  (3) Ribonuclease
    • Ribosomes cannot be degraded and persist in the RBC causing coarse basophilic stippling. (Fig. 5-14).

Pb poisoning: coarse basophilic stippling

  (4) RBC membrane-associated enzymes
    • Increased RBC hemolysis
c. Clinical and laboratory findings
  (1) Abdominal colic with diarrhea
    • Lead is visible in gastrointestinal tract on plain abdominal radiographs.
  (2) Encephalopathy in children
    • δ-ALA damages neurons, increases vessel permeability (cerebral edema), and causes demyelination.
  (3) Growth retardation in children
    (a) Pb deposits in the epiphysis of growing bone
    (b) X-ray shows increased density in the epiphyses.

Pb poisoning: Pb deposits in epiphyses

  (4) Peripheral neuropathy in adults

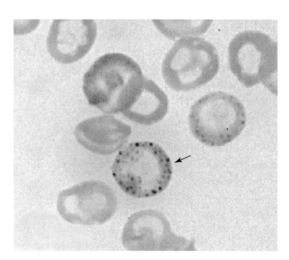

5-14: *Peripheral blood with coarse basophilic stippling of RBCs in lead poisoning. The arrow shows a mature RBC containing dark granules representing ribosomes. Lead denatures ribonuclease; therefore, ribosomes persist in the cytoplasm in routine Wright-Giemsa–stained slides. (From Naeim F: Atlas of Bone Marrow and Blood Pathology. Philadelphia, WB Saunders, 2001, Fig. 2-22M.)*

- Examples—foot drop (peroneal nerve palsy), wrist drop (radial nerve palsy), and claw hand (ulnar nerve palsy)
        (5) Pb line along the gums (adults)
        (6) Nephrotoxic damage to proximal renal tubules
- Fanconi syndrome: proximal renal tubular acidosis (loss of bicarbonate in urine), aminoaciduria, phosphaturia, and glucosuria
        (7) Increased incidence of gout
- Pb decreases renal excretion of uric acid.
        (8) Increased FEP and δ-ALA
        (9) Increased whole blood and urine Pb levels
- Best screen and confirmatory test for Pb poisoning
        (10) Slight increase in reticulocyte count
- Due to hemolysis of RBCs
    d. Treatment
- Succimer, EDTA, dimercaprol
  6. Laboratory findings in sideroblastic anemia
    a. Increased serum iron, iron saturation, ferritin
    b. Decreased TIBC
    c. Ringed sideroblasts in bone marrow aspirate
  G. **Summary table of microcytic anemias** (Table 5-2)

IV. **Macrocytic Anemias**
- Macrocytic anemias are subdivided into megaloblastic (e.g., folate or vitamin B_{12} deficiency) and nonmegaloblastic anemia (e.g., macrocytosis related to alcohol intoxication).
  A. **Megaloblastic macrocytic anemias**
    1. Vitamin B_{12} metabolism
      a. Sources of vitamin B_{12}
- Meat, eggs, and dairy products

Vitamin B_{12}: present in animal products

TABLE 5-2 Summary of Microcytic Anemias

Test	Iron Deficiency	ACD	α, β-Thal Minor	Pb Poisoning
MCV	↓	↓/N	↓	↓
Serum iron	↓	↓	N	↑
TIBC	↑	↓	N	↓
% Saturation	↓	↓	N	↑
Serum ferritin	↓	↑	N	↑
RDW	↑	N	N	N
RBC count	↓	↓	↑	↓
Hb electrophoresis	N	N	α-Thal: normal β-Thal: ↓ HbA; ↑ HbA$_2$, HbF	
Ringed sideroblasts	None	None	None	Present
Coarse basophilic stippling	None	None	None	Present

ACD, anemia chronic disease; Hb, hemoglobin; MCV, mean corpuscular volume; N, normal; Pb, lead; RDW, red blood cell distribution width; Thal, thalassemia; TIBC, total iron-binding capacity.

IF: necessary for vitamin B_{12} reabsorption

b. Parietal cells (body and fundus of stomach)
  (1) Synthesize intrinsic factor (IF) and hydrochloric acid
  (2) Chief cells secrete pepsinogen.
c. Gastric acid
  (1) Converts pepsinogen to pepsin
  (2) Pepsin frees vitamin B_{12} from ingested proteins.
d. R-binders
  (1) Proteins synthesized in salivary glands
  (2) Free vitamin B_{12} is bound to R-binders.
  (3) Protect vitamin B_{12} from acid destruction
e. Pancreatic enzymes in the duodenum
  (1) Cleave off the R-binders
  (2) Releases vitamin B_{12} for binding to IF
f. Vitamin B_{12}-IF complex
  • Reabsorbed in the terminal ileum after attaching to receptors for IF
g. Transcobalamin II
  (1) Reabsorbed vitamin B_{12} binds to transcobalamin II.
  (2) Delivered to metabolically active cells
  (3) Stored in the liver (6- to 9-year supply)

Vitamin B_{12} deficiency: pernicious anemia most common cause

2. Causes of vitamin B_{12} deficiency (Table 5-3)
3. Folate metabolism
  a. Sources
    (1) Green vegetables (most abundant source)

TABLE 5-3
Causes of Vitamin B_{12} Deficiency

Classification	Causes	Discussion
Decreased intake	Pure vegan diet	Breast fed infants of pure vegans may develop deficiency
	Malnutrition	Lack of animal products
Malabsorption	↓ Intrinsic factor	Autoimmune destruction of parietal cells (i.e., pernicious anemia) or gastrectomy
	↓ Gastric acid	Cannot activate pepsinogen to release vitamin B_{12} from protein
	↓ Intestinal reabsorption	Crohn's disease or celiac disease involving terminal ileum (loss of absorptive cells)
		Bacterial overgrowth (bacterial utilization of available vitamin B_{12})
		Chronic pancreatitis (cannot cleave off R-binder)
		Fish tapeworm, infiltrative disorder small bowel (e.g., malignant lymphoma)
Increased utilization	Pregnancy/lactation	Deficiency is more likely if the patient is a pure vegan
	Hyperthyroidism	Increased metabolism of cells
	Disseminated malignancy	Deficiency is more likely if the malignancy has a rapid cell turnover (e.g., leukemia, lymphoma)

(2) Animal proteins

(3) Polyglutamate form in food

  • Heating food for 5 to 10 minutes destroys folate.

  b. Converted to monoglutamates by intestinal conjugase

  • Intestinal conjugase is inhibited by phenytoin.

  c. Reabsorption

(1) Reabsorbed in the jejunum

  • Blocked by alcohol and oral contraceptives

(2) Converted to methyltetrahydrofolate

  • Circulating form of folate

(3) There is a 3- to 4-month supply of folate in the liver.

4. Causes of folate deficiency (Table 5-4)

5. Pathogenesis of macrocytic anemia in folate and vitamin B_{12} deficiency

  a. Impaired DNA synthesis

(1) Delayed nuclear maturation

  • Block in cell division produces large, nucleated hematopoietic (megaloblastic) cells.

(2) All rapidly dividing cells are affected.

  • Examples—RBCs, leukocytes, platelets, intestinal epithelium

(3) Cellular RNA and protein synthesis continues unabated.

  • Cytoplasmic volume continues to expand.

  b. Ineffective erythropoiesis

(1) Megaloblastic precursors are located outside the bone marrow sinusoids

(2) Phagocytosed and destroyed by macrophages or undergo apoptosis

(3) Produces pancytopenia (i.e., anemia, neutropenia, and thrombocytopenia)

Intestinal conjugase: inhibited by phenytoin

Monoglutamate reabsorption: inhibited by alcohol and oral contraceptives

Folate deficiency: alcohol most common cause

Table 5-4
Causes of Folate Deficiency

Classification	Causes	Discussion
Decreased intake	Malnutrition, infants/elderly Chronic alcoholics Excessive heating of food, goat's milk	Most common cause of folate deficiency
Malabsorption	Celiac disease Diffuse small bowel disease (e.g., malignant lymphoma) Bacterial overgrowth	Usually occurs in association with other vitamin deficiencies (fat and water soluble)
Drug inhibition	5-Fluorouracil Methotrexate, trimethoprim Phenytoin Oral contraceptives, alcohol	Inhibits thymidylate synthase Inhibit dihydrofolate reductase Inhibits intestinal conjugase Inhibit uptake of monoglutamate in jejunum. Alcohol also inhibits the release of folate from the liver.
Increased utilization	Pregnancy/lactation Disseminated malignancy Severe hemolytic anemia	Increased utilization of folate in DNA metabolism

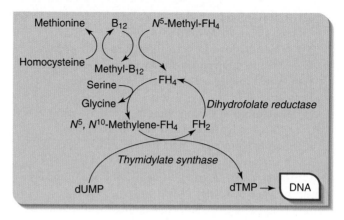

5-15: *Schematic of vitamin B_{12} and folate in DNA synthesis. Refer to text for discussion. dTMP, deoxythymidine monophosphate; dUMP, deoxyuridine monophosphate; FH_2, dihydrofolate; FH_4, tetrahydrofolate; N^5-methyl-FH_4, N^5-methyltetrahydrofolate. (From Pelley JW, Goljan EF: Rapid Review Biochemistry, 2nd ed. St. Louis, Mosby, 2007, Fig. 4-3.)*

6. Vitamin B_{12} and folate in DNA synthesis (Fig. 5-15)
   a. Vitamin B_{12} removes methyl group from methyltetrahydrofolate (N^5-methyl-FH_4) to produce tetrahydrofolate (FH_4)
   b. Methyl group from methyl-B_{12} is transferred to homocysteine to produce methionine.
      (1) Deficiency of folate or vitamin B_{12} increases plasma homocysteine.
      (2) Deficiency of vitamin B_{12} causes N^5-methyl-FH_4 to be trapped in its circulating form.
        • May increase the serum folate in 30% of cases

> Folate deficiency is the most common cause of increased serum homocysteine levels in the United States. Homocysteine damages endothelial cells leading to vessel thrombosis.

   c. Thymidylate synthase transfers methylene group from $N^{5,10}$-methylene FH_4 to deoxyuridine monophosphate (dUMP) to produce deoxythymidine monophosphate (dTMP).
        • 5-Fluorouracil irreversibly inhibits thymidylate synthase.
   d. Dihydrofolate (FH_2) is reduced back to FH_4 by dihydrofolate reductase.
        • Inhibitors of dihydrofolate reductase are methotrexate, trimethoprim.
7. Vitamin B_{12} and odd-chain fatty acid metabolism
   a. Propionyl CoA
      (1) Converted to methylmalonyl CoA by propionyl CoA carboxylase
      (2) Biotin is a cofactor.
   b. Methylmalonyl CoA

↑ Homocysteine: folate (most common) and vitamin B_{12} deficiency

Thymidylate synthase: inhibited by 5-fluorouracil

Dihydrofolate reductase: inhibited by methotrexate, trimethoprim

(1) Converted to succinyl CoA by methylmalonyl CoA mutase
(2) Vitamin B_{12} is a cofactor.

Vitamin B_{12}: odd-chain fatty acid metabolism

  c. Vitamin B_{12} deficiency
    (1) Increases propionyl CoA proximal to enzyme block
    (2) Propionyl CoA replaces acetyl CoA in fatty acids in neuronal membranes.
      • Produces demyelination
8. Clinical findings in vitamin B_{12} deficiency
  a. Findings in pernicious anemia

Pernicious anemia: autoimmune disease

    (1) Achlorhydria (absent hydrochloric acid)
      • Due to autoimmune destruction of parietal cells
    (2) Maldigestion of food
      • Due to chronic atrophic gastritis and achlorhydria
    (3) Increased incidence of gastric cancer of body and fundus
      • Due to chronic atrophic gastritis and achlorhydria
    (4) Hypergastrinemia
      • Due to loss of acid inhibition of gastrin
    (5) Antibodies directed against proton pump in parietal cells
      • Present in 85% to 90% of cases
    (6) Antibodies that block binding of vitamin B_{12} to IF
      (a) Present in 60% to 75% of cases
      (b) Most specific test for pernicious anemia
    (7) Antibodies that prevent binding of vitamin B_{12}-IF complexes to terminal ileal receptors
      • Present in 30% to 50% of patients
  b. Glossitis
    • Smooth, sore tongue with atrophy of papillae
  c. Neurologic disease
    (1) Peripheral neuropathy with motor and sensory dysfunction
    (2) Posterior column dysfunction
      • Decrease in vibratory sensation and proprioception (joint sense)
    (3) Lateral corticospinal tract dysfunction with spasticity
    (4) Dementia

Macrocytic anemia + neurologic disease: vitamin B_{12} deficiency

  d. Increased risk for atherosclerosis and thrombosis
    • Due to increase in homocysteine
  e. Association with other autoimmune diseases
    • Examples—Graves' disease, Hashimoto's thyroiditis, Addison's disease
9. Laboratory findings in vitamin B_{12} deficiency
  a. Decreased serum vitamin B_{12}
  b. Increased serum homocysteine
  c. Increased unconjugated bilirubin
    • Due to ineffective erythropoiesis
  d. Increased methylmalonic acid
    (1) Present in 95% of cases
    (2) Most sensitive test
  e. Increased lactate dehydrogenase

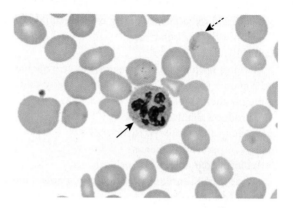

5-16: *Peripheral blood with hypersegmented neutrophil in vitamin B$_{12}$ deficiency. Note the hypersegmented neutrophil with eight lobes (solid arrow). Neutrophils normally have less than five nuclear lobes. Also note the enlarged, egg-shaped RBCs (dashed arrow) (macro-ovalocytes) characteristic of macrocytic anemias associated with problems in DNA synthesis (i.e., vitamin B$_{12}$ and folate deficiency). (From Hoffbrand AV: Color Atlas: Clinical Hematology, 3rd ed. St. Louis, Mosby, 2000, Fig. 3.15A.)*

↑ Methylmalonic acid: most sensitive test for vitamin B$_{12}$ deficiency

Hypersegmented neutrophil: marker for folate and/or vitamin B$_{12}$ deficiency

    (1) Present in 85% of cases
    (2) Due to ineffective erythropoiesis and hemolysis of RBCs
  f. Peripheral blood findings
    (1) Pancytopenia
    (2) Egg-shaped macrocytes
    (3) Hypersegmented neutrophils (>5 nuclear lobes; Fig. 5-16)
      • Present *before* anemia and is the *last* finding to disappear with treatment
  g. Bone marrow findings
    (1) Marrow aspiration is *not* usually necessary to secure the diagnosis.
    (2) Megaloblastic nucleated cells (Fig. 5-17)
      (a) Primitive open (lacy) chromatin in all stages of RBC normoblast and leukocyte development as well as in megakaryocytes
      (b) Giant "band" neutrophils are a prominent finding.
  h. Schilling test

Schilling test: defines the cause of vitamin B$_{12}$ deficiency

    (1) Definitive test that identifies certain causes of vitamin B$_{12}$ deficiency
    (2) Oral dose of ^{57}Co-labeled cobalamin is followed by a 24-hour urine collection to see how much ^{57}Co is reabsorbed and excreted in the urine.
    (3) Dietary cause of vitamin B$_{12}$ deficiency
      • Greater than 7.5% of the standard oral dose of ^{57}Co is excreted in a 24-hour urine collection
    (4) Pernicious anemia
      (a) Less than 7.5% is excreted after oral administration of ^{57}Co.
      (b) Greater than 7.5% is excreted after oral administration of ^{57}Co plus IF.
    (5) Malabsorption other than pernicious anemia

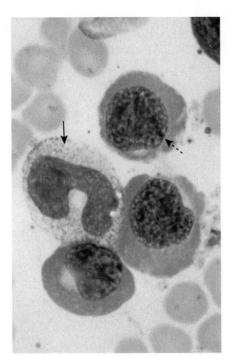

5-17: *Megaloblastic cells in the bone marrow. Early, megaloblastic erythroid cell (interrupted arrow) shows an enlarged nucleus with lacy-appearing nuclear chromatin. The solid arrow shows a giant band neutrophil. (From Wickramasinghe SE, McCullough J: Blood and Bone Marrow Pathology. Philadelphia, Churchill Livingstone, 2003, Fig. 12.1B.)*

- Less than 7.5% is excreted after oral administration of ^{57}Co with or without the addition of IF.
10. Clinical findings in folate deficiency
    - Similar to vitamin B_{12} deficiency with the *exception* of neurologic disease

> Decreased maternal intake of folate *prior* to conception increases the risk for open neural tube defects in the fetus.

11. Laboratory findings in folate deficiency
    a. Peripheral blood and bone marrow findings
       - Similar to vitamin B_{12} deficiency
    b. Decreased serum folate and RBC folate (best screening test)
       (1) Serum folate reflects folic acid intake over the last several days.
           - Decreased serum folate precedes a decrease in RBC folate.
       (2) RBC folate reflects folate available when RBCs were maturing in the marrow.
           - Better indicator of folate stores
12. Table comparing vitamin B_{12} deficiency and folate deficiency (Table 5-5)

RBC folate: best indicator of folate stores

**Table 5-5
Comparison of
Vitamin B$_{12}$
Deficiency and
Folate Deficiency**

Laboratory/Clinical Findings	Pernicious Anemia	Other B$_{12}$ Deficiency	Folate Deficiency
Mean corpuscular volume	↑	↑	↑
Autoantibodies	↑	Absent	Absent
Chronic atrophic gastritis	Present	Absent	Absent
Achlorhydria	Present	Absent	Absent
Serum gastrin levels	↑	Normal	Normal
Gastric carcinoma risk	↑	Absent	Absent
Plasma homocysteine	↑	↑	↑
Urine methylmalonic acid	↑	↑	Normal
Neurological disease	Present	Present	Absent

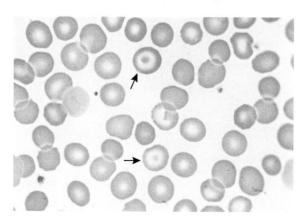

5-18: *Round macrocytes in chronic alcoholism. Note the round macrocytes with marked target cell formation (arrows). The targetoid appearance is due to excess RBC membrane, which bulges in the center of the cell and locally concentrates Hb. (From Wickramasinghe SE, McCullough J: Blood and Bone Marrow Pathology. Philadelphia, Churchill Livingstone, 2003, Fig. 6-2F.)*

Alcohol liver disease:
round macrocytic target
cells

B. **Nonmegaloblastic macrocytosis**
   1. General differences from megaloblastic macrocytic anemias
      a. Macrocytes are round rather than oval.
      b. Hypersegmented neutrophils are *not* present.
      c. Leukocytes and platelets are quantitatively normal.
      d. Absence of glossitis and neuropathy
      e. Anemia may not be present.
      f. Alcohol excess is the most common cause for all types of anemia.
   2. Liver disease associated with alcohol
      a. MCV range: 105 ± 10 μm^3
      b. Thin, round, macrocytic target cells (Fig. 5-18)
         • Excess RBC membrane due to increased membrane cholesterol
      c. Life-span of the RBCs is *not* decreased.
   3. Direct toxic effect of alcohol
      (1) MCV ranges from 100 to 110 μm^3.

(2) Vacuolization of RBC precursors in bone marrow

(3) Abstinence from alcohol reverses the macrocytosis and anemia.

V. **Normocytic Anemias: Corrected Reticulocyte Count or Index <3%**
  - Anemias under this classification include acute blood loss, early iron deficiency or anemia of chronic disease (ACD), aplastic anemia, and renal disease.
  A. **Acute blood loss**
    1. Epidemiology
      a. External blood loss
        - Examples—gastrointestinal bleed (e.g., peptic ulcer), ruptured esophageal varices
      b. Internal blood loss
        - Examples—ruptured abdominal aortic aneurysm, ruptured spleen
    2. Clinical and laboratory findings
      a. Signs of volume depletion
        (1) Decreased blood pressure
        (2) Tachycardia with diminished pulse

> Blood pressure drops further and pulse increases when the patient is raised from a supine to sitting position (positive tilt test). Loss of blood volume is accentuated when sitting up because it imposes a gravitational effect on venous return to the right side of the heart.

        (3) Cold, clammy skin
          - Due to vasoconstriction of peripheral arterioles from catecholamines and angiotensin II

        Signs volume depletion: ↓ blood pressure, ↑ pulse

      b. Hb, Hct, and RBC count
        (1) *No* initial change in concentration
          - Loss of whole blood leads to an equal loss of RBCs and plasma.
        (2) Eventual shift of interstitial fluid to the vascular compartment
          (a) Causes hemodilution and a drop in Hb, Hct, and RBC count
          (b) Infusion of 0.9% normal saline immediately uncovers the RBC deficit.

        Acute blood loss: initially normal Hb, Hct, RBC count

        (3) Decreased oxygenation causes the release of EPO.
          - Requires 5 to 7 days before a reticulocyte response is observed
      c. Neutrophilic leukocytosis
        (1) First hematologic change in acute blood loss
        (2) Due to mobilization of the marginating neutrophil pool (see Chapter 6)
          - Catecholamines inhibit activation of neutrophil adhesion molecules.

        Acute blood loss: neutrophilic leukocytosis first hematologic change

      d. External blood loss may result in iron deficiency.
  B. **Early iron deficiency or ACD**
    1. Anemia is normocytic *before* it becomes microcytic.
    2. Serum ferritin is most useful in distinguishing the two anemias.
      - Decreased in iron deficiency and increased in ACD

TABLE 5-6
Causes of Aplastic Anemia

Classification	Examples/Discussion
Idiopathic	Approximately 50–70% of cases are idiopathic One fourth of cases are in individuals <20 years of age One third of cases are in individuals >60 years of age

Drugs	Most common known cause of aplastic anemia
	Dose-related causes are usually reversible
	    Examples: alkylating agents, antimetabolites (e.g., vincristine)
	Idiosyncratic reactions are frequently irreversible.
	    Examples: phenylbutazone, chlorpromazine, chloramphenicol, streptomycin

Chemical agents	Toxic chemicals in industry and agriculture (e.g., benzene, insecticides– DDT, parathion) Chemotherapy agents kill rapidly proliferating cells that are malignant or normal (e.g., vincristine, busulfan)
Infection	May involve all hematopoietic cell lines (pancytopenia) or erythroid cell line alone (pure RBC aplasia) Examples: EBV; CMV; parvovirus B19; non-A, non-B hepatitis
Physical agent	Whole-body ionizing radiation (therapeutic or nuclear accident)
Miscellaneous	Hypersplenism in cirrhosis of the liver Thymoma (may be associated with pure RBC aplasia) Paroxysmal nocturnal hemoglobinuria Fanconi anemia: AR disorder with a defect in DNA repair; marrow hypofunction and multiple congenital anomalies

AR, autosomal recessive; CMV, cytomegalovirus; EBV, Epstein-Barr virus.

Aplastic anemia: most cases idiopathic; drugs most common known cause

C. **Aplastic anemia**
1. Causes (Table 5-6)
2. Pathogenesis
    a. Antigenic alteration of common myeloid stem cell
        • Causes activation of T cells with release of cytokines (TNF, interferon-γ) that suppress stem cell growth and development
    b. Defective or deficient stem cells (acquired or hereditary causes)
3. Clinical findings
    a. Fever
        • Due to infection associated with neutropenia
    b. Bleeding
        • Due to thrombocytopenia
    c. Fatigue
        • Due to anemia
4. Laboratory findings
    a. Pancytopenia
    b. Reticulocytopenia
    c. Hypocellular bone marrow (Fig. 5-19)
5. Treatment
    a. Immunosuppressive therapy
        • Example—antithymocyte globulin and cyclosporine
    b. Bone marrow transplantation
    c. Complete recovery occurs in <10% of cases.

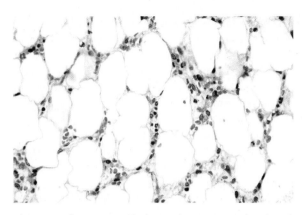

5-19: *Bone marrow biopsy in aplastic anemia. The biopsy shows a marrow largely replaced by adipose cells. Scattered lymphocytes are present in-between adipose cells. (From Kumar V, Fausto N, Abbas A: Robbins and Cotran's Pathologic Basis of Disease, 7th ed. Philadelphia, WB Saunders, 2004, Fig. 13-27B.)*

D. **Chronic renal failure (CRF)**
  1. Pathogenesis
      a. Decreased EPO production
        • Most common cause
      b. Inhibitor of erythropoiesis
        • Removed by dialysis
      c. Decreased RBC survival
        (1) Abnormal pentose phosphate shunt with decreased glutathione
        (2) Reversible defect in Na^+/K^+-ATPase pump
        (3) Unknown extracorpuscular cause
      d. Blood loss, folate deficiency
  2. Laboratory findings
      a. Normocytic normochromic anemia
        • May be microcytic if iron deficiency is present or macrocytic if folate deficiency is present
      b. Reticulocytopenia (corrected reticulocyte count <3%)
      c. Presence of burr cells
        (1) RBCs with a smooth, undulating membrane
        (2) Correlate roughly with the degree of azotemia
      d. Platelet dysfunction
        (1) Thrombocytopenia
        (2) Defects in platelet aggregation that is reversible with dialysis
          • Prolonged bleeding time (see Chapter 7)

Anemia CRF: ↓ EPO most common cause

Burr cells: sign of CRF

VI. **Normocytic Anemias: Corrected Reticulocyte Count or Index ≥3%**
  • Anemias include the hemolytic anemias due to defects within the RBC (intrinsic) or factors outside the RBC (extrinsic). Mechanisms of hemolysis are extravascular (macrophage phagocytosis) or intravascular (destroyed within the vessel).
  A. **Pathogenesis of hemolytic anemias**

1. Intrinsic or extrinsic hemolytic anemias
   a. Intrinsic refers to a defect in the RBC causing the anemia.
      - Examples—membrane defects, abnormal Hb, enzyme deficiency
   b. Extrinsic refers to something outside the RBC causing hemolysis.
      - Examples—stenotic aortic valve, immune destruction
2. Mechanisms of hemolysis
   a. Extravascular hemolysis
      (1) Phagocytosis of RBCs by fixed macrophages
         - Located in the spleen (most common site), liver, and bone marrow
      (2) RBCs phagocytosed:
         (a) Those coated by IgG plus C3b or C3b alone
            - Examples—warm and cold immune hemolytic anemias
         (b) Abnormally shaped RBCs
            - Examples—spherocytes, sickle cells
      (3) Increase in serum unconjugated bilirubin
         - End product of macrophage degradation of Hb
      (4) Increased serum lactate dehydrogenase (LDH)
         - Derives from hemolyzed RBCs
   b. Intravascular hemolysis
      (1) Hemolysis occurs within blood vessels.
      (2) Causes of hemolysis
         (a) Enzyme deficiency
            - Example—deficiency of glucose-6-phosphate dehydrogenase
         (b) Complement destruction
            - Examples—paroxysmal nocturnal hemoglobinuria, IgM-mediated immune hemolysis
         (c) Mechanical damage
            - Example—calcific aortic stenosis producing macroangiopathic hemolytic anemia
      (3) Increased plasma and urine Hb
         - Other breakdown products of free Hb include hemopexin and methemalbumin.
      (4) Hemosiderinuria
         - Renal tubules convert iron in Hb to hemosiderin.
      (5) Decreased serum haptoglobin

> Haptoglobin is an APR that combines with Hb to form a complex that is phagocytosed and degraded by macrophages causing a decrease in serum haptoglobin. The amount of haptoglobin and Hb in the complexes is so small that unconjugated bilirubin from this source is *not* significantly increased.

      (6) Increased serum LDH
         - From hemolyzed RBCs
B. **Hereditary spherocytosis**
   1. Pathogenesis

Extravascular hemolysis: macrophage phagocytosis; unconjugated hyperbilirubinemia

Intravascular hemolysis: ↓ serum haptoglobin, hemoglobinuria, hemosiderinuria

   a. Autosomal dominant disorder
   b. Intrinsic defect with extravascular hemolysis
   c. Membrane protein defect

      (1) Causes reduced membrane stability
         • Macrophages remove pieces of the RBC membrane leading to spherocyte formation
      (2) Mutation in ankyrin
         • Most common defect
      (3) Mutation in band 3, spectrin (α and β), or band 2 account for other defects.

   d. Increased permeability of spherocytes to sodium
      • Due to membrane protein defect and dysfunctional Na^+/K^+-ATPase pump
2. Clinical findings
   a. Jaundice
      • Due to increased unconjugated bilirubin
   b. Increased incidence of calcium bilirubinate gallstones
      • Due to increased concentration of conjugated bilirubin in bile
   c. Splenomegaly
      • Due to "work" hyperplasia of splenic macrophages
   d. Aplastic crisis

      (1) May occur in children especially after a viral infection
      (2) Parvovirus is frequently involved.
         • Infects multipotent myeloid stem cells
3. Laboratory findings
   a. Spherocytosis (Fig. 5-20)
   b. Normocytic anemia with reticulocytosis ≥3%
      • Approximately 25% of patients have no anemia, because RBC hyperplasia in the bone marrow keeps pace with hemolysis (compensated hemolysis).

5-20: *Peripheral blood with spherocytes in hereditary spherocytosis. The arrows show round, dense RBCs without central areas of pallor. The mean corpuscular hemoglobin concentration (MCHC) may be increased in spherocytosis. (From Damjanov I, Linder J: Pathology: A Color Atlas. St. Louis, Mosby, 2000, Fig. 5.7.)*

c. Increased MCHC
- Depends on the number of spherocytes in the peripheral blood

Hereditary spherocytosis:
↑ RBC osmotic fragility

d. Increased RBC osmotic fragility
- Increased permeability to sodium and water renders spherocytes subject to rupture in mildly hypotonic salt solutions.

4. Treatment is splenectomy.
- Spherocytes remain in the peripheral blood.

C. **Hereditary elliptocytosis**
1. Pathogenesis
   a. Autosomal dominant disorder
   b. Defective spectrin and band 4.1
2. Clinical findings
   a. Majority have no anemia (compensated hemolysis)
   - Others have a mild hemolytic anemia
   b. Splenomegaly

Hereditary elliptocytosis:
>25% elliptocytes in
peripheral blood

3. Laboratory findings
   a. Elliptocytes compose >25% of RBCs in peripheral blood (Fig. 5-21).
   b. No anemia to mild normocytic anemia

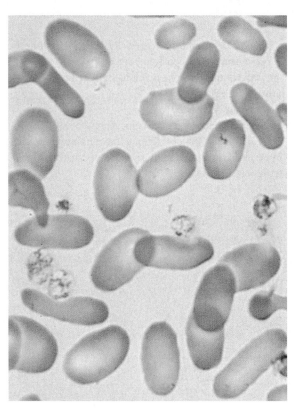

5-21: *Peripheral blood with elliptocytes. In hereditary elliptocytosis, elliptocytes constitute more than 25% of the RBCs, as in this smear. Elliptocytes are also present in iron deficiency anemia. (From Damjanov I, Linder J: Pathology: A Color Atlas. St. Louis, Mosby, 2000, Fig. 5.8A.)*

      c. Mild reticulocytosis

      d. Increased osmotic fragility

   4. Treatment

     • Splenectomy in symptomatic patients

D. **Paroxysmal nocturnal hemoglobinuria (PNH)**

   1. Pathogenesis

      a. Acquired membrane defect in common myeloid stem cells

        (1) Mutation causes loss of anchor for decay accelerating factor (DAF)

        (2) DAF normally neutralizes complement attached to RBCs, neutrophils, and platelets

      b. Intravascular complement destruction of RBCs, neutrophils, and platelets

        (1) Intravascular destruction occurs at night.

        (2) Mild respiratory acidosis causes complement to attach to these cells.

   2. Clinical findings

      a. Episodic hemoglobinuria

        • May cause iron deficiency due to loss of iron in urine

      b. Increased incidence of vessel thrombosis

        (1) Due to release of aggregating agents from destroyed platelets

        (2) Examples—thrombosis of hepatic vein, portal vein, cerebral vessels

      c. Increased risk for acute myelogenous leukemia

   3. Laboratory findings

      a. Screening test is the sucrose hemolysis test (sugar water test).

        • Sucrose enhances complement destruction of RBCs.

      b. Confirmatory test is the acidified serum test (Ham test).

        • Acidified serum activates the alternative pathway causing hemolysis.

      c. New genetic techniques can identify the mutation.

      d. Peripheral blood findings

        (1) Pancytopenia

        (2) Reticulocytosis (5–10%)

        (3) Decreased leukocyte alkaline phosphatase

      e. Decreased serum haptoglobin

      f. Increased serum/urine Hb

        • Hemosiderinuria may occur.

E. **Sickle cell anemia**

   1. Epidemiology

      a. Autosomal recessive disorder

      b. Most common hemoglobinopathy in black population

      c. Heterozygote condition (sickle cell trait, HbAS)

        • Present in 8% to 10% of black population

      d. Homozygous condition (HbSS) produces anemia

      e. Protective against *Plasmodium falciparum* malaria

   2. Pathogenesis

      a. Extravascular hemolysis of sickle cells

        • Minor component of intravascular hemolysis

Margin notes:

PNH: loss of anchor for DAF

PNH: intrinsic defect, intravascular hemolysis

PNH: screen—sucrose hemolysis test; confirm—acidified serum test

Sickle cell anemia: intrinsic defect, extravascular hemolysis

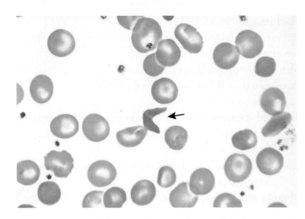

5-22: *Peripheral blood smear with a sickle cell and target cells in sickle cell anemia. The arrow shows a dense, sickle cell. Other cells have a bull's-eye appearance and represent target cells, which are commonly present in hemoglobinopathies. (From Kumar V, Fausto N, Abbas A: Robbins and Cotran's Pathologic Basis of Disease, 7th ed. Philadelphia, WB Saunders, 2004, Fig. 13-9B.)*

b. Missense point mutation
   • Substitution of valine for glutamic acid at sixth position of β-globin chain.
c. Sickling
   (1) HbS molecules aggregate and polymerize into long needle-like fibers.
      • RBCs assume a sickle or boat-like shape (Fig. 5-22).
   (2) Sickle Hb (HbS) > 60% is the most important factor for sickling.

Sickling: ↑ HbS, ↑deoxyHb

> In HbAS, HbS accounts for 40–45% of the total Hb. Therefore, spontaneous sickling does *not* occur in the peripheral blood unless there is severe hypoxemia. However, sickling may occur in the peritubular capillaries in the renal medulla because of reduced O_2 tension.

   (3) Increase in deoxyhemoglobin increases sickling; factors increasing deoxyhemoglobin:
      (a) Acidosis
         • Increases O_2 release from RBCs (right shifts O_2-binding curve)
      (b) Volume depletion
         • Intracellular dehydration increases the concentration of deoxyhemoglobin.
      (c) Decreased O_2 tension
         • Example—hypoxemia
   (4) Inflammation of microvasculature increases sickling.
      • Inflammation causes sluggish blood flow causing decreased O_2 tension.

    d. Reversible and irreversible sickling
      (1) Initial sickling is reversible with oxygenation.
      (2) Repeated bouts of sickling causes irreversible sickling.
        • Due to membrane damage
      (3) Repeated bouts of sickling increases expression of adhesion molecules on sickle cells and normal RBCs.
        • Increases adherence of RBCs to endothelial cells in the microcirculation
      (4) Microvascular occlusions (vaso-occlusive crises) produce ischemic damage.
    e. HbF prevents sickling.
      (1) Increased HbF at birth prevents sickling in HbSS for 5 to 6 months.
      (2) Hydroxyurea increases the synthesis of HbF.

> Sickling: HbF prevents sickling

3. Clinical findings in HbSS
    • Vaso-occlusive crises and severe anemia are primarily responsible for the clinical findings.
    a. Dactylitis
      • Painful swelling of hands and feet in infants (usually 6–9 months old) is due to infarction in the bones.

> Dactylitis: most common presentation in infants

    b. Acute chest syndrome
      (1) Vaso-occlusion of pulmonary capillaries
      (2) Chest pain, lung infiltrates, hypoxemia
      (3) Most common cause of death in adults

> Acute chest syndrome: most common cause of death in adults

    c. Stroke
      • Vaso-occlusion of cerebral vessels
    d. Aseptic necrosis (infarction) of femoral head
    e. Autosplenectomy
      (1) Spleen is enlarged but dysfunctional by 2 years of age.
        • Nuclear remnants (Howell-Jolly bodies) appear in RBCs indicating loss of macrophage function (Fig. 5-23).
      (2) Spleen is fibrosed and diminished in size in young adults.

> Howell-Jolly bodies: sign of splenic dysfunction

    f. Increased susceptibility to infections
      (1) Pathogenesis
        (a) Dysfunctional spleen
          • Functioning spleen is required to remove *Streptococcus pneumoniae* and *Salmonella paratyphi* from the circulation.
        (b) Impaired opsonization of encapsulated bacteria
      (2) Children are at risk for *Streptococcus pneumoniae* sepsis.
        • Most common cause of death in children
      (3) Increased incidence of osteomyelitis due to *Salmonella paratyphi*

> Pathogens: *Streptococcus pneumoniae* sepsis, *Salmonella paratyphi* osteomyelitis

    g. Aplastic crisis
      (1) Erythropoiesis temporally shuts down
      (2) Reticulocytopenia
      (3) Association with parvovirus
    h. Sequestration crisis
      (1) Occurs in children with splenomegaly

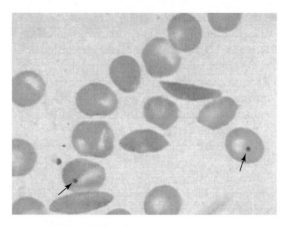

5-23: *Peripheral blood smear with sickle cells and Howell-Jolly bodies in sickle cell anemia. Note the three dense boat-shaped sickle cells and two RBCs (arrows) containing a single dark, round inclusion representing a nuclear remnant. The presence of Howell-Jolly bodies in sickle cell disease indicates splenic dysfunction. (From Henry JB: Clinical Diagnosis and Management by Laboratory Methods, 20th ed. Philadelphia, WB Saunders, 2001, Plate 26-2A.)*

Aplastic vs. sequestration crisis: reticulocytopenia in former, reticulocytosis in latter

    (2) Rapid splenic enlargement with entrapment of RBCs causes hypovolemia.

    (3) Reticulocytosis

  i. Increased risk for calcium bilirubinate gallstones

    (1) Jet black stones

    (2) Due to increased conjugated bilirubin in bile from chronic extravascular hemolysis

4. Clinical findings in HbAS

  a. O₂ tension is low enough to induce sickling in peritubular capillaries in renal medulla

Sickle cell trait: microhematuria; no anemia

  b. Microhematuria may occur

    • Due to infarctions

  c. Potential for renal papillary necrosis

    • Causes a loss of concentration and dilution (see Chapter 4, III)

5. Laboratory findings

  a. Sickle cell screen

    • Sodium metabisulfite reduces O₂ tension, which induces sickling.

  b. Hb electrophoresis

HbAS: HbA 55–60%, HbS 40–45%
HbSS: HbS 90–95%, HbF 5–10%, no HbA

    (1) HbAS: HbA 55–60%, HbS 40–45% (Fig. 5-11E)

    (2) HbSS: HbS 90–95%, HbF 5–10%, no HbA (Fig. 5-11F)

  c. Peripheral blood findings

    (1) Normal peripheral blood in HbAS

    (2) HbSS has sickle cells, target cells, increased RDW.

  d. Prenatal screening

    • Analysis of fetal DNA to detect the point mutation

G6PD deficiency: most common enzyme deficiency causing hemolysis

F. **Glucose-6-phosphate dehydrogenase (G6PD) deficiency**

  • G6PD is the rate-limiting enzyme of the pentose phosphate shunt.

1. Epidemiology

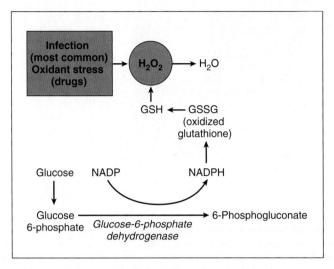

5-24: *Pentose phosphate shunt. The enzyme G6PD catalyzes the irreversible reaction that converts glucose 6-phosphate to 6-phosphogluconate. NADPH is produced in this reaction and reduces oxidized glutathione (GSSG) to glutathione (GSH). GSH neutralizes peroxide and converts it to water. (From Goljan EF: Pathology (Saunders Text and Review Series). Philadelphia, WB Saunders, 1998, Fig. 12-10.)*

     a. X-linked recessive disorder
     b. Common in Greeks, Italians, black population
       • Present in 10% of the black population.
     c. Protective against *Plasmodium falciparum* malaria
  2. Pathophysiology
     a. Intrinsic defect with primarily intravascular hemolysis
       • Mild extravascular hemolytic component
     b. Decrease in G6PD; results in (Fig. 5-24)
       (1) Decreased synthesis of NADPH
       (2) Decreased production of glutathione (GSH)
         • GSH neutralizes hydrogen peroxide, an oxidant product in RBC metabolism.
     c. Decrease in GSH increases oxidant damage by peroxide (Fig. 5-25).
       (1) Peroxide causes clumping of Hb in the RBCs (called Heinz bodies).
         • Heinz bodies in proximity to RBC membranes are removed by splenic macrophages producing bite cells.
       (2) Peroxide damages RBC membranes causing intravascular hemolysis.
     d. Variants of G6PD deficiency
       (1) Half-life of G6PD in the Mediterranean variant is markedly reduced.
         • Produces a very severe, chronic hemolytic anemia
       (2) Half-life of G6PD in the black variant is moderately reduced.
         • Produces an episodic type of hemolytic anemia after exposure to oxidant stresses

G6PD deficiency: intrinsic defect, primarily intravascular hemolysis

G6PD deficiency: oxidant damage with Heinz bodies and bite cells

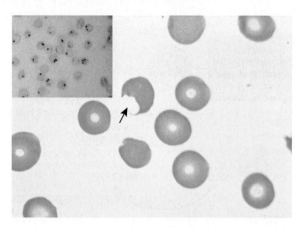

5-25: *Peripheral blood smear with a bite cell and inset showing Heinz bodies in glucose-6-phosphate dehydrogenase deficiency. The arrow shows a bite cell with part of the RBC membrane removed. The inset shows a peripheral blood with a supravital stain visualizing punctate inclusions representing denatured hemoglobin (Heinz bodies). (From Kumar V, Fausto N, Abbas A: Robbins and Cotran's Pathologic Basis of Disease, 7th ed. Philadelphia, WB Saunders, 2004, Fig. 13-8; inset from Wickramasinghe SE, McCullough J: Blood and Bone Marrow Pathology. Philadelphia, Churchill Livingstone, 2003, Fig. 8-8.)*

  e. Oxidant stresses leading to hemolysis
   (1) Infection (most common)

> Decrease in NADPH impairs neutrophils and monocyte killing of bacteria by the O_2-dependent myeloperoxidase system, which requires NADPH as a cofactor for NADPH oxidase.

   (2) Drugs
    • Primaquine, chloroquine, dapsone, sulfonamides
   (3) Fava beans (mainly in Mediterranean variant)
 3. Clinical findings
  a. Sudden onset of back pain with hemoglobinuria
   • Occurs 2 to 3 days after oxidant stress
  b. Jaundice is *not* prominent.
 4. Laboratory findings
  a. Normocytic anemia with reticulocytosis
  b. Heinz body preparation
   (1) Supravital stain identifies Heinz bodies.
   (2) Best screen *during* active hemolysis
  c. RBC enzyme analysis
   • Confirmatory test *after* hemolysis has subsided
  d. Peripheral blood findings
   • Bite cells (macrophage removal of membrane)
 G. **Pyruvate kinase (PK) deficiency**
  1. Epidemiology
   a. Autosomal recessive disease
   b. Most common enzyme deficiency in Embden-Meyerhof pathway

G6PD deficiency: active hemolysis screen with Heinz body prep

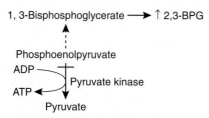

1, 3-Bisphosphoglycerate $\longrightarrow$ ↑ 2,3-BPG

Phosphoenolpyruvate

ADP

ATP

Pyruvate kinase

Pyruvate

5-26: *Schematic of pyruvate kinase (PK) reaction. PK converts phosphoenolpyruvate to pyruvate, which results in the net production of 2 ATPs. Deficiency of PK results in the loss of ATP and an increase in the synthesis of 2,3-bisphosphoglycerate (BPG), which is proximal to the enzyme block. An increase in 2,3-BPG right shifts the O_2-binding curve, causing greater release of O_2 to tissue.*

      (1) Pyruvate kinase normally converts phosphoenolpyruvate to pyruvate leading to a net gain of 2 ATP (Fig. 5-26).

      (2) The 2 ATP are the major energy source for a RBC.

  c. Second most common enzyme deficiency causing hemolytic anemia

2. Pathogenesis

  a. Intrinsic defect with extravascular hemolysis

  b. Lack of ATP results in membrane damage

     • Leads to loss of K^+ and dehydration of the RBC (thorny projections)

3. Clinical findings

  a. Hemolytic anemia with jaundice beginning at birth

  b. Increase in 2,3-bisphosphoglycerate (BPG) proximal to enzyme block

      (1) Right shift of the O_2-binding curve

      (2) Causes increased release of O_2 to tissue

        • Beneficial effect that slightly offsets the clinical effects of anemia

  c. Increased incidence of gallstones (calcium bilirubinate)

4. Laboratory findings

  a. Normocytic anemia with reticulocytosis

  b. RBCs with thorny projections (echinocytes; (Fig. 5-27)

  c. RBC enzyme assay is the confirmatory test.

H. **Immune hemolytic anemias**

1. Classification (Table 5-7)

  a. Autoimmune

      (1) Most common type of immune hemolytic anemia

      (2) More common in women than men

        • Systemic lupus erythematosus (SLE) is the most common cause of autoimmune hemolytic anemia (AIHA).

      (3) 70% are warm type (IgG antibodies) and 30% are cold type (IgM antibodies) of AIHA

  b. Drug-induced

     • Second most common type of immune hemolytic anemia

  c. Alloimmune (e.g., hemolytic disease of the newborn)

2. Pathogenesis

  a. Extrinsic hemolytic anemias with extravascular or intravascular hemolysis

  b. IgG- or C3b-mediated hemolysis

PK deficiency: intrinsic defect, extravascular hemolysis

PK deficiency: ↑ 2,3 BPG right-shifts OBC

Immune hemolytic anemia: autoimmune warm type most common cause

Drug-induced: drug adsorption (penicillin), immunocomplex (quinidine), autoantibody (methyldopa)

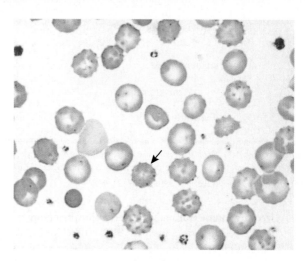

5-27: *Peripheral blood smear in pyruvate kinase deficiency. The arrow shows one of many RBCs with thorny projections extending from the RBC membrane. (From Wickramasinghe SE, McCullough J: Blood and Bone Marrow Pathology. Philadelphia, Churchill Livingstone, 2003, Fig. 8-10.)*

TABLE 5-7
Classification of Immune Hemolytic Anemias

Types	Examples/Discussion
Autoimmune	
Warm antibody type (IgG)	Primary or idiopathic (no underlying cause)
	Secondary
	Systemic lupus erythematosus
	Hodgkin's lymphoma
	Chronic lymphocytic leukemia
Cold antibody type (IgM)	Primary or idiopathic
	Secondary
	Mycoplasma pneumoniae (anti-I antibodies)
	Infectious mononucleosis (anti-i antibodies)
	Chronic lymphocytic leukemia
	Paroxysmal cold hemoglobinuria (IgG *not* IgM antibody)
Drug-induced	Drug adsorption (e.g., penicillin): IgG antibody is directed against the drug attached to the RBC; type II hypersensitivity reaction
	Immunocomplex (e.g., quinidine): drug-IgM immunocomplex deposits on the RBC causing intravascular hemolysis; type III hypersensitivity reaction
	Autoantibody induction (e.g., α-methyldopa): drug alters Rh antigens causing synthesis of autoantibodies against Rh antigens; type II hypersensitivity reaction.
Alloimmune	Hemolytic transfusion reaction (Chapter 8)
	ABO hemolytic disease of newborn (Chapter 8)
	Rh hemolytic disease of newborn (Chapter 8)

(1) Extravascular hemolytic anemia
  - Spherocytes are produced if only small portions of the RBC membrane are removed by macrophages.
(2) IgG coated RBCs
  - Phagocytosed by splenic macrophages
(3) C3b coated RBCs
  - Phagocytosed by liver macrophages
(4) IgG- and C3b-coated RBCs
  - Phagocytosed by both liver and splenic macrophages
c. IgM-mediated hemolysis
  (1) Incomplete activation of complement system
    (a) RBCs coated by C3b
    (b) Extravascular hemolysis by liver macrophages
  (2) Complete activation of complement system
    (a) RBCs coated by terminal complement components
    (b) Intravascular hemolysis

> IgG mediated: extravascular hemolysis; spherocytosis

> IgM mediated: intravascular or extravascular hemolysis

3. Clinical findings
  a. Jaundice
    - Unconjugated hyperbilirubinemia due to extravascular hemolysis
  b. Hepatosplenomegaly
    - Work hyperplasia of splenic and liver macrophages plus sequestration
  c. Raynaud's phenomenon
    (1) Agglutination of RBCs in digital vessels
    (2) Digits turn white then blue and then red with rewarming
    (3) May occur in cold-types of AIHA
  d. Paroxysmal cold hemoglobinuria (PCH)
    (1) Acquired disease
      - Idiopathic or associated with syphilis
    (2) IgG cold antibody with bithermal activity
      - Donath-Landsteiner antibody
      (a) Antibody is directed against the P blood group antigen
      (b) At cold temperatures
        - Binds to RBCs and fixes complement
      (c) At 37°C
        - Detaches from RBCs and activates complement causing intravascular hemolysis
    (3) Hemolytic anemia occurs when moving from a cold to warm environment.

> PCH: IgG cold antibody with bithermal activity; intravascular hemolysis

4. Laboratory findings
  a. Positive direct antihuman globulin test (DAT; Coombs' test)
    (1) Majority have a positive DAT (Fig. 5-28A).
    (2) DAT detects RBCs sensitized with IgG and/or C3b.
  b. Positive indirect antihuman globulin test (indirect Coombs' test; Fig. 5-28B)
    - Detects antibodies in the serum (e.g., anti-D antibodies)
  c. Unconjugated hyperbilirubinemia
    - Extravascular hemolysis

> DAT: most important marker of immune hemolytic anemia

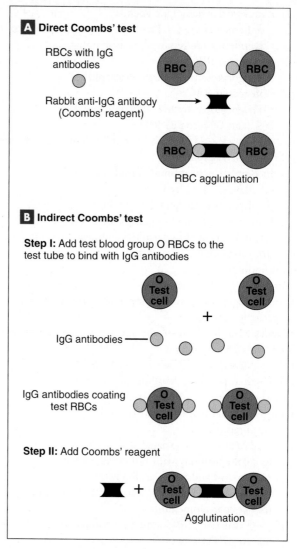

5-28: *Schematic of the direct Coombs' test (**A**) and indirect Coombs' test (**B**). In the direct Coombs' test, RBCs sensitized with IgG (or C3b) are agglutinated when Coombs' reagent (rabbit anti-IgG antibody) is added to the test tube. In the indirect Coombs' test, IgG antibodies in the serum must first bind to O test RBCs added to the test tube. Addition of Coombs' reagent causes the sensitized O test RBCs to agglutinate indicating that IgG antibodies are present in the serum. The specificity of the antibodies (e.g., anti-D IgG antibodies) is determined by other tests performed in the blood bank. (From Goljan EF: Pathology [Saunders Text and Review Series]. Philadelphia, WB Saunders, 1998, Fig. 12-11, p. 289.)*

    d. Hemoglobinuria and decreased serum haptoglobin
- Intravascular hemolysis

    e. Peripheral blood findings
      (1) Normocytic anemia with reticulocytosis
- Polychromasia and nucleated RBCs may be present in severe hemolytic anemias.

Table 5-8
Causes of
Microangiopathic
and
Macroangiopathic
Hemolytic Anemia

Types	Examples
Microangiopathic	
Platelet thrombi	Hemolytic uremic syndrome (Chapter 7)
	Thrombotic thrombocytopenic purpura (Chapter 7)
Fibrin thrombi	Disseminated intravascular coagulation (Chapter 7)
	HELLP syndrome: H, hemolytic anemia; EL, elevated transaminases; LP, low platelets; associated with preeclampsia
Miscellaneous	Long-distance running (march hemoglobinuria)
Macroangiopathic	Aortic stenosis (most common cause of MHA)
	Prosthetic heart valves

    (2) Spherocytosis
- Due to macrophage removal of RBC membrane

  5. Treatment
    a. Varies with the type of immune hemolytic anemia
    b. Treatment modalities
- Glucocorticoids, splenectomy, and immunosuppressive therapy

> Intravenous gamma globulin may be necessary in emergency situations. IgG binds to all the Fc receptor sites on macrophages thereby preventing them from phagocytosing the sensitized RBCs.

I. **Micro- and macroangiopathic hemolytic anemias**
  1. Causes (Table 5-8)
  2. Pathogenesis
    a. Extrinsic hemolytic anemia with intravascular hemolysis
    b. Microangiopathic (MIHA)
- Hemolytic process caused by microcirculatory lesions that cause RBC fragmentation (schistocytes; Fig. 5-29)

    c. Macroangiopathic (MAHA)
- Hemolytic process caused by valvular defects (e.g., aortic stenosis)

  3. Laboratory findings
    a. Normocytic anemia with reticulocytosis
    b. Hemoglobinuria and hemosiderinuria
    c. Long-standing hemoglobinuria causes iron deficiency anemia.
- Microcytic indices, decreased serum ferritin, less increase in reticulocytes, thrombocytosis

    d. Decreased serum haptoglobin
    e. Peripheral blood findings
- Schistocytes

J. **Malaria**
  1. Epidemiology
- Female *Anopheles* mosquito transmits *Plasmodium* to humans

  2. Pathogenesis
    a. Extrinsic hemolytic anemia with predominantly intravascular hemolysis
- Minor component of extravascular hemolysis

MAHA: aortic stenosis most common cause

Schistocytes: sign of MHIA and MAHA

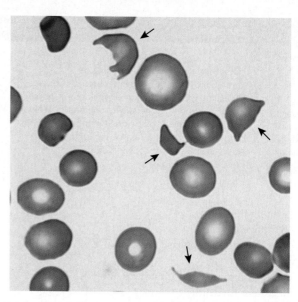

5-29: *Peripheral blood smear with schistocytes in microangiopathic anemia. The arrows show fragmented RBCs (schistocytes) with absence of central pallor. They are produced when they encounter calcium deposits in a stenotic aortic valve, or fibrin thrombi in the microvasculature. (From Kumar V, Fausto N, Abbas A: Robbins and Cotran's Pathologic Basis of Disease, 7th ed. Philadelphia, WB Saunders, 2004, Fig. 13-17.)*

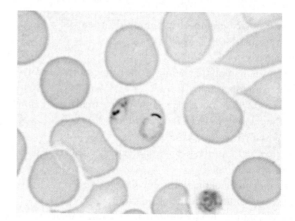

5-30: *Peripheral blood smear showing Plasmodium falciparum ring forms in an RBC. Note the RBC with two ring forms in the cytoplasm. Multiple infestation of an RBC is characteristic of falciparum malaria. (From Hoffbrand AV: Color Atlas: Clinical Hematology, 3rd ed. St. Louis, Mosby, 2000, Fig. 18.4C.)*

Malaria: intravascular hemolysis correlates with fever spikes

  b. Intraerythrocytic parasite causes intravascular hemolysis.
    • Hemolysis correlates with fever spikes.
  3. Clinical findings
    a. Fever and splenomegaly
    b. *Plasmodium vivax*
      (1) Most common type
      (2) Tertian fever pattern (q 48 hours)

Table 5-9
Summary of Normocytic Anemias

Anemia	Pathogenesis of Anemia	Discussion
Reticulocytosis <3%		
Acute blood loss	Loss of whole blood	Initial Hb and Hct normal
		Signs of volume depletion
Early iron deficiency	Decreased iron stores	Normocytic *before* microcytic
		Iron studies abnormal
Early ACD	Hepcidin traps iron in macrophages	Normocytic before microcytic
		Iron studies abnormal
Aplastic anemia	Suppression common myeloid stem cells	Pancytopenia
		Hypocellular marrow
Chronic renal failure	Deficiency of EPO + inhibitors of	Presence of burr cells
	erythropoiesis	Treat with recombinant EPO
Reticulocytosis ≥3%		
Hereditary spherocytosis	AD disorder	Increased osmotic fragility
	Defect in ankyrin	Rx with splenectomy
	Extravascular hemolysis	
Hereditary elliptocytosis	AD disorder	Elliptocytes >25%
	Defect spectrin and band 4.1	
	Extravascular hemolysis	
Paroxysmal nocturnal	Loss of anchor for DAF in myeloid stem cell.	Pancytopenia
hemoglobinuria	Complement destruction of hematopoietic	Positive sugar water test (screen) and
	cells.	acidified serum test (confirmatory test)
	Intravascular hemolysis	
Sickle cell anemia	AR disorder	HbAS: HbA 55–60%; HbS 40-45%
	Valine substitution for glutamic acid	(no anemia)
	β-globin chain	HbSS: HbS 90–95%; HbF 5-10%;
	Extravascular hemolysis	no HbA
G6PD deficiency	XR disorder	Heinz body preparation: screen during
	Deficiency GSH with oxidant damage	active hemolysis
	Intravascular hemolysis	Enzyme assay: confirmatory test when
		hemolysis subsides
Pyruvate kinase deficiency	AR disease	↑ 2,3-BPG right-shifts OBC
	↓ Synthesis of ATP	Dehydrated RBCs with thorny
	Extravascular hemolysis	projections (echinocytes)
Warm AIHA	IgG with or without C3b	Positive direct Coombs'
	Extravascular hemolysis	SLE most common cause
Cold AIHA	IgM with C3b	Positive direct Coombs'
	Extravascular hemolysis	Association with *Mycoplasma*
	Intravascular hemolysis (C5–C9)	*pneumoniae*; EBV; CLL
Drug-induced immune	Drug hapten: penicillin	Positive direct Coombs'
hemolytic anemia	Extravascular hemolysis	
	Immunocomplex: quinidine	
	Intravascular hemolysis	
	Autoantibody: methyldopa	
	Extravascular hemolysis	
Alloimmune hemolytic	Antibodies against foreign RBC antigens	Hemolytic transfusion reaction
anemia	Extravascular hemolysis	ABO and Rh HDN
Paroxysmal cold	Idiopathic or syphilis	Hemolysis occurs when moving from cold
hemoglobinuria	Bithermal IgG antibody	to warm temperature
	Intravascular hemolysis	
Micro-, macroangiopathic	Mechanical destruction of RBCs with	Calcific aortic stenosis most common cause
hemolytic anemia	formation of schistocytes	Chronic hemoglobinuria causes iron
	Intravascular hemolysis	deficiency
Malaria	Transmitted by female *Anopheles* mosquito	Rupture of RBCs corresponds with fever
	Intravascular hemolysis	

AD, autosomal dominant; AR, autosomal recessive; BPG, bisphosphoglycerate; CLL, chronic lymphocytic leukemia; DAF, decay accelerating factor; EBV, Epstein-Barr virus; EPO, erythropoietin; GSH, glutathione; HbAS, sickle cell trait; HbSS, sickle cell disease; OBC, oxygen-binding curve; Rx, treatment; SLE, systemic lupus erythematosus; XR, sex-linked recessive.

      c. *Plasmodium falciparum*
        (1) Most lethal type
        (2) Quotidian fever pattern (daily spikes with no pattern)
      d. *Plasmodium malariae*
        (1) Association with nephrotic syndrome
        (2) Quartan fever pattern (q 72 hours)
   4. Laboratory findings
     a. Thin and thick smears identify organisms in RBCs.
     b. Falciparum malaria has only ring forms (Fig. 5-30) and gametocytes (banana-shaped).
K. **Summary table of normocytic anemias** (Table 5-9)

Questions

To answer questions 1 through 20, see the following list:

A. Alcohol-induced sideroblastic anemia
B. Anemia of chronic disease
C. Anemia chronic renal failure
D. Aplastic anemia
E. Autoimmune hemolytic anemia-cold
F. Autoimmune hemolytic anemia-warm
G. Drug-induced hemolytic anemia
H. Folate deficiency
I. Glucose-6-phosphate dehydrogenase deficiency
J. Hereditary spherocytosis
K. Iron deficiency

L. Lead poisoning
M. Macroangiopathic hemolytic anemia
N. Nonmegaloblastic macrocytosis
O. Paroxysmal cold hemoglobinuria
P. Paroxysmal nocturnal hemoglobinuria
Q. Pyridoxine deficiency
R. Pyruvate kinase deficiency
S. Sickle cell anemia
T. α-Thalassemia
U. β-Thalassemia
V. Vitamin B_{12} deficiency

For each patient described in questions 1 through 20, select the most likely type of anemia that is present.

1. A 68-year-old woman complains of fatigue and chronic diarrhea. Physical examination reveals a beefy red tongue with fissuring along the lateral edges. Vibratory sensation is absent in both lower extremities and there is loss of balance when standing up with her eyes closed that is corrected when the eyes are open. A CBC shows pancytopenia and an MCV of 125 μm^3.

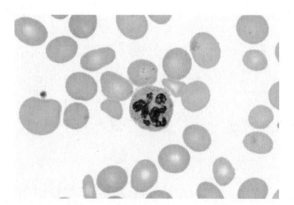

5-31: Refer to question 1. (From Hoffbrand AV: Color Atlas: Clinical Hematology, 3rd ed. St. Louis, Mosby, 2000, Fig. 3.15A.)

Figure 5-31 shows the peripheral blood smear. Laboratory studies show a marked increase in serum gastrin and lactate dehydrogenase.

2. A 40-year-old black American medical missionary who recently returned from Africa is diagnosed with leprosy. After 3 days of therapy, he develops fever, low back pain, and pink urine. A CBC reveals the following: Hb 8 g/dL, WBC count 10,000/mm³, and a platelet count 350,000/mm³. A corrected reticulocyte count is increased. Direct and indirect Coombs' test results are negative. Figure 5-32 shows a representative portion of the peripheral blood smear. A supravital stain of the peripheral blood RBCs shows punctate inclusions in the cytoplasm and RBC membrane. There is a positive urine dipstick for blood; however, the urine sediment shows no RBCs.

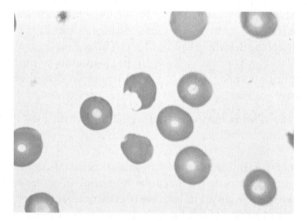

5-32: Refer to question 2. (From Kumar V, Fausto N, Abbas A: Robbins and Cotran's Pathologic Basis of Disease, 7th ed. Philadelphia, WB Saunders, 2004, Fig. 13-8.)

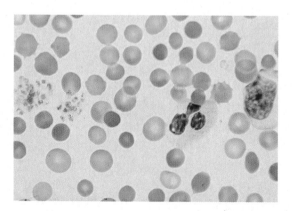

5-33: Refer to question 3. (From Damjanov I, Linder J: Pathology: A Color Atlas. St. Louis, Mosby, 2000, Fig. 5.7.)

3. A 30-year-old man complains of fever and right upper quadrant pain. Physical examination reveals scleral icterus, right upper quadrant tenderness, and splenomegaly. A CBC shows the following: total WBC count 18,000/mm³, Hb 9.5 g/dL, MCV 82 μm³, and MCHC 38%. Figure 5-33 shows the peripheral blood smear. The corrected reticulocyte count is increased. The total bilirubin is 3.0 mg/dL and is entirely composed of unconjugated bilirubin. An ultrasound reveals numerous stones in the gallbladder. At surgery, black gallstones are noted in the gallbladder.

4. A 35-year-old woman who works as a painter in a pottery factor complains of fatigue, abdominal pain, diarrhea, and burning feet and muscle weakness in the upper and lower extremities. The MCV is slightly decreased. Hb is 10.5 g/dL. Figure 5-34 shows the peripheral blood smear.

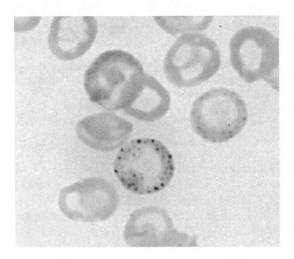

5-34: *Refer to question 4. (From Naeim F: Atlas of Bone Marrow and Blood Pathology. Philadelphia, WB Saunders, 2001, Fig. 2-22M.)*

5. A 35-year-old woman complains of fatigue and chronic diarrhea with greasy stools. Physical examination reveals pale conjunctivae, glossitis, and a normal neurologic exam. A CBC shows a macrocytic anemia with neutropenia and thrombocytopenia. The peripheral blood reveals macro-ovalocytes and a few hypersegmented neutrophils. A stool for occult blood is negative. Serum antigliadin antibodies are present.

6. A 70-year-old man complains of substernal chest pain with exertion that is relieved by resting. Physical examination reveals pale conjunctivae and a harsh grade IV systolic ejection murmur with radiation into the carotid arteries. A CBC shows the following: MCV 80 μm³, Hb 7.0 g/dL, WBC count 5000/mm³, and a platelet count of 500,000/mm³. Figure 5-35 shows the peripheral blood smear. The corrected reticulocyte count is increased. There is a positive urine

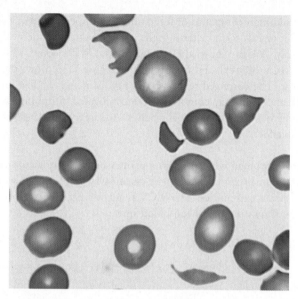

5-35: *Refer to question 6. (From Kumar V, Fausto N, Abbas A: Robbins and Cotran's Pathologic Basis of Disease, 7th ed. Philadelphia, WB Saunders, 2004, Fig. 13-17.)*

dipstick for blood; however, RBCs are not present in the sediment. Serum haptoglobin levels are 0.

7. A 24-year-old black American female complains of exercise intolerance. She has a long history of dysfunctional uterine bleeding. The fecal occult blood test is negative. A CBC shows the following: Hb 8.5 g/dL, WBC count 4500/mm³, platelet count 350,000/mm³, MCV 75 μm³, MCHC 28% Hb/cell, and an RDW of 20% (13.2 ± 1.6). Figure 5-36 shows the peripheral blood smear.

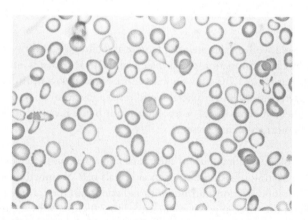

5-36: *Refer to question 7. (From Wickramasinghe SE, McCullough J: Blood and Bone Marrow Pathology. Philadelphia, Churchill Livingstone, 2003, Fig. 11.6.)*

8. A pregnant 21-year-old black American woman has anemia. Physical examination is normal. The CBC shows the following: Hb 8.0 g/dL, RBC count 6.0 million/mm^3, WBC count 4700/mm^3, platelet count 300,000/mm^3, and an MCV of 71 μm^3. Serum ferritin and Hb electrophoresis are both normal.

9. A 50-year-old man with diastolic hypertension develops fever, jaundice, and a hemolytic anemia. The hematocrit is 20% and the uncorrected reticulocyte count is 18%. Spherocytes and polychromasia are present in the peripheral smear. The direct Coombs' test is positive. An indirect Coombs' test reveals antibodies with specificity against the Rh antigens.

10. A 38-year-old woman with systemic lupus erythematosus (SLE) complains of fatigue and yellow discoloration of her eyes. Physical examination reveals scleral icterus, splenomegaly, and generalized, painful lymphadenopathy. A CBC shows a Hb of 5 g/dL and an MCV of 95 μm^3. The corrected reticulocyte count is increased and the direct Coombs' test is positive. The total bilirubin is 3.5 mg/dL, all of which is unconjugated bilirubin.

11. A 35-year-old woman complains of exercise intolerance. Pertinent history is that she is currently in her fourth month of prophylactic therapy with isoniazid for a positive PPD skin test. A CBC shows a moderately severe microcytic anemia. There is an increase in serum ferritin. Figure 5-37 shows a bone marrow aspirate stained with Prussian blue.

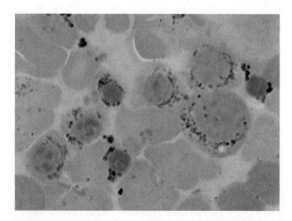

5-37: *Refer to question 11. (From Forbes C, Jackson W: Color Atlas and Text of Clinical Medicine, 2nd ed. St. Louis, Mosby, 2003, Fig. 10.27.)*

12. An asymptomatic 32-year-old man is found to have a mild microcytic anemia. Additional findings include a normal serum ferritin, increase in the RBC count, and a Hb electrophoresis showing a decrease in HbA and an increase in HbA$_2$ and HbF.

13. A 25-year-old man presents with fever, nonproductive cough, and fatigue. Physical examination reveals no signs of consolidation in the lungs; however, a chest x-ray shows an interstitial type of pneumonia. A CBC reveals a Hb of 7 g/dL and a normal MCV, WBC, and platelet count. The peripheral smear shows clumping of RBCs. The corrected reticulocyte count is increased. The direct Coombs' test is positive. An indirect Coombs' test is positive for an antibody with I antigen specificity. A dipstick of urine is positive for blood; however, the urine sediment does not contain RBCs.

14. A 32-year-old man with hereditary spherocytosis develops fever, ulcers in the mouth, and petechial lesions on the trunk and extremities. A CBC shows a severe normocytic anemia with pancytopenia. No reticulocytes are present. Figure 5-38 shows a bone marrow biopsy.

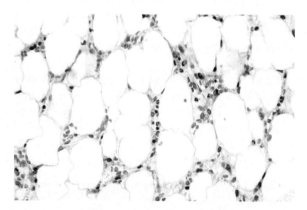

5-38: *Refer to question 14. (From Kumar V, Fausto N, Abbas A: Robbins and Cotran's Pathologic Basis of Disease, 7th ed. Philadelphia, WB Saunders, 2004, Fig. 13-27B.)*

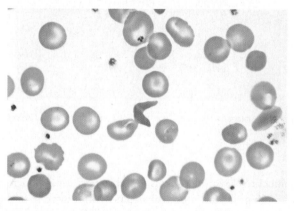

5-39: *Refer to question 15. (From Kumar V, Fausto N, Abbas A: Robbins and Cotran's Pathologic Basis of Disease, 7th ed. Philadelphia, WB Saunders, 2004, Fig. 13-9B.)*

15. A dyspneic 28-year-old black American man presents with fever, nonproductive cough, and chest pain that is exacerbated with inspiration. Physical examination reveals scattered sibilant rhonchi that clear with coughing. A chest x-ray shows patchy areas of consolidation throughout both lung fields. A CBC reveals the following: Hb 7 g/dL, WBC count of 25,000/mm^3, and a platelet count of 550,000/mm^3. Figure 5-39 shows the peripheral blood smear. The corrected reticulocyte count is increased. An arterial Po$_2$ is 40 mm Hg.

16. A 30-year-old man with dyspnea is diagnosed with sarcoidosis. A CBC shows a mild normocytic anemia with hypochromic RBCs. The WBC count and platelet count are normal. The corrected reticulocyte count is 1%. Serum ferritin is increased.

17. A 35-year-old male has a 10-year history of alcohol abuse. Physical examination reveals tender hepatomegaly. A CBC shows macrocytosis without anemia. Round macrocytes, many of which have a target cell appearance, are present in the peripheral blood. No hypersegmented neutrophils are noted. Liver studies show a slight increase in serum aspartate aminotransferase (AST).

18. A 20-year-old man with chronic cholecystitis has a family history of anemia. Physical examination reveals splenomegaly. A CBC shows a normocytic anemia with an increased corrected reticulocyte count. Figure 5-40 shows the peripheral blood smear.

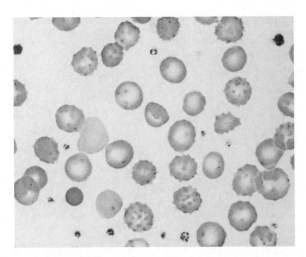

5-40: *Refer to question 18. (From Wickramasinghe SE, McCullough J: Blood and Bone Marrow Pathology. Philadelphia, Churchill Livingstone, 2003, Fig. 8-10.)*

19. A 45-year-old man with secondary syphilis has a normocytic anemia with an increased corrected reticulocyte count. The direct Coombs' test is positive for C3b, but negative for IgG at normal body temperature. The indirect Coombs' test detects an IgG antibody with anti-P specificity.

20. A 38-year-old man complains of fatigue and periodic episodes of red-colored urine during a morning void. Physical examination reveals conjunctival pallor. A CBC shows a pancytopenia with a normal MCV. A dipstick of urine is positive for blood; however, the urine sediment does not contain RBCs. The direct Coombs' test is negative. A sucrose hemolysis test is positive.

21. An asymptomatic 25-year-old black American man who requires a physical examination for health insurance is found to have microscopic hematuria unassociated with RBC casts, dysmorphic RBCs, or proteinuria. The CBC is normal and the urine culture is negative. A renal ultrasound is negative for stones and renal masses. Which of the following tests is most recommended for further evaluation?
A. Cystoscopy
B. Renal biopsy
C. Reticulocyte count
D. Serum ferritin
E. Sickle cell preparation

22. A 48-year-old woman is struck by a car directly in front of an emergency room. Physical examination reveals cold, clammy skin; multiple lacerations and bruises over the upper thighs; and point tenderness over the right and left upper abdomen. The blood pressure and pulse while lying down are 110/72 mm Hg and 124 beats/minute, respectively. The blood pressure drops to 60/40 mm Hg and pulse increases to 150 beats/minute when the patient is raised to a sitting position. Which of the following laboratory findings is most likely present?
A. Decreased Hb
B. Decreased platelet count
C. Increased RDW
D. Normal mean corpuscular volume
E. Normal WBC count

Answers

1. V (vitamin B_{12} deficiency) is correct. The patient has pernicious anemia (PA), which is the most common cause of vitamin B_{12} deficiency. PA is characterized by autoimmune destruction of parietal cells leading to a deficiency of intrinsic factor (required for vitamin B_{12} reabsorption), chronic atrophic gastritis, and achlorhydria. Lack of acid causes a corresponding increase in serum gastrin. Vitamin B_{12} is important in DNA synthesis; therefore, deficiency causes a megaloblastic anemia with delayed nuclear maturation. There is massive ineffective erythropoiesis, granulopoiesis, and thrombopoiesis in the bone marrow with associated apoptosis and macrophage destruction of cells causing pancytopenia and a marked increase in lactate dehydrogenase. Additional hematologic findings include a macrocytic anemia with macro-ovalocytes and hypersegmented neutrophils, which are present in the photograph. Maldigestion leading to diarrhea is common in PA due to lack of gastric acid. Neurologic findings include posterior column disease (decreased vibratory sensation, loss of proprioception) and lateral corticospinal tract disease (spasticity).

2. I (glucose-6-phosphate dehydrogenase deficiency) is correct. G6PD deficiency is an X-linked recessive disease. Owing to the lack of G6PD, there is a corresponding deficiency of glutathione (GSH), which is necessary to neutralize oxidants such as hydrogen peroxide. The hemolytic episode in this patient was precipitated by dapsone, which is a sulfonamide (an oxidizing agent) that is used in the treatment of leprosy. Unneutralized hydrogen peroxide damages Hb causing it to precipitate in the form of Heinz bodies (identified by supravital stains). Peroxide also damages the RBC membrane leading to intravascular hemolysis with hemoglobinuria. Heinz bodies in proximity or attached to the RBC membrane are removed by macrophages producing characteristic bite cells in the peripheral blood (these cells are present in the photograph). A Heinz body preparation is the best initial screening test, because the RBCs lacking G6PD are those that are hemolyzed, and those remaining behind contain the enzyme. Therefore, the enzyme assay is normal during active hemolysis. A RBC enzyme assay to confirm the diagnosis of G6PD deficiency should be obtained when the patient is not actively hemolyzing.

3. J (hereditary spherocytosis) is correct. Hereditary spherocytosis is an autosomal dominant disorder with a deficiency of ankyrin in the RBC membrane. Key findings include an extravascular hemolytic anemia (unconjugated hyperbilirubinemia), splenomegaly, calcium bilirubinate gallstones (black stones), an increase in the MCHC, and the presence of spherocytes without central areas of pallor (present in the photograph). An osmotic fragility test is the screening test of choice. Spherocytes show increased osmotic fragility.

4. **L** (lead poisoning) is correct. The paint used for decorating pottery is often lead-based. Signs of lead poisoning in this patient are a microcytic anemia with coarse basophilic stippling (RBCs with dark inclusions in the photograph), abdominal pain, diarrhea, and peripheral neuropathies (burning feet, muscle weakness). Lead poisoning produces a sideroblastic anemia, because lead denatures key enzymes in heme synthesis within the mitochondria (e.g., ferrochelatase). A bone marrow aspirate to detect ringed sideroblasts (normoblasts with mitochondria containing iron) is unnecessary to confirm the diagnosis, because whole blood lead levels are increased.

5. **H** (folate deficiency) is the correct answer. The patient has celiac sprue (positive anti-gliadin antibodies) complicated by folate deficiency due to involvement of the jejunum where folate is normally reabsorbed. Like vitamin B_{12}, folate is important in DNA synthesis; therefore, deficiency causes a megaloblastic anemia with delayed nuclear maturation. Hematologic findings are similar to vitamin B_{12} deficiency and include pancytopenia, macro-ovalocytes, and hypersegmented neutrophils. Vitamin B_{12} deficiency is excluded by the normal neurologic examination.

6. **M** (macroangiopathic hemolytic anemia) is correct. The patient has intravascular destruction of RBCs due to calcific aortic stenosis (systolic ejection murmur with radiation into the neck). Damage to RBCs whether by a stenotic aortic valve or fibrin/platelet thrombi in the microvasculature (microangiopathic hemolytic anemia) produces fragmented RBCs called schistocytes (present in the photograph). Intravascular hemolysis leads to depletion of haptoglobin, which complexes with free Hb and is removed from the blood by macrophages. Chronic hemoglobinuria may result in iron deficiency, due to loss of iron in Hb. The patient is at the borderline for a microcytic anemia due to iron deficiency, which explains why the corrected reticulocyte count is less than anticipated for a hemolytic anemia. The substernal chest pain in the patient is due to angina related to a combination of anemia and aortic stenosis. In aortic stenosis, there is concentric hypertrophy of the left ventricle. The thick, hypertrophied muscle requires a greater amount of O_2, especially during exercise. Therefore, the decrease in O_2 content related to the anemia and increased demand of the hypertrophied muscle for O_2 leads to angina.

7. **K** (iron deficiency anemia) is correct. The iron deficiency is due to menorrhagia associated with dysfunctional uterine bleeding. Tests that are utilized in the workup of iron deficiency and other iron-related disorders (e.g., anemia of chronic disease) include, serum iron, total iron-binding capacity (TIBC), percent saturation (iron ÷ TIBC × 100), and serum ferritin (most sensitive test). In iron deficiency, serum iron is decreased, TIBC increased, % saturation decreased, and serum ferritin decreased. TIBC is increased, because transferrin synthesis in the liver is inversely related to ferritin iron stores in the bone marrow macrophages. A decrease in serum ferritin leads to an increase in transferrin synthesis, which, in turn, increases the TIBC. The red blood cell distribution width (RDW) determines whether there is significant size variation of the RBCs in the peripheral blood. In iron deficiency, the RDW is increased, because normocytic and microcytic RBCs are present in the peripheral blood. The photograph shows significant size variation and increased central pallor of the RBCs.

8. **T** (α-thalassemia) is correct. α-Thalassemia is an autosomal recessive disease with deletions of one or more of the four genes involved in α-globin chain synthesis. Deletion of one gene is not associated with anemia. A two-gene deletion produces a mild microcytic anemia called α-thalassemia trait (this case). Because HbA (2α, 2β), HbA$_2$ (2α, 2δ), and HbF (2α, 2γ) all require α-globin chains, they are all decreased on a Hb electrophoresis. However, the relative proportions of the normal Hbs remains the same; therefore, the Hb electrophoresis is normal. An increase in the RBC count is a common finding in all the thalassemias and is a useful marker for thalassemia.

9. **G** (drug-induced hemolytic anemia) is correct. The patient has diastolic hypertension that is complicated by a hemolytic anemia (reticulocyte index >3%, see calculation below) most likely due to methyldopa, an antihypertensive drug that alters Rh antigens on the surface of RBCs. IgG autoantibodies develop against the altered Rh antigens, attach to RBCs, and are phagocytosed by splenic macrophages (extravascular hemolysis). Patients develop fever, an unconjugated hyperbilirubinemia, spherocytes in the peripheral blood (membrane removed by macrophages), and polychromasia.

　　Peripheral blood reticulocytes are young RBCs that require 24 hours before they become mature RBCs. Therefore, a reticulocyte count is an excellent test to evaluate effective erythropoiesis, or the bone marrows response to anemia. However, because the reticulocyte count reported as a percentage, it must be corrected for the degree of anemia. The correction is as follows: (patient's hematocrit/45% hematocrit) × percentage reticulocyte count. In this patient, the corrected reticulocyte count is 8% (20/45 × 18% = 8%). If polychromasia is present (blue-tinted reticulocytes requiring 2–3 days to mature), an additional correction must be made to eliminate their contribution to the total reticulocyte count. This is accomplished by dividing the initial corrected reticulocyte count by 2. In this patient, the additional correction is $8/2 = 4.0\%$ (called reticulocyte index). A corrected reticulocyte count $\geq 3\%$ is indicative of a good bone marrow response to anemia, which is an expected finding in hemolytic anemia.

10. **F** (autoimmune hemolytic anemia-warm) is correct. The most common cause of a warm type (IgG-mediated) autoimmune hemolytic anemia is SLE. The RBCs are coated by IgG and C3b causing them to be phagocytosed by splenic and liver macrophages. The end product of heme degradation is unconjugated bilirubin, which explains the presence of unconjugated hyperbilirubinemia. The direct Coombs' test is positive, because the cells are coated by both IgG and C3b.

11. **Q** (pyridoxine deficiency) is correct. The patient has a sideroblastic anemia caused by a deficiency of pyridoxine (vitamin B_6). The most common cause of pyridoxine deficiency is isoniazid therapy for tuberculosis. Sideroblastic anemias are due to defects in heme synthesis in the mitochondria of developing RBC precursors in the bone marrow. Most acquired types of sideroblastic anemia are microcytic. Iron accumulates in the mitochondria producing ringed sideroblasts, which are identified with a Prussian blue stain. The photograph shows a rim of blue staining iron granules around the nucleus of a nucleated RBC precursor. Iron overload occurs, which causes an increase in serum ferritin.

12. **U** (β-thalassemia) is correct. The patient has β-thalassemia minor, which is an autosomal recessive disease with a DNA splicing defect causing a slight decrease in β-globin chain synthesis with subsequent development of a microcytic anemia. A decrease in β-globin chain synthesis decreases the synthesis of HbA (2α, 2β) and increases the synthesis of HbA$_2$ (2α, 2δ), and HbF (2α, 2γ), which do not contain β-globin chains. Because the defect in thalassemia involves globin chain synthesis, serum ferritin is normal.

13. **E** (autoimmune hemolytic anemia-cold) is correct. The patient has *Mycoplasma pneumoniae* atypical pneumonia complicated by a cold (IgM) type of autoimmune hemolytic anemia due to anti-I antibodies. IgM antibodies (cold agglutinins) cause clumping of RBCs in the peripheral blood. The direct Coombs' test is positive, because C3b is coating the cells (IgM falls off the cells at warm temperatures). The patient has an intravascular hemolytic anemia (hemoglobinuria), the latter due to complete activation of the complement system.

14. **D** (aplastic anemia) is correct. The patient has hereditary spherocytosis complicated by an aplastic anemia (pancytopenia) most likely due to parvovirus B19 infecting the common myeloid stem cells in the bone marrow. Aplastic anemia due to a viral infection is usually self-limiting. Ulcerations in the mouth commonly occur with neutropenia and petechiae are due to thrombocytopenia. The photograph shows a hypocellular marrow that is largely replaced by adipose cells.

15. **S** (sickle cell anemia) is correct. The patient has sickle cell disease complicated by the acute chest syndrome. The photograph shows a centrally located sickle cell and occasional target cells. Acute chest syndrome is due to vaso-occlusion of pulmonary capillaries by sickle cells. It presents with fever, lung infiltrates, pleuritic chest pain, and hypoxemia. It is the most common cause of death in adults with sickle cell disease. Neutrophilic leukocytosis is due to the loss of adhesion to endothelium of the marginating neutrophil pool by inhibition of neutrophil adhesion molecules by catecholamines. Thrombocytosis is due to autosplenectomy causing platelets that are normally stored in the spleen to become part of the circulating pool.

16. **B** (anemia of chronic disease) is correct. The patient has sarcoidosis, which is a noninfectious, chronic granulomatous disease that targets the lungs and other organ systems. Chronic inflammation is associated with the release of hepcidin, an acute phase reactant released by the liver. Hepcidin prevents the release of iron from bone marrow macrophages to transferrin leading to an increase in iron stores. Laboratory findings include a decrease in serum iron, total iron-binding capacity, and percent saturation and an increase in serum ferritin. The total iron-binding capacity is decreased, because transferrin synthesis is decreased when ferritin stores are increased.

17. **N** (nonmegaloblastic macrocytosis) is correct. Macrocytosis associated with alcohol may be due to folate deficiency (most common; anemia present), liver disease (no anemia), or a direct toxic effect of alcohol (anemia). In this patient, the macrocytosis is due to liver disease, most likely fatty change. Because alcohol is a mitochondrial toxin, AST located in the mitochondria is preferentially released into the blood over alanine aminotransferase, which is located in the cytosol. The patient has a nonmegaloblastic type of macrocytosis, because there are no hypersegmented neutrophils and the macrocytic cells are round and often show target cell formation. Target cells have an excess of RBC membrane due to an increase in the cholesterol content in the membrane. Folate deficiency produces a megaloblastic type of macrocytic anemia due to diminished DNA synthesis. There is pancytopenia with macroovalocytes and hypersegmented neutrophils.

18. **R** (pyruvate kinase deficiency) is correct. Pyruvate kinase (PK) deficiency is an autosomal recessive hemolytic disease with extravascular hemolysis. PK normally converts phosphoenolpyruvate to pyruvate leading to a net gain of 2 ATP. In PK deficiency, lack of ATP damages the membrane causing a loss of K^+ and dehydration of the RBC (echinocytes with thorny projections, which are present in the photograph). In homozygous variants, hemolytic anemia with jaundice begins at birth. There is an increase in 2,3-bisphosphoglycerate (BPG) proximal to the enzyme block, which right shifts the O_2-binding curve causing increased release of O_2 to tissue. This somewhat offsets the deleterious effects of the anemia. Chronic extravascular hemolysis increases the risk for developing calcium bilirubinate stones leading to cholecystitis. An RBC enzyme assay is the confirmatory test for the anemia.

19. **O** (paroxysmal cold hemoglobinuria) is correct. Paroxysmal cold hemoglobinuria (PCH) is an acquired disease that is most commonly idiopathic. Syphilis is the most common known cause of the disease. The cold-reacting antibody is unusual in that it is an IgG (*not* IgM) antibody with anti-P specificity. The antibody also has bithermal activity. At cold temperatures, it binds to RBCs and fixes complement. However, in a warm environment, the antibody detaches from RBCs and activates complement causing intravascular hemolysis. The direct Coombs' test is positive for only C3b when the test tube is warmed to body temperature. However, when the test tube is refrigerated, the direct Coombs' is positive for IgG and C3b.

20. **P** (paroxysmal nocturnal hemoglobinuria, PNH) is correct. PNH is an acquired membrane defect involving common myeloid stem cells. A gene mutation causes loss of the anchor for decay accelerating factor (DAF), which normally neutralizes complement attached to RBCs, neutrophils, and platelets at night. Loss of DAF causes intravascular complement destruction of RBCs, neutrophils, and platelets leading to pancytopenia and hemoglobinuria. There is an increased incidence of vessel thrombosis due to release of aggregating agents from destroyed platelets. Chronic loss of Hb in the urine may result in iron deficiency. The screening test for PNH is the sucrose hemolysis test (sugar water test). If this test returns positive, the acidified serum test (Ham test) is used to distinguish PNH from other causes of complement-mediated hemolysis of RBCs.

21. **E** (sickle cell preparation) is correct. The patient most likely has sickle cell trait causing the microhematuria. The low oxygen tension in the renal medulla induces sickling in the microvasculature causing microinfarctions that initially present with microhematuria, but may eventuate in renal papillary necrosis and loss of concentration and dilution.

A (cystoscopy) is incorrect. Cystoscopy may be necessary at a future date if the sickle cell preparation returns negative.

B (renal biopsy) is incorrect. Renal biopsy is an invasive test and is unnecessary at this juncture in the workup. Renal stones and a renal tumor have been excluded, so the only other possible cause of hematuria is glomerulonephritis. However, this is unlikely, because proteinuria, RBC casts, and dysmorphic RBCs, the latter a sign of glomerular origin for hematuria, are not present.

C (reticulocyte count) is incorrect. A reticulocyte count is unnecessary, because the patient does not have anemia.

D (serum ferritin) is incorrect. Serum ferritin is used to evaluate iron-related disorders (e.g., iron deficiency, anemia of chronic disease). Although the serum ferritin is decreased before anemia develops in these disorders, microhematuria is not a feature of these disorders.

22. D (normal mean corpuscular volume) is correct. The patient is volume-depleted owing to the drop in blood pressure and increase in pulse when raised from a supine to sitting position (positive tilt test). Because no external sites of bleeding have been described, the patient most likely has internal bleeding from a ruptured spleen or liver. There is no initial change in Hb concentration and the RBC count when there is a loss of whole blood. However, there is an eventual shift of fluid from the interstitial space into the vascular compartment causing hemodilution and a drop in the above parameters. Hb and the RBC count decrease immediately if 0.9% normal saline is infused. The mean corpuscular volume remains normal during all stages of acute blood loss.

A (decreased Hb) is incorrect. Initially, the Hb (and Hct) is normal when a patient has an acute blood loss.

B (decreased platelet count) is incorrect. The platelet count usually remains normal in acute blood loss.

C (increased RDW) is incorrect. The RDW, which reflects size variation in the RBCs, is normal in acute blood loss.

E (normal WBC count) is incorrect. Neutrophilic leukocytosis is the first hematologic change in acute blood loss. It is due to mobilization of the marginating neutrophil pool by inhibition of the neutrophil adhesion molecules by increased catecholamines.

CHAPTER 6

White Blood Cell Disorders

I. **Neutrophil Kinetics and Function**
  A. **Bone marrow pools**
    1. Stem cell pool
    2. Mitotic pool
      • Myeloblast, promyelocyte, myelocyte
    3. Postmitotic (storage) pool
      • Metamyelocyte, band neutrophil, segmented neutrophil

Circulation pool: circulating and marginating pool; usually equal proportions

  B. **Peripheral blood pools**
    1. Circulating pool
      • Neutrophils counted in a CBC
    2. Marginating pool
      • Neutrophils normally adherent to venular endothelium

  C. **Neutrophil events in acute inflammation**
    1. Primary leukocytes in acute inflammation

Neutrophils: primary leukocytes in acute inflammation

    2. Neutrophil rolling
      a. Activation of selectin adhesion molecules
        • Located on the surface of neutrophils and endothelial cells

Selectins: responsible for "rolling" of neutrophils

      b. Neutrophils loosely bind to selectin receptors on endothelial cells.
        • "Roll" along the endothelium of venules
    3. Neutrophil adhesion
      a. Adhesion molecules firmly bind neutrophils to venular endothelium.
      b. Neutrophil adhesion molecules

β_2-Integrins: neutrophil adhesion molecules

        (1) β_2-Integrins (CD11a/CD18)
        (2) Adhesion molecule activation
          • Mediated by C5a and leukotriene B_4 (LTB_4).
        (3) Chemicals that inhibit activation of adhesion molecules
          (a) Catecholeamines, corticosteroids, lithium
          (b) Increases peripheral blood neutrophil count (neutrophilic leukocytosis)
            • Decreases marginating neutrophil pool
        (4) Endotoxins enhance activation of adhesion molecules.
          (a) Decreases peripheral blood neutrophil count (neutropenia)
          (b) Increases marginating neutrophil pool
      c. Endothelial cell adhesion molecules

       (1) Intercellular adhesion molecule (ICAM) and vascular cell adhesion molecule (VCAM)
- Bind to integrins on the surface of neutrophils

       (2) ICAM and VCAM activation
- Mediated by interleukin 1 (IL-1) and tumor necrosis factor (TNF)

    d. Leukocyte adhesion deficiency (LAD)

       (1) Autosomal recessive disorders

       (2) LAD type 1
- Deficiency of CD11a/CD18.

       (3) LAD type 2
- Deficiency of a selectin

       (4) Clinical findings

         (a) Delayed separation of the umbilical cord (>1 month)
- Neutrophil enzymes are important in cord separation.

         (b) Severe gingivitis, poor wound healing, peripheral blood neutrophilic leukocytosis

> Delayed separation umbilical cord: selectin or CD11a/CD18 deficiency

5. Transmigration (diapedesis)

    a. Neutrophils dissolve venular basement membrane and enter interstitial tissue.

    b. Interstitial fluid is rich in proteins and cells.
- Fluid is called an exudate.

    c. Functions of exudate

       (1) Dilute bacterial toxins

       (2) Provides opsonins, antibodies, and complement

6. Chemotaxis

    a. Neutrophils follow chemical gradients that lead to the infection site.

    b. Chemotactic mediators bind to neutrophil receptors.
- Mediators include C5a, LTB_4, bacterial products, and IL-8.

    c. Binding causes the release of calcium.
- Increases neutrophil motility

> Chemotaxis: directed migration of neutrophils

> Job syndrome is an autosomal recessive disorder of neutrophils, characterized by abnormal chemotaxis leading to "cold" soft tissue abscesses due to *Staphylococcus aureus*. Patients have red hair, a leonine face, chronic eczema, and increased IgE (hyperimmune E syndrome).

7. Phagocytosis

    a. Multistep process:

       (1) Opsonization

       (2) Ingestion

       (3) Killing

    b. Opsonization

       (1) Opsonins attach to bacteria
- Examples—IgG, C3b

       (2) Neutrophils have membrane receptors for IgG and C3b.
- Monocytes and macrophages also have these receptors.

> Opsonins: IgG and C3b

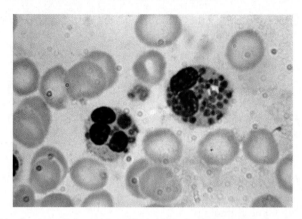

6-1: *Peripheral blood segmented neutrophils in Chédiak-Higashi syndrome. Both segmented neutrophils show giant azurophilic granules in the cytoplasm. (From Wickramasinghe SE, McCullough J: Blood and Bone Marrow Pathology. Philadelphia, Churchill Livingstone, 2003, Fig. 17.1B.)*

Bruton's agammaglobulinemia: opsonization defect

     (3) Opsonization enhances neutrophil recognition and attachment to bacteria.
     (4) Bruton's agammaglobulinemia
        • Opsonization defect due to a decrease in IgG
  c. Ingestion
     (1) Neutrophils phagocytose and trap bacteria in phagocytic vacuoles.
     (2) Primary lysosomes empty hydrolytic enzymes into phagocytic vacuoles.
        • Produces phagolysosomes

Chédiak-Higashi syndrome: cannot form phagolysosomes; giant azurophilic granules

> Chédiak-Higashi syndrome is a autosomal recessive disorder in which there is a defect in membrane fusion, which prevents phagolysosome formation. Azurophilic granules in the primary lysosomes fuse (forms giant granules in leukocytes; Fig. 6-1). In addition, primary lysosomes cannot fuse with the membrane of phagosomes to produce secondary phagolysosomes. Additional defects in chemotaxis (directed migration), degranulation, and bactericidal activity are also present. Patients are very susceptible to *Staphylococcus aureus* infections.

O$_2$-dependent MPO system: most potent microbicidal system

  d. Bacterial killing
     (1) O$_2$-dependent myeloperoxidase (MPO) system (Fig. 6-2)
        (a) Present only in neutrophils and monocytes (*not* macrophages)
        (b) Production of superoxide free radicals (O$_2^{\bullet}$)
           • NADPH oxidase converts molecular O$_2$ to O$_2^{\bullet}$, which releases energy called the respiratory, or oxidative burst.
        (c) Production of peroxide (H$_2$O$_2$)
           • Superoxide dismutase converts O$_2^{\bullet}$ to H$_2$O$_2$.
        (d) Production of hypochlorous acid (HOCl$^{\bullet}$)

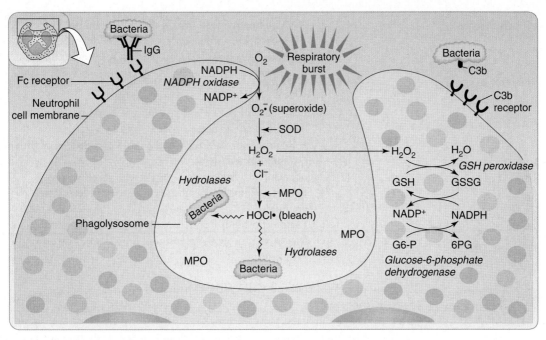

6-2: O_2-dependent myeloperoxidase system. See text for discussion. (From Goljan EF: Rapid Review Pathology, 2nd ed. St. Louis, Mosby, 2007, Fig. 2-3.)

- MPO combines H_2O_2 with chloride (Cl^-) to form hypochlorous free radicals ($HOCl^•$), which kill bacteria.

Chronic granulomatous disease (CGD), an X-linked recessive disorder, is characterized by deficient NADPH oxidase in the cell membranes of neutrophils and monocytes. The reduced production of $O_2^{•-}$ results in an absent respiratory burst. Catalase-positive organisms that produce H_2O_2 (e.g., *Staphylococcus aureus*) are ingested but not killed, because the catalase degrades H_2O_2. Myeloperoxidase is present, but $HOCl^•$ is not synthesized because of the absence of H_2O_2. Catalase-negative organisms (e.g., *Streptococcus* species) are ingested and killed when myeloperoxidase combines H_2O_2 with Cl^- to form $HOCl^•$. The classic screening test for CGD is the nitroblue tetrazolium test (NBT). In this test, leukocytes are incubated with a colorless NBT dye, which is converted to a blue color if the respiratory burst is intact. This test has been replaced by the chemiluminescence test.

Chronic granulomatous disease: absent NADPH oxidase and respiratory burst

MPO deficiency: normal respiratory burst

> Myeloperoxidase (MPO) deficiency, an autosomal recessive disorder, differs from CGD in that both $O_2^{-\bullet}$ and H_2O_2 are produced (normal respiratory burst). However, the absence of MPO prevents synthesis of $HOCl^{\bullet}$.

(e) Deficiency of NADPH (e.g., glucose-6-phosphate dehydrogenase deficiency)
  • Required for NADPH oxidase to work; deficiency produces a microbicidal defect
(2) O_2-independent system
(a) Bacterial killing from substances located in leukocyte granules
(b) Lactoferrin binds iron necessary for bacterial reproduction.
(c) Major basic protein, an eosinophil product, is cytotoxic to helminths.

II. **Qualitative White Blood Cell (WBC) Disorders**
   A. **Pathogenesis**
      1. Defects in leukocyte structure
         • Example—membrane fusion defect in Chédiak-Higashi syndrome (see Section IC)
      2. Defects in leukocyte function (see Section IC)
         a. Leukocyte adhesion defect
            • Example—deficient selectin or CD11a/CD18
         b. Phagocytosis defect
            • Example—decreased IgG (opsonin) in Bruton's agammaglobulinemia
         c. Microbicidal defect
            • Example—deficiency of NADPH oxidase or myeloperoxidase

Qualitative WBC defects: defects in structure and function

   B. **Clinical findings**
      1. Unusual pathogens (e.g., coagulase-negative *Staphylococcus*)
      2. Frequent infections and growth failure in children
      3. Lack of an inflammatory response
         • Example—production of "cold" abscesses (Job syndrome; see Section IC)
      4. Severe gingivitis
         • Example—leukocyte adhesion defect (see Section IC)
   C. **Screening laboratory tests**
      1. Complete blood cell count (CBC)
         a. Rule out structural abnormalities
            • Example—giant azurophilic granules in Chédiak-Higashi syndrome
         b. Rule out shifts in peripheral blood neutrophil pools
            • Example—shift of marginating to circulating pool in leukocyte adhesion defects
      2. Quantitative immunoglobulins
         a. Rule out Job syndrome with increased IgE
         b. Rule out hypogammaglobulinemia with decreased IgG (opsonin)

3. Complement assay
   - Rule out complement deficiency causing opsonization defect (C3b) or chemotaxis defect (C5a)
4. Chemiluminescence
   - Rule out chronic granulomatous disease with absent respiratory burst

III. **Benign Quantitative Leukocyte Disorders**
  A. **Benign leukocyte reactions**
   1. Leukemoid reaction
      a. Absolute leukocyte count usually >50,000/mm^3
         - May involve neutrophils, lymphocytes, or eosinophils
      b. Examples
         (1) Neutrophilic leukemoid reaction
             - Example—perforating appendicitis
         (2) Lymphocytic leukemoid reaction
             - Example—whooping cough
         (3) Eosinophil leukemoid reaction
             - Example—cutaneous larva migrans
      c. Pathogenesis
         - Exaggerated leukocyte response, usually against a microbial pathogen
   2. Leukoerythroblastic reaction
      a. Immature and mature bone marrow cells enter the peripheral blood
      b. Pathogenesis
         (1) Bone marrow infiltrative disease
         (2) Examples—fibrosis, metastatic breast cancer
      c. Peripheral blood findings (Fig. 6-3)
         (1) Myeloblasts, progranulocytes
         (2) Nucleated red blood cells (RBCs)
         (3) Tear drop RBCs, if myelofibrosis is present
  B. **Benign neutrophil disorders**
   1. Neutrophilic leukocytosis
      a. Absolute neutrophil count >7000/mm^3
      b. Pathogenesis
         (1) Increased bone marrow production and release of storage pool neutrophils
             (a) Infection
                 - Examples—acute appendicitis, bacterial lobar pneumonia
             (b) Sterile inflammation with necrosis
                 - Examples—acute myocardial infarction, atherosclerotic stroke
             (c) Acute hemorrhage
                 - First sign of an acute bleed
         (2) Decreased activation of neutrophil adhesion molecules
             (a) Marginating pool becomes part of the circulating neutrophil pool.
             (b) Examples—corticosteroids, catecholamines, lithium
      c. Concept of left shift and toxic granulation

Absolute count = % leukocytes × total WBC count

Leukemoid reaction: benign, exaggerated leukocyte response

Leukoerythroblastic reaction: bone marrow cells in peripheral blood

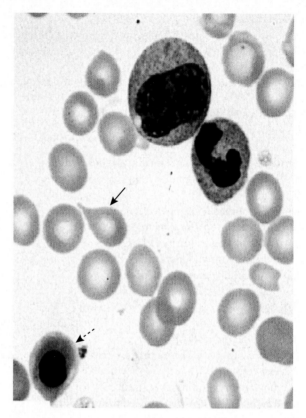

6-3: *Peripheral blood in a patient with myelofibrosis. The solid arrow shows a tear drop RBC. Immature myeloid cells are also present as well a nucleated RBC (broken arrow). (From Naeim F: Atlas of Bone Marrow and Blood Pathology. Philadelphia, WB Saunders, 2001, Fig. 4-10B.)*

      (1) Occurs in acute inflammation (i.e., microbial or sterile)
      (2) Accelerated release of bone marrow storage pool neutrophils (Fig. 6-4)
         • Shift to early neutrophil precursors
         (a) Increased numbers of segmented neutrophils, band neutrophils, and metamyelocytes in peripheral blood
         (b) Defined as >10% band (stab) neutrophils or the presence of earlier precursors (e.g., metamyelocytes)
      (3) Toxic granulation refers to prominence of azurophilic granules.
         • Caused by increased synthesis of lysosomal enzymes
   2. Neutropenia
     a. Absolute neutrophil count < 1500/mm^3
     b. Pathogenesis
       (1) Decreased production
          • Example—aplastic anemia
       (2) Increased destruction
         (a) Paroxysmal nocturnal hemoglobinuria
           • Complement destruction

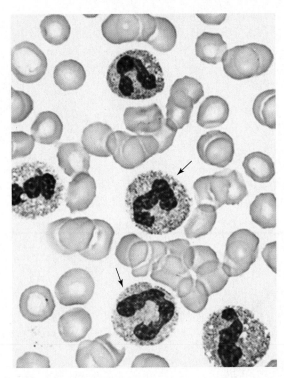

6-4: *Absolute leukocytosis with left shift. Arrows point to band (stab) neutrophils, which exhibit prominence of the azurophilic granules (toxic granulation). Vacuoles in the cytoplasm represent phagolysosomes. (From Hoffbrand AV: Color Atlas: Clinical Hematology, 3rd ed. St. Louis, Mosby, 2000, Fig. 7.11A.)*

      (b) Autoimmune neutropenia
- IgG antibodies directed against neutrophils (e.g., SLE)

      (c) Sequestration in spleen (hypersplenism)
- Splenomegaly in portal hypertension with entrapment of cells in cords of Billroth

    (3) Activation of neutrophil adhesion molecules

      (a) In septic shock, endotoxins activate adhesion molecules.

      (b) Neutrophils shift from the circulating to the marginating pool.

C. **Disorders involving eosinophils** (Fig. 6-5A)

  1. Eosinophilia

    a. Absolute eosinophil count >700/mm^3

    b. Pathogenesis

      (1) Mast cell release of eosinophil chemotactic factor (type I hypersensitivity); examples:

      (a) Bronchial asthma, skin rash due to penicillin, hay fever

      (b) Invasive helminthic infection
- Strongyloidiasis, hookworm

      (2) Increased release of eosinophils from lymph nodes
- Example—Addison's disease with hypocortisolism

  2. Eosinopenia

Eosinophilia: type I hypersensitivity, invasive helminths, hypocortisolism

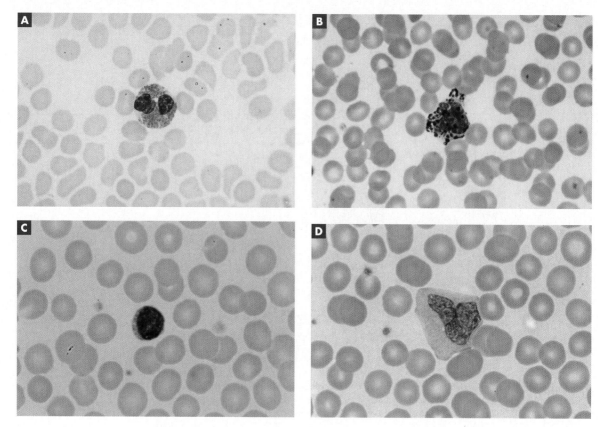

6-5: *Normal morphology of eosinophil (**A**), basophil (**B**), lymphocyte (**C**), and monocyte (**D**). The cytoplasm of an eosinophil (**A**) is packed with reddish orange granules that do not cover the nucleus. Most eosinophils are bilobed or trilobed (this eosinophil). The cytoplasm of a basophil (**B**) is packed with large purplish black granules that cover the usually bilobed nucleus. The cytoplasm of a small lymphocyte (**C**) is scant and surrounds a nucleus that is usually round (sometimes indented) and contains condensed nuclear chromatin. The cytoplasm of a monocyte (**D**) is grayish blue and contains many fine azurophilic granules and one or more clear vacuoles. The nucleus is large, eccentrically located, and either round, kidney- or horseshoe-shaped (monocyte in the picture), or lobulated. The nuclear chromatin is lacy in appearance and is not as condensed as a neutrophil (see Fig. 5-4). (From Wickramasinghe SE, McCullough J: Blood and Bone Marrow Pathology. Philadelphia, Churchill Livingstone, 2003, Fig. 1.1.)*

> a. Example—hypercortisolism
>   • Cushing's syndrome, corticosteroids
> b. Pathogenesis
>   • Corticosteroids sequester eosinophils in lymph nodes.
> D. **Disorders involving basophils; basophilia** (Fig. 6-5B)
>   1. Absolute basophil count > 110/mm^3
>   2. Etiology
>   a. Chronic myeloproliferative disorders
>   b. Examples—polycythemia vera, chronic myelogenous leukemia
> E. **Disorders involving lymphocytes** (Fig. 6-5C)
>   1. Lymphocytosis

Basophilia: consider myeloproliferative disease

a. Absolute lymphocyte count >4000/mm^3 in adults
   • >8000/mm^3 in children
b. Pathogenesis
   (1) Increased production
      • Viral infections—mononucleosis, viral hepatitis
   (2) Decreased entry into lymph nodes
      • Whooping cough (*Bordetella pertussis*)
   (3) Drugs
      • Phenytoin stimulates release of T cells from lymph nodes.

Viral infections: most common cause of lymphocytosis

2. Atypical lymphocytosis
   a. Etiology
   b. Pathogenesis
      (1) Antigenic stimulation of lymphocytes (usually T cells)
      (2) Examples
         (a) Infections—mononucleosis, viral hepatitis, cytomegalovirus, toxoplasmosis
         (b) Drugs—phenytoin
3. Infectious mononucleosis
   a. Caused by Epstein-Barr virus (EBV)
   b. Pathogenesis
      (1) Primarily transmitted by kissing
         • EBV initially replicates in the salivary glands and then disseminates.
      (2) EBV attaches to CD21 receptors on B cells.
         • Causes B-cell proliferation and increased synthesis of antibodies
      (3) Virus remains dormant in B cells
         • Recurrences possible

B cells: CD21 receptor sites for EBV

   c. Clinical findings
      (1) Fatigue, exudative tonsillitis
      (2) Hepatosplenomegaly, generalized lymphadenopathy
         • Danger of splenic rupture in contact sports
      (3) Rash develops if treated with ampicillin.
   d. Laboratory findings
      (1) Atypical lymphocytosis
         (a) Usually >20% of the total WBC count
         (b) Atypical lymphocytes are antigenically stimulated T cells (Fig. 6-6).
      (2) Positive heterophil antibody test
         • Detects IgM antibodies against horse (most common), sheep, and bovine RBCs

Heterophile antibodies: IgM antibodies directed against horse, sheep, bovine RBCs

      (3) Positive antiviral capsid antigen test
         • Most sensitive test
      (4) Increased serum transaminases from hepatitis
         • Jaundice is rare.
4. Lymphopenia
   a. Absolute lymphocyte count < 1500/mm^3 in adults
      • <3000/mm^3 in children

Lymphopenia in HIV: lysis of CD4 helper T cells by the virus

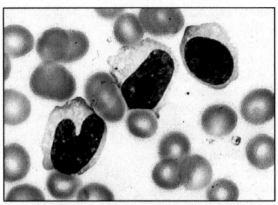
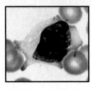
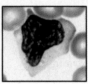
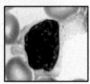

6-6: *Peripheral blood with atypical lymphocytes. The lymphocytes are large and have abundant blue-gray cytoplasm. Nuclei are irregular and have dark chromatin with inconspicuous nucleoli. (From Naeim F: Atlas of Bone Marrow and Blood Pathology. Philadelphia, WB Saunders, 2001, Fig. 13-1.)*

    b. Pathogenesis
       (1) Increased destruction
          (a) Lysis of CD4 helper T cells
             • Example—human immunodeficiency virus
          (b) Apoptosis of lymphocytes
             • Example—corticosteroids
          (c) Immune destruction by IgG antibodies
             • Example—SLE
       (2) Decreased production
          (a) Example—ionizing radiation destroying stem cells
          (b) B and T cell immunodeficiency disorders
             • Example—Bruton's agammaglobulinemia, DiGeorge's syndrome
       (3) Sequestered in lymph nodes
          • Example—corticosteroids
  F. **Disorders involving monocytes; monocytosis** (Fig. 6-5D)
    1. Absolute monocyte count > 800/mm³
    2. Pathogenesis
      a. Response to chronic inflammation or malignancy
      b. Examples
        (1) Chronic inflammation
          • Examples—tuberculosis, Crohn's disease
        (2) Autoimmune disease
          • Example—rheumatoid arthritis
        (3) Malignancy
          • Examples—carcinoma, malignant lymphoma

Corticosteroids produce neutrophilic leukocytosis, eosinopenia, and lymphopenia.

Monocytosis: chronic inflammation, malignancy, autoimmune disease

III. **Acute and Chronic Leukemias**
  A. **Epidemiology**
    1. Malignancy of bone marrow stem cells
       • May involve all cell lines
    2. Risk factors
       a. Chromosomal abnormalities
          • Example—Down syndrome
       b. Ionizing radiation
       c. Chemicals
          • Example—benzene
       d. Alkylating agents
          • Particularly busulfan
    3. Age ranges for common leukemias
       a. Newborn to 14 years old
          • Acute lymphoblastic leukemia (ALL)
       b. 15 to 39 years old
          • Acute myelogenous leukemia (AML)
       c. 40 to 60 years old
          (1) AML (~60% of cases)
          (2) Chronic myelogenous leukemia (~40% of cases)
       d. >60 years old
          • Chronic lymphocytic leukemia (CLL)
  B. **Pathogenesis**
    1. Block in stem cell differentiation
       • Monoclonal proliferation of neoplastic leukocytes behind the block.
    2. Leukemic cells ultimately:
       a. Replace the bone marrow
          • Replace normal hematopoietic cells
       b. Enter the peripheral blood
       c. Metastasize to multiple sites
  C. **Clinical findings in acute leukemia**
    1. Abrupt onset of signs and symptoms
    2. Fever
       • Most often due to infection
    3. Bleeding
       a. Most often due to thrombocytopenia
       b. Qualitative platelet abnormalities
    4. Fatigue
       • Most often due to anemia
    5. Metastatic disease
       a. Hepatosplenomegaly
       b. Generalized lymphadenopathy
       c. Central nervous system (CNS) involvement
          • Very common in ALL
       d. Skin involvement
          • Very common in T cell leukemias

Most common overall leukemia: CLL

      e. Testicular involvement
- Very common in ALL

    6. Bone pain and tenderness
- Due to bone marrow expansion by leukemic cells

    7. Disseminated intravascular coagulation
- Very common in acute promyelocytic leukemia

D. **Laboratory findings in acute leukemia**
1. Peripheral WBC count
   a. <10,000/mm^3 (normal) to >100,000/mm^3
   b. Blast cells and nucleated RBCs
      - Examples—myeloblasts, lymphoblasts, monoblasts
2. Normocytic to macrocytic anemia
   a. Normocytic most often anemia of chronic disease
   b. Macrocytic most often due to folate deficiency
      - Folate stores depleted by increased DNA synthesis
3. Thrombocytopenia
   - Usually <100,000/mm^3
4. Bone marrow findings
   - Hypercellular with >20% blasts

E. **Clinical findings in chronic leukemia**
1. Insidious onset
2. Hepatosplenomegaly
3. Generalized lymphadenopathy

F. **Laboratory findings in chronic leukemia**
1. Peripheral WBC count
   a. Similar to that of acute leukemia
   b. Blast cells
      - Evidence of maturation of cells
2. Normocytic to macrocytic anemia
3. Thrombocytopenia (usually <100,000/mm^3)
   - Exception in CML, in which thrombocytosis occurs in 40% of cases
4. Bone marrow findings
   - Hypercellular with <10% blasts

IV. **Neoplastic Myeloid Disorders**
A. **Overview**
1. Myeloid disorders are neoplastic stem cell disorders.
   - May involve one or more stem cell lines
2. Classification
   a. Chronic myeloproliferative disorders
   b. Myelodysplastic syndrome
   c. Acute myelogenous leukemia

B. **Chronic myeloproliferative disorders**
1. Classification
   a. Polycythemia vera
   b. Chronic myelogenous leukemia

Most important test for diagnosing leukemia: bone marrow examination

Acute versus chronic leukemia: bone marrow aspirate with blast count

Myeloid disorders: neoplastic stem cell disorders

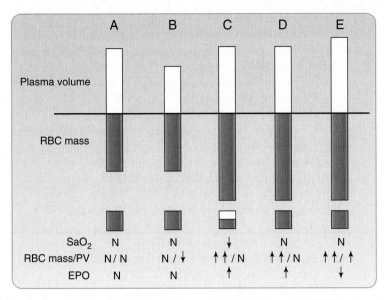

6-7: *Schematic showing RBC count, RBC mass, plasma volume (PV), erythropoietin (EPO) concentration, and O_2 saturation (SaO_2) in polycythemia. Normal (A), relative polycythemia (B), appropriate absolute polycythemia (C), inappropriate absolute polycythemia due to ectopic production of EPO (D), polycythemia vera (E). See text for discussion. N, normal. (From Goljan EF: Rapid Review Pathology, 2nd ed. St. Louis, Mosby, 2007, Fig. 12-3.)*

    c. Myeloid metaplasia with myelofibrosis

    d. Essential thrombocythemia

  2. General characteristics

    a. Splenomegaly

    b. Propensity for reactive bone marrow fibrosis

     • Called the "spent phase"

    c. Propensity for transformation to acute leukemia

  3. Polycythemia characteristics

    a. Increased hemoglobin (Hb), hematocrit (Hct), and RBC count

    b. Plasma volume (PV) varies with the type of polycythemia.

    c. RBC count versus RBC mass (Fig. 6-7A)

     (1) RBC count

      (a) Reported as RBCs (in millions)/mm³ of blood

      (b) Ratio of RBC mass as absolute number to plasma volume (PV)

     (2) RBC mass

      (a) Reported as RBC volume (in mL)/kg

      (b) Absolute number of RBCs in peripheral blood

  4. Nonmyeloproliferative types of polycythemia

    a. Relative polycythemia (Fig. 6-7B)

     (1) Increased RBC count due to a decrease in PV

      • Example—volume depletion from excessive sweating

> RBC count = RBC mass/PV

(2) RBC mass is normal.
- *No* increase in bone marrow production of RBCs

(3) Erythropoietin (EPO) and O_2 saturation (SaO_2) are normal.

Relative polycythemia: ↑ RBC count; ↓ PV; normal RBC mass, SaO_2, EPO

b. Appropriate absolute polycythemia
  (1) Increase in bone marrow production of RBCs
   - Increased RBC count and RBC mass
  (2) Hypoxic stimulus for EPO release (Fig. 6-7C)
   - Examples—primary lung disease, cyanotic congenital heart disease
  (3) Decreased SaO_2
  (4) Increased RBC count, RBC mass, EPO
  (5) Normal PV

Appropriate absolute polycythemia: ↑ RBC mass, EPO; normal PV; ↓ SaO_2

c. Inappropriate absolute polycythemia; ectopic secretion EPO (Fig. 6-7D)
  (1) *No* hypoxic stimulus for EPO release
  (2) Examples—renal cell carcinoma, hepatocellular carcinoma
  (3) Increased RBC count, RBC mass, EPO
  (4) Normal PV and SaO_2

Inappropriate absolute polycythemia (ectopic secretion EPO): ↑ RBC mass, EPO; normal PV, SaO_2

5. Polycythemia vera (Fig. 6-7E)
  a. Pathogenesis
   (1) Clonal expansion of the common myeloid stem cell
   (2) Increased RBCs, granulocytes (neutrophils, eosinophils, basophils), mast cells, platelets
  b. Clinical findings
   (1) Splenomegaly
   (2) Thrombotic events
    (a) Due to hyperviscosity
    (b) Examples—hepatic vein, coronary artery
   (3) Signs of increased histamine
    - Released from mast cells
    (a) Ruddy face
    (b) Pruritus after bathing
    (c) Peptic ulcer disease
     - Histamine stimulates production of gastric acid.
   (4) Gout
    - Increased breakdown of nucleated cells with release of purines (converted to uric acid)
  c. Laboratory findings in polycythemia vera
   (1) Increased RBC mass and PV
    - Only polycythemia with an increase in PV
   (2) Absolute neutrophilic leukocytosis
    - Leukocytes $> 12,000/mm^3$
   (3) Thrombocytosis
    - Platelets $> 400,000/mm^3$
   (4) Decreased EPO
    (a) Increased O_2 content inhibits EPO release
    (b) Only polycythemia with decreased EPO

TABLE 6-1
Laboratory
Findings in
Polycythemias

Polycythemia	RBC Mass	Plasma Volume	SaO$_2$	EPO
Relative polycythemia (e.g., volume depletion)	Normal	↓	Normal	Normal
Appropriate polycythemia (e.g., COPD, cyanotic congenital heart disease)	↑	Normal	↓	↑
Inappropriate polycythemia: ectopic EPO (e.g., renal cell carcinoma)	↑	Normal	Normal	↑
Polycythemia vera	↑	↑	Normal	↓

COPD, chronic obstructive pulmonary disease; EPO, erythropoietin; RBC, red blood cell; SaO$_2$, oxygen saturation.

     (5) Normal SaO$_2$
     (6) Hypercellular bone marrow
       • Fibrosis in later stages
   d. Summary table of polycythemias (Table 6-1)
 6. Chronic myelogenous leukemia (CML)
   a. Epidemiology
     (1) Usually occurs between 40 and 60 years of age
     (2) Risk factors
       • Exposure to ionizing radiation and benzene
   b. Pathogenesis
     (1) Neoplastic clonal expansion of the pluripotential stem cell
       • Capacity to differentiate into a lymphoid or common myeloid stem cell
     (2) t9;22 translocation of *ABL* proto-oncogene
       (a) Proto-oncogene fuses with break cluster region (BCR) on chromosome 22.
       (b) Produces a *BCR-ABL* fusion gene
   c. Clinical findings
     (1) Hepatosplenomegaly and generalized lymphadenopathy
       • Due to metastasis
     (2) Blast crisis
       (a) Usually occurs in ~5 years
       (b) Increase in numbers of myeloblasts or lymphoblasts
       (c) Myeloblasts do *not* contain Auer rods (see IV.D).
   d. Laboratory findings
     (1) Peripheral WBC count 50,000 to 200,000 cells/mm^3 (Fig. 6-8)
       • Myeloid series in all stages of development
     (2) Normocytic to macrocytic anemia
     (3) Platelet count
       (a) Thrombocytosis (40% of cases)
       (b) Thrombocytopenia in the remainder of cases
     (4) Bone marrow findings
       (a) Myeloblasts <10%
       (b) Hypercellular

Polycythemia vera: only polycythemia with ↑ PV and ↓ EPO

Philadelphia chromosome = chromosome 22 with translocation

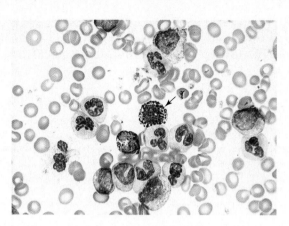

6-8: *Peripheral blood in chronic myelogenous leukemia. Marked leukocytosis shows neutrophils at different stages of development (segmented and band neutrophils, metamyelocytes and myelocytes). The cell in the center (arrow) depicts a basophil with dark granules in the cytosol and overlying the nucleus. Basophilia is prominent in chronic myeloproliferative diseases. (From Damjanov I, Linder J: Pathology: A Color Atlas. St. Louis, Mosby, 2000, Fig. 5.26.)*

 (5) Positive Philadelphia chromosome (95% of cases)

  (a) It is *not* specific for CML.

   • May be positive in ALL

  (b) It is *not* lost during therapy unless α-interferon is used.

 (6) *BCR-ABL* fusion gene (100% of cases)

  • Fusion gene is the most sensitive and specific test for CML.

 (7) Decreased leukocyte alkaline phosphatase (LAP)

  • LAP is absent in neoplastic granulocytes and present in benign granulocytes.

7. Myelofibrosis and myeloid metaplasia

 a. Pathogenesis

  (1) Marrow fibrosis

   • Occurs earlier than in other types of myeloproliferative disease.

  (2) Neoplastic cells are produced in the spleen (primary site) and liver.

   • Extramedullary hematopoiesis (EMH)

 b. Clinical findings

  (1) Massive splenomegaly

   • Portal hypertension with ascites

  (2) Splenic infarcts

  (3) Left-sided pleural effusions

   • Accompanies splenic infarcts

 c. Laboratory findings

  (1) Bone marrow fibrosis due to stimulation of fibroblasts (Fig. 6-9)

  (2) Peripheral WBC count 10,000 to 50,000 cells/mm³

  (3) Normocytic anemia

   (a) Tear drop cells

    • Damaged RBCs released from fibrotic marrow

   (b) Leukoerythroblastic reaction (see Fig. 6-3)

  (4) Platelet count is variable.

BCR-ABL fusion gene: most sensitive and specific test for CML

Myelofibrosis and myeloid metaplasia: EMH; marrow fibrosis

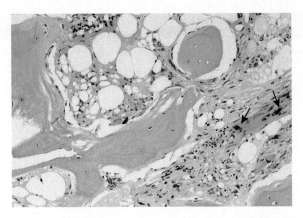

6-9: *Bone marrow biopsy with myelofibrosis. Marrow cells are markedly reduced in number and replaced by fibroblasts and collagen. The large nucleated cells (arrows) are megakaryocytes, which release cytokines that stimulate collagen production. (From Wickramasinghe SE, McCullough J: Blood and Bone Marrow Pathology. Philadelphia, Churchill Livingstone, 2003, Fig. 5.24.)*

8. Essential thrombocythemia
   a. Pathogenesis
      (1) Neoplastic stem cell disorder with proliferation of megakaryocytes
      (2) Platelets are markedly increased.
         • Platelets are dysfunctional.
   b. Clinical findings
      (1) Bleeding
         • Usually gastrointestinal with concomitant iron deficiency
      (2) Splenomegaly
   c. Laboratory findings
      (1) Thrombocytosis
         (a) Platelets > 600,000/mm^3
         (b) Platelet morphology is abnormal.
      (2) Mild neutrophilic leukocytosis
      (3) Hypercellular bone marrow with abnormal megakaryocytes
C. **Myelodysplastic syndrome (MDS)**
   1. Epidemiology
      • Usually occurs in men between 50 and 80 years old
   2. Pathogenesis
      a. Group of neoplastic stem cell disorders
         (1) Chromosomal abnormalities in 50% of cases
         (2) Examples—5q$^-$, trisomy 8
      b. Frequently progresses to AML (30% of cases)
         • "Preleukemia"
   3. Laboratory findings
      a. Severe pancytopenia
         (1) Normocytic to macrocytic anemia
            • Dimorphic RBC population (microcytic and macrocytic)
         (2) Leukoerythroblastic reaction
      b. Bone marrow findings

Essential thrombocythemia: bleeding more common than thrombosis

**TABLE 6-2
French–American–
British
Classification of
Acute
Myelogenous
Leukemia (AML)**

Class	Discussion
M0: Minimally differentiated AML	No Auer rods
M1: AML without differentiation	Rare Auer rods
M2: AML with maturation	Most common type (30–40% of cases) Auer rods present 15- to 59-yr age bracket
M3: Acute promyelocytic	Numerous Auer rods DIC is invariably present t(15;17) translocation Abnormal retinoic acid metabolism: high doses of vitamin A may induce remission by maturing cells
M4: Acute myelomonocytic	Auer rods uncommon
M5: Acute monocytic	No Auer rods Gum infiltration
M6: Acute erythroleukemia	Bizarre, multinucleated erythroblasts Myeloblasts present
M7: Acute megakaryocytic	Myelofibrosis in bone marrow Increased incidence in Down syndrome <3 yr old

DIC, disseminated intravascular coagulation.

(1) Ringed sideroblasts (some cases)
- Nucleated RBCs with excess iron
(2) Myeloblasts <20%
- If >20%, MDS has progressed into AML

D. **Acute myelogenous leukemia (AML)**
1. Epidemiology
a. Usually occurs between 15 and 59 years of age
b. French-American-British (FAB) classification is used (Table 6-2)
2. Cytogenetic abnormalities are common
- Example—t(15;17) in acute promyelocytic leukemia (M3)
3. Clinical findings
a. Disseminated intravascular coagulation (DIC) is common.
- Invariable in acute promyelocytic leukemia
b. Gum infiltration is common in acute monocytic leukemia (M5)
4. Auer rods
a. Splinter-shaped to rod-shaped structures in the cytosol of myeloblasts
- Auer rods are fused azurophilic granules (Fig. 6-10).
b. Only present in acute myelogenous leukemia (M2 and M3)
- They are *not* present in myeloblasts in chronic myelogenous leukemia.

AML: Auer rods in the
cytoplasm of myeloblasts

V. **Lymphoid Leukemias**
A. **Acute lymphoblastic leukemia (ALL)**
1. Epidemiology

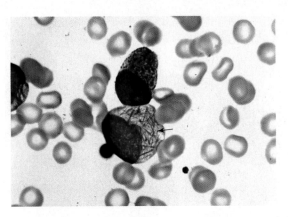

6-10: *Peripheral blood with promyelocyte filled with Auer rods in acute promyelocytic leukemia. The promyelocyte has numerous splinter-shaped inclusions in the cytoplasm (arrow) representing Auer rods. (From Damjanov I, Linder J: Pathology: A Color Atlas. St. Louis, Mosby, 2000, Fig. 5.21.)*

    a. Most common leukemia in children
       (1) Newborn to 14 years of age
       (2) 75% occur between 2 and 6 years of age
    b. Subtypes
       (1) Early pre–B-cell ALL (80% of cases)
       (2) Pre–B-, B-, and T-cell ALL

> Early pre–B-cell ALL: most common acute leukemia in children

2. Pathogenesis
    • Clonal lymphoid stem cell disease
3. Early pre–B-cell ALL
    a. Positive marker studies for common ALL antigen (CALLA, CD10)
    b. Positive marker studies for terminal deoxynucleotidyl transferase (TdT)
    c. t(12;21) translocation
       • Offers a favorable prognosis
    d. Greater than 90% achieve complete remission
       • At least two thirds can be considered cured.

> Early pre—B-cell ALL: CD10 and TdT positive

4. T-cell ALL
    • CD10 negative and TdT positive
5. Clinical findings
    a. Metastatic sites similar to those of AML
    b. B-cell types
       • Commonly metastasize to the CNS and testicles
    c. T-cell type
       • In adolescents/young adults it presents as an anterior mediastinal mass or acute leukemia.
6. Laboratory findings
    a. Peripheral WBC count 10,000 to 100,000/mm^3
       • Numerous lymphoblasts (Fig. 6-11)
    b. Normocytic anemia
    c. Thrombocytopenia

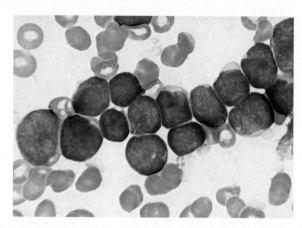

6-11: *Peripheral blood in acute lymphoblastic leukemia. Lymphoblasts show condensed nuclear chromatin, small nucleoli, and scant cytoplasm. (From Kumar V, Fausto N, Abbas A: Robbins and Cotran's Pathologic Basis of Disease, 7th ed. Philadlephia, WB Saunders, 2004, Fig. 14-5A.)*

Adult T-cell leukemia:
association with HTLV-1

     d. Bone marrow findings
- \>20% lymphoblasts

B. **Adult T-cell leukemia**
1. Epidemiology
    a. Associated with human T-cell leukemia virus (HTLV-1)
    b. May present as a malignant lymphoma
2. Pathogenesis
    a. Activation of *TAX* gene
- Inhibits *TP53* suppressor gene
    b. Monoclonal proliferation of CD4 helper T cells
3. Clinical findings
    a. Hepatosplenomegaly
    b. Generalized lymphadenopathy
    c. Skin infiltration
- Common finding in all T-cell malignancies
    d. Lytic bone lesions
      (1) Due to lymphoblast release of osteoclast-activating factor
      (2) Associated with hypercalcemia
4. Laboratory findings
    a. Peripheral WBC count 10,000 to 50,000/mm^3
      (1) Positive CD4 marker study
      (2) Negative for TdT
    b. Normocytic anemia
    c. Thrombocytopenia

C. **Chronic lymphocytic leukemia (CLL)**
1. Epidemiology
    a. Occurs in individuals >60 years old
    b. Most common overall leukemia

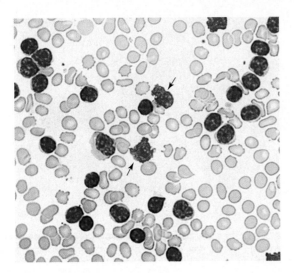

6-12: *Peripheral blood in chronic lymphocytic leukemia. There are an increased number of lymphocytes with dense nuclear chromatin and scant cytoplasmic borders. The lymphocytes are extremely fragile and produce characteristic "smudge" cells (arrows) during preparation of a slide. (From Hoffbrand AV: Color Atlas: Clinical Hematology, 3rd ed. St. Louis, Mosby, 2000, Fig. 10.11, p 179.)*

     c. Most common cause of generalized lymphadenopathy in the same age bracket

  2. Pathogenesis
     a. Neoplastic disorder of virgin B cells
     b. Neoplastic B cells cannot differentiate into plasma cells.

  3. Clinical findings
     a. Generalized lymphadenopathy
     b. Metastatic sites similar to those of AML
     c. Increased incidence of immune hemolytic anemia
       • Both warm (IgG) and cold (IgM) types

  4. Laboratory findings
     a. Peripheral WBC count 15,000 to 200,000/mm^3
       (1) Neutropenia
       (2) Numerous "smudge" cells (fragile leukemic cells) (Fig. 6-12)
     b. Normocytic anemia (50% of cases)
     c. Thrombocytopenia (40% of cases)
     d. Bone marrow findings
       • Lymphoblasts <10%
     e. Hypogammaglobulinemia is common.

D. **Hairy cell leukemia**
  1. B-cell leukemia
     • Most common in middle-aged men
  2. Clinical findings
     a. Splenomegaly (90% of cases)
     b. Absence of lymphadenopathy
       • Only leukemia *without* lymphadenopathy

CLL: most common cause of generalized lymphadenopathy in individuals > 60 years old

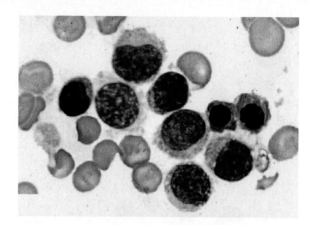

6-13: *Peripheral blood in hairy cell leukemia. Clusters of neoplastic cells show dense chromatin and cytoplasmic projections. (From Naeim F: Atlas of Bone Marrow and Blood Pathology. Philadelphia, WB Saunders, 2001, Fig. 8-20A.)*

TABLE 6-3
Summary of Acute and Chronic Lymphoid Leukemias

Leukemia	Discussion
Acute lymphoblastic (Early pre-B type)	Most common leukemia in children Newborn to 14 yr old CALLA (CD10) and TdT positive t(12;21) offers a good prognosis
Chronic lymphocytic	Virgin B cell leukemia Patients > 60 yr old Most common cause of generalized lymphadenopathy in same age bracket Hypogammaglobulinemia
Adult T cell	HTLV-1 association. Leukemic cells CD4 positive and TdT negative Skin infiltration Lytic bone lesions with hypercalcemia
Hairy cell	B cell leukemia Cytoplasmic projections TRAP stain positive Splenomegaly, absence of lymphadenopathy Pancytopenia Dramatic response to purine nucleosides

CALLA, common acute lymphoblastic leukemia antigen; HTLV, human T cell leukemia; TdT, terminal deoxynucleotidyl transferase; TRAP, tartrate-resistant acid phosphatase.

    c. Hepatomegaly (20% of cases)
    d. Autoimmune vasculitis and arthritis
   3. Laboratory findings
    a. Pancytopenia

Hairy cell leukemia: positive TRAP stain

      • Leukemic cells have hair-like cytoplasmic projections (Fig. 6-13)
    b. Positive tartrate-resistant acid phosphatase stain (TRAP)
 E. **Summary table of the lymphoid leukemias** (Table 6-3)

Questions

Use the following choices to answer questions 1 through 6:

A. Acute lymphoblastic leukemia
B. Acute promyelocytic leukemia (M3)
C. Adult T-cell leukemia
D. Chronic lymphocytic leukemia
E. Chronic myelogenous leukemia (CML)
F. Hairy cell leukemia

For each clinical description, select the type of leukemia that is best described.

1. A 22-year-old man presents with ecchymoses, petechiae, generalized nontender lymphadenopathy, and painful hepatosplenomegaly. A CBC reveals a hemoglobin (Hb) of 7 g/dL, normal mean corpuscular volume (MCV), a total WBC count of 38,000/mm^3, and a platelet count of 35,000/mm^3. Abnormal cells are present in the peripheral blood (see photograph in Fig. 6-14). The prothrombin time and partial thromboplastin time are both prolonged, serum fibrinogen level is decreased, and the D-dimer test is positive.

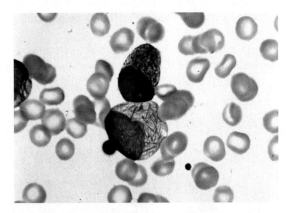

6-14: *Refer to question 1. (From Wickramasinghe SE, McCullough J: Blood and Bone Marrow Pathology. Philadelphia, Churchill Livingstone, 2003, Fig. 11.6.)*

2. A 59-year-old man complains of painful joints, fullness in the right upper quadrant, and a rash. Physical examination reveals palpable purpura and hepatosplenomegaly. There is no evidence of lymphadenopathy. His CBC shows

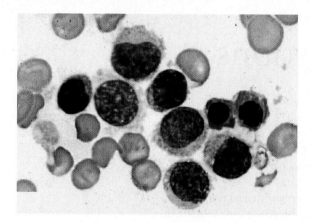

6-15: Refer to question 2. (From Forbes C, Jackson W: Color Atlas and Text of Clinical Medicine, 2nd ed. St. Louis, Mosby, 2003, Fig. 10.27.)

a Hb of 8 g/dL, platelet count of 75,000/mm^3, and a WBC count of 3500/mm^3. Abnormal cells are present in the peripheral blood (see Fig. 6-15). A bone marrow biopsy reveals a monomorphic infiltrate of cells with abundant cytoplasm. The patient is scheduled for a splenectomy.

3. A 38-year-old Japanese man presents with epistaxis, a generalized eczematous type of skin rash, generalized nontender lymphadenopathy, and hepatosplenomegaly. A complete blood count (CBC) reveals a Hb of 7.2 g/dL, a total WBC count of 37,000/mm^3, and a platelet count of 48,000/mm^3. Occasional blast cells are present in the peripheral blood smear and on bone marrow examination. Lytic bone lesions are noted on a routine chest radiograph.

4. A 49-year-old man presents with fever, weight loss, petechiae, generalized nontender lymphadenopathy, and massive hepatosplenomegaly. A CBC exhibits

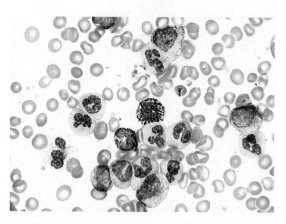

6-16: Refer to question 4. (From Goljan EF: Rapid Review Pathology, 2nd ed. St. Louis, Mosby, 2007, Fig. 11-4.)

a Hb of 7.1 g/dL, MCV of 105 µm³, a WBC count of 110,000/mm³, and a platelet count of 600,000/mm³. Figure 6-16 shows the peripheral blood findings. The leukocyte alkaline phosphatase score is very low. A special chromosome study is pending.

5. A 68-year-old woman presents with fatigue, generalized, nontender lymphadenopathy, hepatosplenomegaly, and scattered petechiae and ecchymoses over the anterior chest. A CBC report shows a Hb of 9.5 g/dL, WBC count of 92,000/mm³, and a platelet count of 73,000/mm³. Figure 6-17 shows the peripheral blood smear. The total serum protein concentration is 4.5 g/dL.

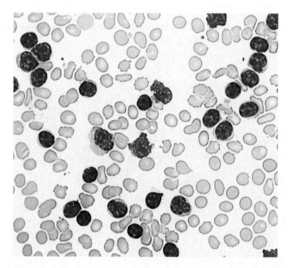

6-17: Refer to question 5. (From Hoffbrand AV: Color Atlas: Clinical Hematology, 3rd ed. St. Louis, Mosby, 2000, Fig. 10.11, p 179.)

6. A 6-year-old boy presents with fever, fatigue, epistaxis, and pain over the sternum. Physical examination reveals generalized, nontender lymphadenopathy, hepatosplenomegaly, sternal tenderness to percussion, and widespread petechiae and ecchymoses. The CBC report indicates shows a Hb of 6 g/dL, WBC count of 46,000/mm³, and a platelet count of 30,000/mm³. Figure 6-18 shows the peripheral blood smear. A bone marrow aspirate reveals sheets of cells similar to those that are present in the peripheral blood. The blast count is >20%.

7. A 3-year-old boy with blond hair has recurrent *Staphylococcus aureus* infections. The CBC shows an absolute neutrophilic leukocytosis. Figure 6-19 shows a leukocyte abnormality in the peripheral blood smear. The chemiluminescence test is normal. What is the pathogenesis of his disorder?
   A. Adhesion molecule defect
   B. Enzyme defect

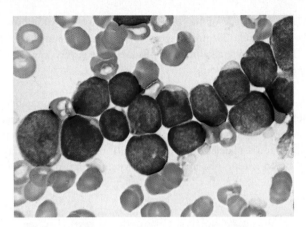

6-18: Refer to question 6. (From Kumar V, Fausto N, Abbas A: Robbins and Cotran's Pathologic Basis of Disease, 7th ed. Philadlephia, WB Saunders, 2004, Fig. 14-5A.)

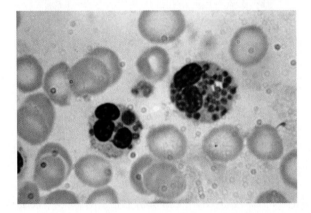

6-19: Refer to question 7. (From Naeim F: Atlas of Bone Marrow and Blood Pathology. Philadelphia, WB Saunders, 2001, Fig. 1-15B.)

    C. Membrane fusion defect
    D. Opsonization defect
    E. Respiratory burst defect

8. A 62-year-old man who is a nonsmoker presents with a sudden onset of bloody diarrhea followed by abdominal pain and vomiting. Over the past few months he has had problems with recurrent headaches, blurry vision, and generalized pruritus after bathing. He had a bout of gouty arthritis involving his right big toe approximately 1 month ago. The blood pressure is 90/72 mm Hg and the pulse is 160 beats/minute. The retinal veins are congested and flame hemorrhages are present. The abdomen is distended and abdominal bowel sounds are absent. Hepatosplenomegaly is present. The CBC shows a Hb of 20 g/dL, WBC count of 25,000/mm³ with left shift and toxic granulation, and a platelet count of 625,000/mm^3. Which of the following groups of laboratory test results are expected?

	RBC Mass	Plasma Volume	SaO$_2$	EPO
A.	Increased	Normal	Normal	Increased
B.	Increased	Normal	Decreased	Increased
C.	Increased	Increased	Normal	Decreased
D.	Normal	Decreased	Normal	Normal

EPO, erythropoietin; Sao$_2$, oxygen saturation.

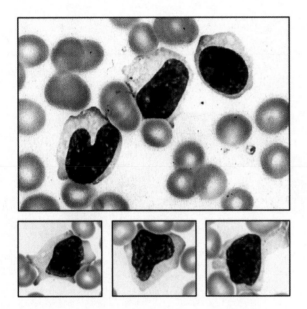

6-20: Refer to question 9. (From Hoffbrand AV: Color Atlas: Clinical Hematology, 3rd ed. St. Louis, Mosby, 2000, Fig. 1.62.)

9. A 20-year-old woman complains of extreme fatigue and a sore throat. Physical examination reveals an exudative tonsillitis and palatal petechiae. There is generalized painful lymphadenopathy and tender hepatosplenomegaly. The hemoglobin and platelet count are normal. Figure 6-20 shows examples of leukocytes that account for greater than 20% of the differential count. Serum transaminases are markedly increased; however, the total bilirubin is normal. Which of the following tests is most indicated?

A. Bone marrow aspirate
B. Heterophile antibody test
C. Lymph node biopsy
D. Marker studies for CALLA antigen
E. Reticulocyte count

Refer to the following illustrations to answer questions 10 through 14:

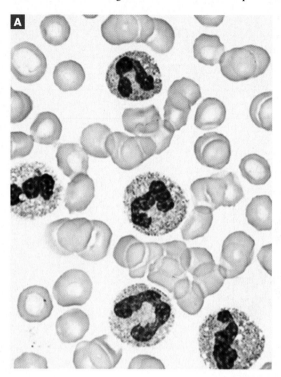

6-21: *Refer to questions 10 through 14. (From Wickramasinghe SE, McCullough J: Blood and Bone Marrow Pathology. Philadelphia, Churchill Livingstone, 2003, Fig. 6.6.)*

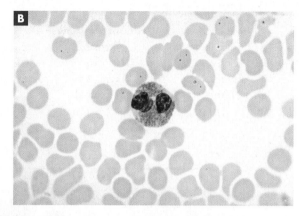

6-22: *Refer to questions 10 through 14. (From Goljan EF: Rapid Review Pathology, 2nd ed. St. Louis, Mosby, 2007, Fig. 11-2A.)*

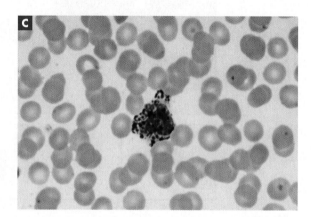

6-23: *Refer to questions 10 through 14. (From Goljan EF: Rapid Review Pathology, 2nd ed. St. Louis, Mosby, 2007, Fig. 11-2B.)*

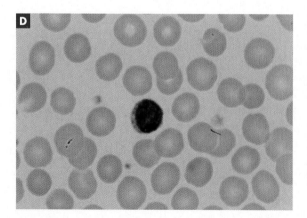

6-24: *Refer to questions 10 through 14. (From Goljan EF: Rapid Review Pathology, 2nd ed. St. Louis, Mosby, 2007, Fig. 11-2C.)*

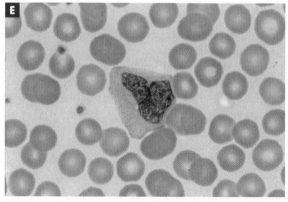

6-25: *Refer to questions 10 through 14. (From Goljan EF: Rapid Review Pathology, 2nd ed. St. Louis, Mosby, 2007, Fig. 11-2D.)*

For each of the clinical scenarios in questions 10 through 14 select the leukocyte in the photographs that is most likely to be increased. Each lettered option may be selected once, more than once, or not at all.

10. A 24-year-old man who raises hogs has a habit of eating raw bacon. He complains of muscle tenderness, particularly in the deltoid muscles.

11. A 56-year-old man with polycythemia vera has flushing of his face.

12. A 45-year-old woman has severe rheumatoid arthritis.

13. A 4-year-old child has whooping cough.

14. A 28-year-old man has a perforated acute appendicitis.

15. A 10-year-old boy has minimal change disease. In addition to generalized edema and ascites, he has a moon-shaped face and truncal obesity with purple stretch marks. Which of the following leukocyte alterations would most likely be present?

	Neutrophil Count	Lymphocyte Count	Eosinophil Count
A.	Decreased	Decreased	Decreased
B.	Decreased	Increased	Increased
C.	Decreased	Increased	Normal
D.	Increased	Decreased	Decreased
E.	Normal	Normal	Increased

Answers

1. **B** (acute promyelocytic leukemia, M3) is correct. The patient most likely has acute progranulocytic leukemia (M3), which is the most common leukemia associated with disseminated intravascular coagulation (DIC). Signs of DIC in this patient include prolonged prothrombin and partial thromboplastin times, decreased fibrinogen, and a positive D-dimer test (i.e., cross-linked dimers indicating fibrinolysis of fibrin clots). The ecchymoses and petechiae in the patient are due to thrombocytopenia partly from replacement of the bone marrow by leukemic cells and partly due to trapping of platelets in fibrin thrombi in DIC. The peripheral blood smear shows a neoplastic promyelocyte containing numerous splinter-shaped Auer rods in the cytoplasm. Acute promyelocytic leukemia is associated with a t(15;17) translocation, which produces an abnormality in retinoic acid in the myeloid series causing the cells to remain blocked at the promyelocyte state. High doses of retinoic acid often induce remission by causing a temporary maturation of the cells.

2. **F** (hairy cell leukemia) is correct. The patient has hairy cell leukemia. The peripheral smear shows lymphocytes with dense chromatin and cytoplasmic projections. His leukemia is complicated by arthritis, palpable purpura (a small vessel vasculitis), and pancytopenia. Lymphadenopathy is absent. Splenomegaly is the most consistent finding. The spleen is the most important site for proliferation of the neoplastic cells, which explains the importance of splenectomy in treatment. The malignant B cells characteristically have a positive tartrate-resistant acid phosphatase (TRAP) stain.

3. **C** (adult T-cell leukemia) is correct. Adult T-cell leukemia is associated with the human T-lymphocyte virus (HTLV)-1. This is a common leukemia in Japan and occurs sporadically in the United States. Lymphoblasts secrete osteoclast-activating factor, which produces lytic bone lesions and the potential for hypercalcemia. T-cell infiltration of the skin is commonly present.

4. **E** (chronic myelogenous leukemia) is correct. The patient has chronic myelogenous leukemia (CML). The slightly macrocytic anemia and hypersegmented neutrophils are caused by folate deficiency due to increased

DNA synthesis. The peripheral blood smear shows neutrophils at different stages of development and increased numbers of basophils. CML is one of the few leukemias associated with thrombocytosis with the remaining cases showing thrombocytopenia. Because all the neutrophils are neoplastic, they do not take up the leukocyte alkaline phosphatase (LAP) stain like normal mature neutrophils; therefore, the LAP score, which grades 100 cells on the intensity of the stain (0 to +4), is low. The Philadelphia chromosome [chromosome 22 in the t(9;22) translocation] is present in most cases; however, detection of the *bcr-fusion* gene has 100% positive predictive value for diagnosing CML. Most patients progress to a terminal blast crisis after 3 years, which may be associated with myeloblasts or lymphoblasts.

5. **D** (chronic lymphocytic leukemia) is correct. The patient has chronic lymphocytic leukemia (CLL), which is the most common leukemia in patients over 60 years of age. CLL is also the most common cause of generalized lymphadenopathy in patients in the same age bracket. CLL is a malignancy of virgin B cells, which do not respond to antigenic stimulation. This produces hypogammaglobulinemia and increased susceptibility to infections. The peripheral smear shows numerous lymphocytes with dense nuclear chromatin and inconspicuous nucleoli. Occasional smudge cells are present.

6. **A** (acute lymphoblastic leukemia) is correct. The patient has acute lymphoblastic leukemia (ALL), the most common cancer and leukemia in children. The type of ALL is the most important prognostic factor. The most common type is early pre–B-ALL where the lymphoblasts are positive for CALLA (common ALL) antigen (CD10) and TdT (terminal deoxynucleotidyl transferase, pre–B-cell and T-cell marker). This type has the best prognosis. The peripheral blood smear shows increased numbers of lymphocytes with dense chromatin and small nucleoli.

7. **C** (membrane fusion defect) is correct. The patient has Chédiak-Higashi syndrome (CHS), which is a autosomal recessive disorder. There is a defect in membrane fusion, which prevents phagolysosome formation. Azurophilic granules in the primary lysosomes fuse to form giant granules in the leukocytes (present in the photograph). In addition, primary lysosomes cannot fuse with the membrane of phagosomes to produce secondary phagolysosomes. Additional defects in chemotaxis (directed migration), degranulation, and bactericidal activity are also present. Melanosomes are frequently defective as well resulting in blond hair. Patients are very susceptible to *Staphylococcus aureus* infections.

A (adhesion molecule defect) is incorrect. Adhesion molecule defects prevent neutrophil adhesion to venular endothelium. This causes the marginating pool to enter the circulating pool causing an increase in the absolute neutrophil count. Furthermore, the defect prevents transmigration of neutrophils into tissue. This produces problems with the umbilical cord sloughing off and wound healing, which are not present in this patient.

B (enzyme defect) is incorrect. In CHS, the problem is in membrane fusion, which is not associated with an enzyme deficiency.

D (opsonization defect) is incorrect. Opsonins like IgG and C3b coat bacteria. Neutrophils, monocytes, and macrophages have receptors for these opsonins, which facilitates phagocytosis. Deficiency of opsonins produces a defect in phagocytosis; however, there are no giant granules in leukocytes.

E (respiratory burst defect) is incorrect. The respiratory burst occurs when molecular oxygen is converted to superoxide free radicals. This requires the presence of NADPH oxidase in the membrane of neutrophils or monocytes and NADPH as a cofactor. The chemiluminescence test measures the energy given off by this reaction. The test is abnormal if there is a deficiency of NADPH oxidase (e.g., chronic granulomatous disease) or NADPH (e.g., glucose-6-phosphate dehydrogenase deficiency). In CHS, the respiratory burst is intact.

8. **C** is correct. The patient has polycythemia vera (PV), a neoplastic disease involving the common myeloid stem cell in the bone marrow. Patients have an increase in all the hematopoietic cells (*except* lymphocytes). Hyperviscosity due to the increase in RBC mass is the most serious component of the disease. It is responsible for thrombosis of the superior mesenteric vein with small bowel infarction (bloody diarrhea) in this patient and retinal vein engorgement with hemorrhage. Hypervolemia (increased plasma volume) differentiates PV from other causes of polycythemia where PV is either normal or decreased. The headaches and pruritus after bathing are due to histamine release from the increase in mast cells in tissue and basophils in the blood stream. Hyperuricemia due to increased cell turnover and release of purines is also a commonly observed finding in PV. It is responsible for the gouty arthritis experienced by the patient. The classic laboratory abnormalities in PV are RBC mass increased, plasma volume increased, Sao_2 normal, erythropoietin decreased (O_2 content is increased and suppresses EPO). In addition to the increase in RBC mass, there is neutrophilic leukocytosis and thrombocytosis.

A is incorrect. Increased RBC mass, normal plasma volume, normal Sao_2, and an increase in EPO is consistent with an inappropriate absolute polycythemia due to ectopic production of EPO. Examples include renal disease (e.g., renal cell carcinoma) and hepatocellular carcinoma.

B is incorrect. Increased RBC mass, normal plasma volume, decreased Sao_2, and increased EPO is consistent with an appropriate absolute polycythemia associated hypoxic stimulation of EPO leading to RBC hyperplasia in the bone marrow. Examples include respiratory disorders (e.g., chronic obstructive lung disease, restrictive lung disease), cardiovascular disorders (e.g., cyanotic congenital heart disease), and miscellaneous disorders (e.g., high altitude).

D is incorrect. A normal RBC mass, decreased plasma volume, normal Sao_2, and normal EPO is consistent with a relative polycythemia due to volume depletion. This produces hemoconcentration of RBCs in the blood leading to an increase in the RBC count; however, the RBC mass (absolute number of RBCs in the peripheral blood) is normal.

9. **B** (heterophile antibody test) is correct. The patient most likely has infectious mononucleosis due to the Epstein-Barr virus (EBV). It is primarily transmitted by kissing. EBV attaches to CD21 receptors on B cells and causes B-cell proliferation and increased synthesis of heterophile antibodies. These are IgM antibodies directed against horse, bovine, and sheep RBCs. Clinical findings include fatigue, exudative tonsillitis, hepatosplenomegaly, and generalized lymphadenopathy. Atypical lymphocytosis is present in the peripheral blood. The slide shows a number of different types of antigenically stimulated lymphocytes that are large and have abundant cytoplasm ("ballerina skirt") appearance. Anicteric hepatitis is invariably present along with marked transaminasemia. Jaundice is rare.

A (bone marrow aspirate) is incorrect. There is no anemia or thrombocytopenia and the patient does not have immature leukocytes in the peripheral blood; therefore, a bone marrow aspiration is unwarranted.

C (lymph node biopsy) is incorrect. The patient has generalized painful lymphadenopathy, which is a marker of inflammation rather than malignancy. In addition, the CBC is unremarkable except for atypical lymphocytosis; therefore, leukemia with metastasis to lymph nodes is unlikely.

D (marker studies for CALLA antigen) is incorrect. CALLA antigen is a marker for early pre–B-cell acute lymphoblastic leukemia. It is not indicated in this patient.

E (reticulocyte count) is incorrect. A reticulocyte count is useful when a patient has anemia, because it reflects the bone marrow response to the anemia. The patient does not have anemia.

10. **B** (eosinophil) is correct. The patient has trichinosis (*Trichinella spiralis*), which is contracted by eating raw or undercooked pork. The larvae penetrate muscle producing muscle pain and tenderness. Invasive helminths produce eosinophilia (type I hypersensitivity).

11. **C** (basophil) is correct. In polycythemia, all cell lines except lymphocytes are increased. An increase in basophils and mast cells causes the release of histamine, which produces flushing of the face (called plethora), headaches, and pruritus after bathing. All of the myeloproliferative diseases have basophilia.

12. **E** (monocyte) is correct. Monocytosis is the primary leukocyte alteration in chronic inflammation (e.g., rheumatoid arthritis).

13. **D** (lymphocyte) is correct. *Bordetella pertussis* is the cause of whooping cough. The lymphotoxin decreases entry of lymphocytes into lymph nodes causing lymphocytosis, with lymphocyte counts often >50,000/mm^3 (lymphoid leukemoid reaction).

14. **A** (neutrophil) is correct. A perforated acute appendicitis produces neutrophilic leukocytosis with left shift (shift to early neutrophil precursors) and toxic granulation (prominent azurophilic granules), which is evident in the photograph.

15. **D** is the correct answer. The patient has minimal change disease, which is the most common cause of the nephrotic syndrome in children. In all cases, the 24-hour urine test for protein is >3.5 g/24 hours, which leads to hypoalbuminemia and generalized edema and ascites. The patient also has a moon facies and truncal obesity with purple stretch marks indicating that he is on high doses of corticosteroids. Corticosteroids inhibit neutrophil adhesion molecules causing the release of the marginating neutrophil pool into the circulating neutrophil pool. This produces an absolute neutrophilic leukocytosis. Corticosteroids also are a signal for apoptosis of lymphocytes and sequester lymphocytes and eosinophils in lymph nodes leading to lymphopenia and eosinopenia, respectively.

A is incorrect. A decrease in the neutrophil, lymphocyte, and eosinophil count is seen in aplastic anemia with destruction of the common myeloid stem cell.

B is incorrect. A decrease in the neutrophil count and increase in the lymphocyte and eosinophil count is present in hypocortisolism (e.g., Addison's disease).

C is incorrect. A decrease in the neutrophil count, increase in the lymphocyte count, and decrease in the eosinophil count is most often present in a viral infection.

E is incorrect. A normal neutrophil and lymphocyte count with an increase in the eosinophil count is present in type I hypersensitivity reactions due to asthma, hay fever, and invasive helminth infections.

Hemostasis Disorders

I. **Normal Hemostasis**

A. **Anticoagulants in small blood vessels**
- Small blood vessels include capillaries, venules, arterioles.
  1. Heparin-like molecules
     a. Enhance antithrombin III (ATIII) activity
     b. Neutralize the following activated coagulation factors
        - Factors XII, XI, IX, X, thrombin
  2. Proteins C and S
     a. Vitamin K–dependent factors
     b. Inactivate factors V and VIII
     c. Enhance fibrinolysis
  3. Prostaglandin I_2 (prostacyclin, PGI_2)
     a. Synthesized by endothelial cells
     b. Vasodilator; inhibits platelet aggregation
     c. Effect of aspirin
        - Does *not* inhibit synthesis of PGI_2.
  4. Tissue plasminogen activator (tPA)
     a. Synthesized by endothelial cells
     b. Activates plasminogen to release plasmin
     c. Functions of plasmin
        (1) Degrades coagulation factors
        (2) Lyses fibrin clots (thrombi)

B. **Procoagulants in small vessel injury**
  1. Extrinsic and intrinsic coagulation systems (see below)
  2. Tissue thromboplastin (factor III)
     a. Released from injured tissue
     b. Activates factor VII
        - Extrinsic coagulation system
  3. Von Willebrand factor (vWF)
     a. Synthesized by endothelial cells and megakaryocytes
        - Platelets carry vWF in their α-granules.
     b. Functions of vWF
        (1) Platelet adhesion molecule
           (a) Binds platelets to exposed collagen
           (b) Platelets have glycoprotein (Gp)Ib receptors for vWF.

Heparin: enhances ATIII activity

Proteins C and S: inactivate factors V and VIII, enhance fibrinolysis

PGI_2: vasodilator, inhibits platelet aggregation

tPA: activates plasminogen to release plasmin

Tissue thromboplastin: activates factor VII in extrinsic coagulation system vWF: platelet adhesion; prevents degradation of VIII : C

(2) Complexes with factor VIII:coagulant (VIII:C) in the circulation
  (a) Prevents degradation of factor VIII:C
  (b) Decrease in vWF secondarily decreases VIII:C activity.

> When VIII:C is activated by thrombin, it dissociates from the VIII:vWF complex and performs its procoagulant function in the intrinsic coagulation cascade system.

4. Thromboxane A_2 (TXA$_2$)
  a. Synthesized by platelets
    (1) Thromboxane synthase converts PGH_2 to TXA$_2$.
    (2) Aspirin irreversibly inhibits platelet cyclooxygenase.
      • Prevents formation of PGH_2
    (3) Other nonsteroidal anti-inflammatory drugs reversibly inhibit platelet cyclooxygenase.
  b. Functions of TXA$_2$

TXA$_2$: vasoconstrictor; enhances platelet aggregation

    (1) Vasoconstrictor
    (2) Enhances platelet aggregation
C. **Platelet structure and function**
  1. Derivation
    • Cytoplasmic fragmentation of megakaryocytes
  2. Locations
    a. Peripheral blood
      • Live for ~9 to 10 days
    b. Spleen is a storage site.
      • Contains about one third of the total platelet pool
  3. Platelet receptors
    a. GpIb receptors for vWF
    b. GpIIb:IIIa receptors for fibrinogen
      (1) Ticlopidine and clopidogrel
        (a) Inhibit ADP-induced expression of platelet GpIIb:IIIa receptors
        (b) Prevent fibrinogen binding and platelet aggregation
        (c) Commonly used when patients are allergic to aspirin

Platelet receptors: GpIb (binds to vWF) GpIIb:IIIa (binds to fibrinogen)

      (2) Abciximab
        (a) Monoclonal antibody directed against GpIIb:IIIa receptor
        (b) Commonly used to prevent thrombosis after coronary artery balloon angioplasty or stent placement
  4. Platelet factor 3 (PF3)
    • Phospholipid substrate required for the clotting sequence
  5. Platelet structure
    a. Contractile element
      (1) Called thrombosthenin
      (2) Important in clot retraction
    b. Dense bodies; important components:
      (1) Adenosine diphosphate (ADP)
        • Aggregating agent

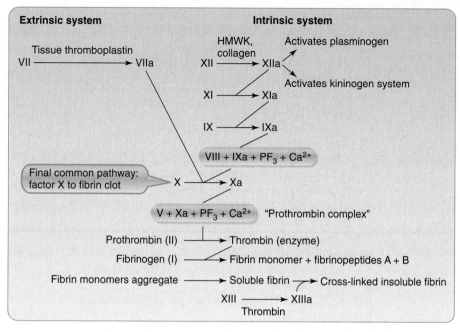

7-1: *Coagulation cascade. Factor VII is in the extrinsic system. Factors XII, XI, IX, and VIII are in the intrinsic system. Both the extrinsic and intrinsic coagulation systems use the final common pathway (factors X, V, II, I) for the formation of a fibrin clot. a, activated; HMWK, high-molecular-weight kininogen; PF₃, platelet factor 3. (From Goljan EF: Rapid Review Pathology, 2nd ed. St. Louis, Mosby, 2007, Fig. 14-1.)*

       (2) Calcium
         • Binding agent for vitamin K–dependent factors
    c. α-Granules; important components:
       (1) vWF, fibrinogen
       (2) Platelet factor 4 (PF4)
         • Heparin neutralizing factor
  6. Platelet function
    a. Fill in gaps between endothelial cells in small vessels
       (1) Prevents leakage of RBCs into the interstitium
       (2) Thrombocytopenia causes leakage of RBCs into interstitium.
         • Pinpoint areas of hemorrhage are called petechiae.
    b. Hemostatic plug formation in small vessel injury
D. **Coagulation system** (Fig. 7-1)
  1. Coagulation cascade
    a. Extrinsic system
      • Factor VII
    b. Intrinsic system
      • Factors XII, XI, IX, VIII
  2. Extrinsic system
    a. Tissue thromboplastin activates factor VII.
    b. VIIa activates X in the final common pathway.

Extrinsic system:
factor VII

3. Intrinsic system
  a. Factor XII (Hageman factor) is activated by
    (1) Exposed subendothelial collagen
    (2) High-molecular-weight kininogen (HMWK)
  b. Functions of factor XIIa
    (1) Activates factor XI
    (2) Activates plasminogen
      • Produces plasmin
    (3) Activates kininogen system
      • Produces kallikrein and bradykinin
  c. Factor XIa activates factor IX to form factor IXa
    (1) Four-component complex is formed:
      (a) IXa, VIII, PF3, calcium
      (b) PF3 and calcium are platelet-derived
    (2) Complex activates factor X
    (3) Calcium binds factor IXa
      • IXa is a vitamin K–dependent coagulation factor.
4. Final common pathway
  a. Includes factors X, V, prothrombin (II), and fibrinogen (I)
  b. Prothrombin complex
    (1) Four-component system:
      • Xa, V, PF3, calcium
    (2) Calcium binds factor Xa
      • Xa is a vitamin K–dependent coagulation factor.
    (3) Complex cleaves prothrombin to thrombin
      • Thrombin is an enzyme.
  c. Primary functions of thrombin
    (1) Acts on fibrinogen; cleavage products:
      (a) Fibrin monomers
      (b) Fibrinopeptides A and B
    (2) Activates factor XIII
      (a) Factor XIIIa converts soluble fibrin monomers to insoluble fibrin.
      (b) Enhances protein-protein cross-linking
        • Cross-linking strengthens the fibrin clot.
5. Vitamin K–dependent factors
  a. Factors II, VII, IX, X, proteins C and S
  b. Synthesized in the liver
    • Nonfunctional precursor proteins
  c. Function of vitamin K
    (1) Most vitamin K is synthesized by colonic bacteria.
      • Vitamin K produced is nonfunctional.
    (2) Vitamin K is activated in the liver by epoxide reductase.
    (3) Activated vitamin K γ-carboxylates the vitamin K–dependent factors.
      • Carboxylated factors can bind to calcium and PF3 in the above cascade sequence.

Margin notes:

Intrinsic system: factors XII, XI, IX, VIII

Final common pathway: factors X, V, II, I

Factor XIII: cross-links fibrin monomers

Vitamin K: activated in the liver by epoxide reductase

Calcium: binds γ-carboxylated vitamin K–dependent factors

Warfarin is an anticoagulant that inhibits epoxide reductase, rendering vitamin K inactive. This prevents any further γ-carboxylation of the vitamin K–dependent coagulation factors. Full anticoagulation does *not* immediately occur, because previously γ-carboxylated factors are still circulating. Carboxylated prothrombin has the longest half-life; therefore, full anticoagulation requires at least 3 to 4 days before all functional prothrombin has disappeared. Patients are initially placed on both heparin and warfarin, because heparin immediately anticoagulates the patient by enhancing ATIII activity. Heparin is withdrawn in 3 to 4 days and the patient remains on warfarin.

Warfarin: inhibits epoxide reductase; vitamin K is nonfunctional

6. Coagulation factors consumed in the formation of a fibrin clot
   • Fibrinogen (I), factors V and VIII, and prothrombin (II)

When blood is drawn into a clot tube (no anticoagulant is added), a fibrin clot is formed that traps RBCs, platelets, and leukocytes. When the tube is spun down in a centrifuge, the supranate is called serum, which, unlike plasma, is missing fibrinogen, prothrombin (II), factor V, and factor VIII. These factors are completely used up in the formation of the fibrin clot.

E. **Fibrinolytic system**
   1. Activation
      a. Plasminogen is activated by tPA.
         • The enzyme plasmin is released.
      b. Other activators of plasminogen
         (1) Factor XIIa
         (2) Streptokinase
            • Derived from streptococci
         (3) Anistreplase
            • Complex of streptokinase and plasminogen
         (4) Urokinase
            • Derived from human urine
   2. Functions of plasmin (see I.A)
   3. α₂-Antiplasmin
      a. Synthesized in the liver
      b. Inactivates plasmin
   4. Alteplase and reteplase
      • Recombinant forms of tPA used in thrombolytic therapy
   5. Aminocaproic acid
      a. Competitively blocks plasminogen activation
      b. Inhibits fibrinolysis
F. **Small vessel hemostasis response to injury** (Fig. 7-2)
   1. Vascular phase
      a. Transient vasoconstriction
         • Occurs directly after injury

7-2: *Small-vessel hemostasis response to injury. See text for discussion. TXA₂, thromboxane A₂; vWD, von Willebrand disease; vWF, von Willebrand factor. (From Goljan EF: Rapid Review Pathology, 2nd ed. St. Louis, Mosby, 2007, Fig. 14-2.)*

    b. Tissue thromboplastin activates factor VII.
    c. Exposed collagen activates factor XII.
  2. Platelet phase
    a. Platelet adhesion
      • Platelet GpIb receptors adhere to exposed vWF.
    b. Platelet release reaction
      (1) Release of ADP
      (2) Induces conformation change of the GpIIb:IIIa receptors
        • Allows them to bind fibrinogen
    c. Platelet synthesis and release of TXA₂
      (1) Vessels constrict.
        • Reduces blood flow
      (2) Platelet aggregation is further enhanced.
    d. Temporary platelet plug stops bleeding.
      (1) Aggregated platelets have fibrinogen attached to GpIIb:IIIa receptors.
      (2) Platelet plug is an unstable plug and can easily be dislodged.
  3. Coagulation phase
    a. Thrombin eventually is produced from localized activation of coagulation system.
      • Converts fibrinogen in temporary plug to insoluble fibrin monomers
    b. Stable platelet plug is formed.
  4. Fibrinolytic phase
    a. Plasmin cleaves insoluble fibrin monomers holding platelet plug together.
    b. Blood flow is reestablished.

Platelet sequence: adhesion, release reaction, synthesis of TXA₂, temporary plug

TABLE 7-1
Causes of
Prolonged
Bleeding Time

Cause	Nature of Defect	Comments
Aspirin or NSAIDs	Platelet aggregation defect Inhibition of platelet COX, which ultimately inhibits synthesis of TXA_2 from PGH_2	Normal platelet count
Bernard-Soulier syndrome	Platelet adhesion defect Autosomal recessive disease Absent GpIb platelet receptors for vWF	Thrombocytopenia, giant platelets Life-long bleeding problem
Glanzmann's disease	Platelet aggregation defect Autosomal recessive disease Absent GpIIb:IIIa fibrinogen receptors	Life-long bleeding problem
Renal failure	Platelet aggregation defect Inhibition of platelet phospholipid by toxic products	Reversed with dialysis and desmopressin acetate
Scurvy	Vascular defect Caused by vitamin C deficiency Defective collagen resulting from poor cross-linking of α-chains	May cause ecchymoses and hemarthroses
Thrombocytopenia	Decreased platelet number	Increased bleeding time when platelet count < 90,000/mm^3
von Willebrand disease	Platelet adhesion defect Autosomal dominant disorder Absent or defective vWF Decreased VIII:C and VIII:Ag	Other factor VIII coagulation defects

COX, cyclooxygenase; NSAID, nonsteroidal anti-inflammatory drug; TXA_2, thromboxane A_2; VIII:Ag, factor VIII antigen; VIII:C, factor VIII coagulant; vWF, von Willebrand factor.

II. **Hemostasis Testing**
   A. **Platelet tests**
      1. Platelet count
         a. Normal count is 150,000 to 400,000/mm^3.
         b. Normal count does *not* guarantee normal platelet function.
      2. Bleeding time
         a. Evaluates platelet phase of small vessel injury (see Fig. 7-2)
            (1) Platelet adhesion, release reaction, synthesis of TXA_2, formation of temporary platelet plug
            (2) Normal reference interval is 2 to 7 minutes.
         b. Disorders causing a prolonged bleeding time (Table 7-1)
      3. Platelet aggregation test
         a. Evaluates platelet aggregation in a test tube
         b. Aggregating agents used
            • ADP, epinephrine, collagen, and ristocetin

Bleeding time: test of platelet function up to formation of temporary plug

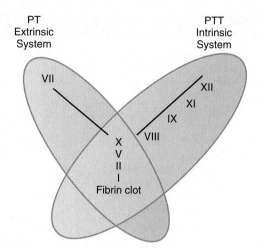

7-3: *Prothrombin time (PT) and partial thromboplastin time (PTT). See text for discussion. (From Goljan EF: Rapid Review Pathology, 2nd ed. St. Louis, Mosby, 2007, Fig. 14-3.)*

      c. Aspirin is most common cause of decreased aggregation.
- Inhibits synthesis of TXA_2

    4. Tests for vWF

      a. Ristocetin cofactor assay

        (1) Evaluates vWF function

        (2) Abnormal assay

          (a) Classic von Willebrand disease
- Deficiency of vWF

          (b) Bernard-Soulier disease
- Absent GpIb receptor

      b. vWF antigen assay

        (1) Measures the quantity of vWF
- Does *not* evaluate functional capability of vWF

        (2) Decreased in classic von Willebrand disease

      c. Agar gel electrophoresis

        (1) Evaluates the size distribution of circulating vWF multimers
- High-molecular-weight multimers are the most active form of vWF.

        (2) Useful in differentiating subtypes of von Willebrand disease

  B. **Coagulation tests** (Fig. 7-3)

    1. Prothrombin time (PT)

      a. Evaluates the extrinsic system to formation of the fibrin clot
- Factors VII, X, V, II, and I are included.

      b. Normal reference interval for PT is 12 to 14 seconds.
- Only prolonged if a factor level is 30% to 40% of normal

      c. International normalized ratio (INR)
- Standardizes the PT for use in warfarin therapy

      d. Uses of PT

        (1) Follow patients taking warfarin for anticoagulation

---

Ristocetin cofactor assay: functional assay of vWF

PT: evaluates factors VII, X, V, II, I

    (2) Evaluate liver synthetic function
- Increased PT indicates severe liver dysfunction.

    (3) Detect factor VII deficiency

2. Partial thromboplastin time (PTT)
  a. Evaluates the intrinsic system to formation of a fibrin clot
- Factors XII, XI, IX, VIII, X, V, II, and I are included.

  b. Normal reference interval for PTT is 25 to 40 seconds.
- Only prolonged if a factor level is 30% to 40% of normal

  c. Uses of PTT
    (1) Follow heparin therapy
      (a) Heparin enhances ATIII activity.
      (b) PTT is *not* required to follow low-molecular-weight heparin therapy.
    (2) Detect factor deficiencies in the intrinsic system

> Whether the patient is anticoagulated with heparin or warfarin, both the PT and PTT are prolonged, because both inhibit factors in the final common pathway (e.g., factors X, II). Experience has shown that the PT performs better in monitoring warfarin, and the PTT performs better in monitoring heparin.

C. **Fibrinolytic system tests**
1. Fibrin(ogen) degradation products (FDPs)
- Test detects products associated with plasmin degradation of fibrinogen and insoluble fibrin in fibrin thrombi.

2. D-dimer assay
  a. Only detects cross-linked insoluble fibrin monomers in a fibrin clot
- Cross-linked fibrin monomers are called D-dimers.

  b. Does *not* detect fibrinogen degradation products (not cross-linked)
- Test is negative if only fibrinogen degradation products are present.

  c. Uses of D-dimer assay
    (1) Thrombolytic therapy for coronary artery thrombosis
- Thrombus is composed of platelets held together by fibrin.

    (2) Screening test for pulmonary thromboembolism
- Thrombus is composed of RBCs, platelets, WBCs held together by fibrin.

    (3) Screening test for disseminated intravascular coagulation (DIC)
- Thrombus is composed of RBCs, platelets, WBCs held together by fibrin (see Section IV).

III. **Platelet Disorders**
  A. **Classification**
    1. Quantitative disorders
      a. Thrombocytopenia
      b. Thrombocytosis
    2. Qualitative (functional) disorders

PTT: evaluates factors XII, XI, IX, VIII, X, V, II, I

FDPs: increased with lysis of fibrinogen and fibrin in fibrin thrombi

D-dimer assay: specific for lysis of fibrin clots (thrombi)

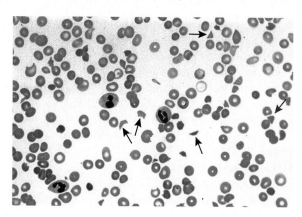

7-4: *Peripheral blood smear in a patient with thrombotic thrombocytopenic purpura (TTP). Note the absence of platelets in the smear and the presence of fragmented red blood cells (arrows) called schistocytes. (From Wickramasinghe SE, McCullough J: Blood and Bone Marrow Pathology. Philadelphia, Churchill Livingstone, 2003, Fig. 26.9.)*

B. **Pathogenesis**
  1. Thrombocytopenia (Table 7-2)
     • Decreased number of platelets
     a. Decreased production
        • Examples—aplastic anemia, leukemia
     b. Increased destruction
        (1) Immune causes
           • Examples—idiopathic thrombocytopenic purpura, drugs
        (2) Nonimmune causes
           • Examples—thrombotic thrombocytopenic purpura (Fig. 7-4), DIC
     c. Sequestration in the spleen
        • Hypersplenism in portal hypertension
  2. Thrombocytosis
     • Increased platelet count
     a. Primary thrombocytosis
        • Examples—essential thrombocythemia, polycythemia vera
     b. Secondary (reactive) thrombocytosis
        • Examples—chronic iron deficiency, infections, splenectomy, malignancy
  3. Qualitative platelet disorders
     a. Acquired
        • Example—aspirin
     b. Hereditary
        • Example—von Willebrand disease
C. **Clinical findings**
  1. Epistaxis (nosebleeds)
     • Most common symptom

Acute ITP: most common cause of thrombocytopenia in children

Aspirin: most common cause of a qualitative platelet defect

TABLE 7-2
Disorders
Producing
Thrombocytopenia

Acute idiopathic thrombocytopenic purpura (ITP)	Most common cause thrombocytopenia in children 2 to 6 years of age IgG antibodies directed against GpIIb:IIIa receptors (type II reaction) Abrupt onset 1 to 3 weeks after a viral infection Absence of lymphadenopathy and splenomegaly Responds well to corticosteroids
Chronic ITP	Most common cause thrombocytopenia in adults Most common in women 20 to 40 years of age IgG antibodies directed against GpIIb:IIIa receptors (type II reaction) Insidious onset Often resistant to steroids and requires splenectomy. IV γ-globulin temporarily stops serious bleeding (IgG blocks macrophage Fc receptors) Newborn infants of mothers with ITP may have transient thrombocytopenia due to transplacental passage of IgG antibodies Secondary causes: SLE, HIV, lymphoproliferative diseases
Neonatal alloimmune thrombocytopenia (NAIT)	Accounts for 20% of cases of thrombocytopenia in neonates Fetomaternal incompatibility for platelet specific antigens (e.g., Pl^{A1}). Pl^{A1} absent from 2% of population. Pl^{A1} negative mother develops IgG antibodies during pregnancy or from a previous pregnancy or transfusion. Transplacental passage of IgG antibodies bind to fetal Pl^{A1} positive platelets leading to macrophage destruction of platelets (type II hypersensitivity) May produce petechial hemorrhages in first few days of life or CNS hemorrhages in severe cases
Post-transfusion purpura	Primarily occurs in multiparous women Patient receiving blood has antibodies against Pl^{A1} or other platelet antigens that are present on donor platelets. Severe thrombocytopenia with destruction of donor and patient platelets occurs 7 to 10 days after a blood transfusion.
Heparin-induced thrombocytopenia	Most common cause thrombocytopenia in hospitalized patients Macrophage removal of platelets surfaced by IgG antibody directed against heparin attached to PF4 (type II hypersensitivity); occurs 5–14 days after Rx; must stop heparin; release of PF4 (anti-heparin factor) after platelet destruction may result in vessel thrombosis
Thrombotic thrombocytopenic purpura (TTP) (see Fig. 7-4)	Occurs in adult females Acquired or genetic deficiency in vWF-cleaving metalloprotease in endothelial cells; increase in circulating multimers of vWF increases platelet adhesion to areas of endothelial injury at arteriole-capillary junctions Platelets are consumed owing to production of platelet thrombi in areas of injury (*not* DIC) Enhanced by other factors that damage endothelial cells (e.g., ticlopidine, hypertension) Clinical pentad: fever, thrombocytopenia, renal failure, microangiopathic hemolytic anemia with schistocytes (damage by platelet thrombi), CNS deficits Treated with plasmapheresis Mortality rate 10% to 20%
Hemolytic uremic syndrome (HUS)	Primarily occurs in children Endothelial damage at arteriole-capillary junction is due to Shiga-like toxin of 0157:H7 serotype of *E. coli* Organisms proliferate in undercooked beef Clinical findings similar to TTP; however, CNS findings are less frequent Mortality rate 3% to 5%

CNS, central nervous system; DIC, disseminated intravascular coagulation; HIV, human immunodeficiency virus; IV, intravenous; PF4, platelet factor 4; Rx, treatment; SLE, systemic lupus erythematosus; vWF, von Willebrand factor.

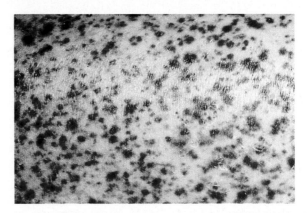

7-5: *Petechiae in a patient with chronic thrombocytopenic purpura showing pinpoint hemorrhages. Petechiae do not blanch with pressure. (From Wickramasinghe SE, McCullough J: Blood and Bone Marrow Pathology. Philadelphia, Churchill Livingstone, 2003, Fig. 26.10.)*

    2. Petechiae
- Pinpoint areas of hemorrhage in subcutaneous tissue (Fig. 7-5).

    3. Ecchymoses (purpura)
- Areas of subcutaneous hemorrhage the size of a quarter

> Ecchymoses (purpura) are caused by a variety of disorders that are unrelated to platelet dysfunction. Palpable purpura (purpura that can be palpated) is a sign of acute inflammation associated with a small vessel vasculitis. Hemorrhage is due to rupture of the weakened blood vessel. Senile purpura is a normal finding in elderly patients and is due to damage to the connective tissue of the dermis, which fails to support the vasculature, rendering it more susceptible to mild trauma (Fig. 7-6). The ecchymoses develop in areas of trauma (e.g., back of the hands, forearms, shins).

    4. Bleeding from superficial scratches
- No temporary platelet plug is present to stop bleeding.

    5. Other findings
- a. Menorrhagia, hematuria
- b. Bleeding from tooth extraction sites
- c. Gastrointestinal and intracranial bleeding

IV. **Coagulation Disorders**
    A. **Classification of coagulation disorders**
        1. Acquired
           a. Single coagulation factor deficiencies
- Example—hemophilia A

           b. Multiple coagulation factor deficiencies
- Examples—cirrhosis, DIC, vitamin K deficiency

        2. Hereditary
- Usually a single coagulation factor deficiency

Coagulation disorders: most are due to decreased production of a coagulation factor

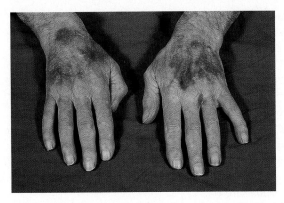

7-6: *Senile purpura showing large, irregular areas of hemorrhage on the backs of both hands. See text for discussion. (From Forbes C, Jackson W: Color Atlas and Text of Clinical Medicine, 2nd ed. St. Louis, Mosby, 2003, Fig. 10-112.)*

B. **Pathogenesis**
1. Decreased production
   - Examples—hemophilia A, cirrhosis
2. Pathologic inhibition
   - Example—acquired circulating antibodies (inhibitors) against coagulation factors
3. Excessive consumption
   - Example—disseminated intravascular coagulation

C. **Clinical findings**
1. Late rebleeding after surgery
   a. Temporary platelet plug is the only mechanical block preventing bleeding.
   b. Because of lack of thrombin, fibrinogen (*not* fibrin) holds the plug together.
   c. Plug is easily dislodged with movement.
2. Findings in severe factor deficiencies
   a. Hemarthroses
   b. Retroperitoneal and deep muscle bleeding
3. Findings similar to platelet disorders
   a. Ecchymoses, epistaxis
   b. Menorrhagia, hematuria
   c. Bleeding from tooth extraction sites
   d. Gastrointestinal and intracranial bleeding

D. **Hemophilia A**
1. Epidemiology
   a. X-linked recessive
      (1) Females are asymptomatic carriers
      (2) Transmit the mutant gene on the X chromosome to 50% of their boys

Hemophilia A: X-linked recessive

b. Absent family history of hemophilia
  • Most likely due to a new mutation (30% of cases)
  c. Female carriers with symptomatic disease
    (1) Inactivation of more maternal than paternal X chromosomes
    (2) Become homozygous-like for the mutant gene on the X chromosome
2. Pathogenesis
  • Decreased synthesis of factor VIII:C in the intrinsic system
3. Clinical findings
  a. Signs and symptoms correlate with the level of factor VIII:C activity
    • Activity <1% correlates with severe disease (e.g., spontaneous hemarthroses).
  b. Bleeding problems may occur in newborns (10–15% of cases)
    • Excessive bleeding after circumcision or umbilical cord separation

> Hemophilia B (Christmas disease) is an X-linked recessive disorder involving a deficiency of factor IX. It is clinically indistinguishable from hemophilia A.

  c. Laboratory findings
    (1) Increased PTT
    (2) Normal PT
    (3) Decreased factor VIII:C activity
    (4) Decreased factor VIII:antigen (VIII:Ag)
      • Factor VIII protein
    (5) Detection of female carriers
      • DNA techniques are most sensitive.

Hemophilia A: ↓ VIII:C, VIII:Ag

4. Treatment
  a. Mild cases respond to desmopressin acetate.
    • Increases VIII:C activity
  b. Severe cases require infusion of recombinant factor VIII
    • *No* risk for contracting HIV
E. **Classical von Willebrand disease (vWD)**
  1. Epidemiology
    a. Autosomal dominant disorder
    b. Most common hereditary coagulation disorder

vWD: most common hereditary coagulation disorder

  2. Pathogenesis
    • Decreased vWF and factor VIII:C activity
  3. Clinical findings
    a. Menorrhagia, epistaxis, easy bruisability
    b. Association with angiodysplasia of the right colon
  4. Laboratory findings
    a. Increased PTT
    b. Normal PT
    c. Increased bleeding time
      • Due a platelet adhesion defect
    d. Abnormal ristocetin cofactor assay

vWD: combined platelet and coagulation factor disorder

vWD: ↑ PTT, bleeding time

      e. Decreased vWF antigen

      f. Decreased VIII:Ag and VIII:C activity

   5. Treatment

      a. Desmopressin acetate

        • Increases vWF and VIII:C activity

      b. Oral contraceptive

        • Estrogen has a similar action as desmopressin

F. **Circulating anticoagulants (inhibitors)**

   1. Pathogenesis

      a. Coagulation factor is destroyed by antibodies.

      b. Most common type is caused by antibodies against factor VIII:C.

        • Example—occurs post-partum and after treatment with recombinant factor VIII

   2. Clinical findings

      • Similar to decreased production types of deficiencies

   3. Laboratory findings

      a. Prolonged PT or PTT depending on the factor deficiency

        • Does *not* differentiate immune destruction versus decreased production

      b. Mixing studies

        (1) Normal plasma is mixed with patient plasma in a test tube.

        (2) *No* correction of PT or PTT

          • Indicates immune destruction

        (3) Correction of PT and PTT

          • Indicates decreased production

> Circulating anticoagulant: PT and PTT *not* corrected with mixing study

G. **Vitamin K deficiency**

   1. Function of vitamin K (see Section ID)

   2. Causes of vitamin K deficiency

      a. Decreased synthesis of vitamin K by colonic bacteria

        (1) Newborns lack bacterial colonization of the bowel.

          (a) Vitamin K levels normally decrease between days 2 and 5.

          (b) Danger of severe bleeding

            • Example—intracerebral hemorrhage

          (c) Newborns require an intramuscular injection of vitamin K at birth.

            • Breast milk contains very little vitamin K.

        (2) Prolonged treatment with antibiotics

          (a) Antibiotics sterilize the bowel

            • Decreased production of vitamin K

          (b) Most common cause of vitamin K deficiency in a hospitalized patient

> Vitamin K deficiency in hospitalized patient: due to antibiotic therapy

      b. Decreased small bowel reabsorption of vitamin K

        (1) Malabsorption of fat causes malabsorption of fat-soluble vitamins.

        (2) Examples—celiac disease, chronic pancreatitis, bile salt deficiency

      c. Decreased activation of vitamin K

        (1) Warfarin inhibits epoxide reductase

          (a) Vitamin K–dependent factors are nonfunctional.

(b) Rat poison contains warfarin.

(c) Children may have exposure to warfarin from elders living in the family.

(2) Cirrhosis

(a) Decreased activation of vitamin K

(b) Decreased synthesis of vitamin K–dependent coagulation factors

(c) Prolonged PT

- *Not* corrected with intramuscular injection of vitamin K

3. Clinical findings

  a. Gastrointestinal bleeding

  b. Bleeding into subcutaneous tissue

  c. Bleeding at the time of circumcision

  d. Intracranial hemorrhage

4. Treatment

  a. Bleeding is not severe.

    (1) Treat with intramuscular injection of vitamin K

    (2) Corrects bleeding in a few hours

  b. Bleeding is severe.

    (1) Treat with fresh frozen plasma

- Vitamin K–dependent factors are γ-carboxylated.

    (2) Immediate correction

H. **Hemostasis disorders in liver disease**

1. Pathogenesis

  a. Decreased synthesis of coagulation factors

- Produces bleeding problems

    (1) Multiple coagulation factor deficiencies

    (2) Decreased γ-carboxylation of vitamin K–dependent factors

  b. Decreased synthesis of anticoagulants

    (1) Produces vessel thrombosis

    (2) Examples—ATIII, proteins C and S

  c. Decreased clearance of FDPs and D-dimers

    (1) Produces bleeding problems

    (2) Interfere with platelet aggregation and polymerization of fibrin

  d. Decreased clearance of tPA

- Produces bleeding (see Section V)

  e. Decreased synthesis of α_2-antiplasmin

- Produces bleeding (see Section V)

2. Laboratory findings

  a. Increased PT and PTT

  b. Increased FDPs and D-dimers

  c. Increased bleeding time

I. **Disseminated intravascular coagulation (DIC)**

1. Causes of DIC

  a. Sepsis

- *Escherichia coli* (most common) and *Neisseria meningitidis*

  b. Disseminated malignancy

      (1) Acute promyelocytic leukemia

      (2) Pancreatic cancer

        • Release of procoagulants in mucin

      (3) Crush injuries, rattlesnake envenomation, amniotic fluid embolism

2. Pathogenesis

  a. Activation of the coagulation cascade

    • Release of tissue thromboplastin and endothelial cell injury

  b. Fibrin thrombi develop in the microcirculation.

    (1) Thrombi obstruct blood flow.

    (2) Consumption of coagulation factors I, II, V, VIII.

    (3) Trapping of platelets in fibrin thrombus

  c. Activation of the fibrinolytic system

    (1) Activation of plasminogen by factor XII

    (2) Produces a secondary fibrinolysis

3. Clinical findings

  a. Thrombohemorrhagic disorder

    (1) Ischemia from occlusive fibrin thrombi

    (2) Bleeding from anticoagulation

      • Factors I, II, V, and VIII are consumed in fibrin thrombi.

  b. Shock

    • Due to blood loss

  c. Diffuse oozing of blood from multiple sites

    • Examples—gastrointestinal tract; breaks in skin; needle puncture sites

  d. Petechiae and ecchymoses

4. Laboratory findings

  a. Coagulation

    (1) Increased PT and PTT

    (2) Decreased fibrinogen

  b. Platelets

    (1) Thrombocytopenia

    (2) Increased bleeding time

  c. Fibrinolysis

    • Presence of FDPs and D-dimers

  d. Normocytic anemia

    (1) Schistocytes

      • Microangiopathic hemolytic anemia (Chapter 5)

    (2) Reticulocytosis

5. Treatment

  a. Treat the underlying disease

    • Most important

  b. Transfuse blood components

    (1) Fresh frozen plasma

      • Corrects multiple coagulation factor deficiencies

    (2) Packed RBCs

      • Correct anemia

    (3) Platelet concentrates

      • Correct thrombocytopenia

Margin notes:

DIC: consumption of coagulation factors

DIC: thrombo-hemorrhagic disorder

D-dimers: best screen for DIC

V. **Fibrinolytic Disorders**
   A. **Primary fibrinolysis**
      1. Causes
         a. Open heart surgery with cardiopulmonary bypass
            • Cardiopulmonary bypass decreases α_2-antiplasmin and increases tPA.
         b. Radical prostatectomy
            • Increased release of urokinase
         c. Diffuse liver disease
            • Decreased synthesis of α_2-antiplasmin
      2. Pathogenesis
         a. FDPs interfere with platelet aggregation.
         b. Plasmin degrades coagulation factors.
            • Produces multiple factor deficiencies
      3. Clinical findings
         • Severe bleeding
      4. Laboratory findings
         a. Increased PT and PTT
            • Due to multiple factor deficiencies
         b. Increased bleeding time
            • FDPs interfere with platelet aggregation.
         c. Positive test for FDPs
            • Plasmin is degrading fibrinogen *not* fibrin.
         d. Negative D-dimer assay
            • *No* fibrin thrombi are present.
         e. Normal platelet count
   B. **Secondary fibrinolysis**
      1. Compensatory reaction
         • Occurs in the presence of intravascular coagulation
      2. Increase in both FDPs and D-dimers

VI. **Summary of Laboratory Test Results in Hemostasis Disorders** (Table 7-3)

VII. **Thrombosis Syndromes**
   A. **Acquired thrombosis syndromes**
      1. Antiphospholipid syndrome (APLS)
         a. Epidemiology
            • Associations include SLE and HIV.
         b. Pathogenesis
            (1) Presence of antiphospholipid antibodies (APAs)
               • Directed against phospholipids bound to plasma proteins including coagulation factors
            (2) APAs include:
               (a) Anticardiolipin antibody
                  • Also reacts with the cardiolipin reagent in the rapid plasma reagin (RPR) test for syphilis
               (b) Lupus anticoagulant

Primary fibrinolysis: positive test for FDPs, negative D-dimer assay

Anticardiolipin antibody: produce a false positive syphilis serology

TABLE 7-3
Laboratory
Findings in
Common
Hemostasis
Disorders

Disorder	Platelet Count	Bleeding Time	PT	PTT
Thrombocytopenia ITP, TTP, HUS	↓	↑	Normal	Normal
von Willebrand disease	Normal	↑	Normal	↑
Hemophilia A	Normal	Normal	Normal	↑
DIC	↓	↑	↑	↑
Primary fibrinolysis	Normal	↑	↑	↑
Aspirin or NSAIDs	Normal	↑	Normal	Normal
Warfarin or heparin	Normal	Normal	↑	↑

DIC, disseminated intravascular coagulation; HUS; hemolytic uremic syndrome; ITP, idiopathic thrombocytopenic purpura; NSAIDs, nonsteroidal anti-inflammatory drugs; PT, prothrombin time; PTT, partial thromboplastin time; TTP, thrombotic thrombocytopenic purpura.

   c. Clinical findings
     (1) Arterial and venous thrombosis syndromes
     (2) Repeated abortions
       • Due to thrombosis of placental bed vessels
     (3) Strokes, thromboembolism
   d. Laboratory findings
     (1) Increased APAs
       (a) Both APAs present in 60% of cases.
       (b) One or the other is present in 40% of cases.
     (2) Prolonged PTT
       (a) Variable finding
         • Depends on amount of phospholipid used in PTT test system
       (b) Usually associated with presence of lupus anticoagulant
  2. Other acquired causes of thrombosis
   a. Postoperative state
     (1) Stasis of blood flow
     (2) Fibrin thrombus
       • Develops in deep veins of lower extremity
   b. Malignancy
     (1) Increase in coagulation factors
     (2) Thrombocytosis
     (3) Release of procoagulants from tumors
       • Particularly pancreatic cancers
   c. Folate or vitamin B_{12} deficiency
     • Due to increased plasma homocysteine levels
   d. Oral contraceptives; estrogen
     (1) Increases the synthesis of coagulation factors
     (2) Decreases synthesis of ATIII
   e. Hyperviscosity
     (1) Polycythemia syndromes
       • Hyperviscosity due to increase in RBCs

Stasis of blood flow: most common acquired cause of thrombosis

(2) Waldenström's macroglobulinemia
- Hyperviscosity due to increase in IgM

B. **Hereditary thrombosis syndromes**
1. Epidemiology
   a. Autosomal dominant syndromes
   b. Deep venous thrombosis and pulmonary emboli occur at an early age.
   c. Venous thromboses often occur in unusual places.
      - Examples—hepatic vein, dural sinus
2. Factor V Leiden
   a. Most common hereditary thrombosis syndrome
   b. Mutant form of factor V
      - Cannot be degraded by protein C and S
3. Antithrombin III (ATIII) deficiency
   a. Functions of ATIII
      (1) Activity is enhanced by heparin
      (2) Neutralizes activated serine proteases
         - Examples—XII, XI, IX, X, thrombin
   b. *No* prolongation of PTT after injecting a standard dose of heparin
   c. Treatment
      (1) Infuse a greater dose of heparin than normal
         (a) PTT eventually increases
         (b) Due to enhancement of residual ATIII
      (2) Patient is sent home on warfarin
4. Protein C and S deficiency
   a. Pathogenesis
      - Cannot inactivate factors V and VIII
   b. Treatment
      (1) Begin with heparin and a very low dose of warfarin
         - Reduces the risk for developing hemorrhagic skin necrosis
      (2) Patient is sent home on warfarin

Factor V Leiden: most common hereditary thrombosis syndrome

Hemorrhagic skin necrosis: associated with warfarin therapy in protein C deficiency

> Heterozygote carriers of protein C deficiency may develop hemorrhagic skin necrosis when placed on warfarin. Normally, heterozygote carriers have ~50% protein C activity. Protein C has a short half-life (~6 hours). When patients are placed on warfarin, protein C activity falls to zero activity in 6 hours. This produces a hypercoagulable state due to increased activity of factors V and VIII. Fibrin thrombi develop in the cutaneous vessels leading to skin necrosis.

Questions

For each of the clinical scenarios in questions 1 through 9 select the set of hemostasis test abnormalities in this table that is most likely present. Each lettered option may be selected once, more than once, or not at all.

	Platelet Count	Bleeding Time	PT	PTT
A.	↓	↑	Normal	Normal
B.	Normal	↑	Normal	↑
C.	Normal	Normal	Normal	↑
D.	↓	↑	↑	↑
E.	Normal	↑	↑	↑
F.	Normal	↑	Normal	Normal
G.	Normal	Normal	↑	↑

PTT, partial thromboplastin time; PT, prothrombin time.

1. A 3-year-old boy ingests an unknown quantity of rat poison. He is bleeding from the nose, mouth, and gastrointestinal tract. Multiple ecchymoses are also present.

2. A 70-year-old man requires a transurethral resection of the prostate gland for urinary retention secondary to benign prostate hyperplasia. Prior to surgery, his platelet count, bleeding time, PT, and PTT are all normal. Following surgery he develops severe bleeding from the penis that requires blood transfusions.

3. A 70-year-old woman in a nursing home has an indwelling urinary catheter. She suddenly develops high fever, warm skin, and bounding pulses. Shortly thereafter, she has bleeding from the mouth, nose, gastrointestinal tract, and venipuncture sites. Multiple petechiae and ecchymoses develop over the trunk and extremities. A blood culture uncovers *Escherichia coli*.

4. A 50-year-old woman has severe osteoarthritis in the hip and vertebral column. She is taking a nonsteroidal anti-inflammatory drug for pain.

5. A 25-year-old woman has history of menorrhagia since menarche at age 12. She has been diagnosed with anovulatory dysfunctional uterine bleeding. Additional complaints are easy bruisability, excessive bleeding from superficial cuts from shaving her legs, and frequent nosebleeds. Her bleeding problems improve significantly when she is taking an oral contraceptive and recur to the same level of severity when she discontinues the medication.

6. A 20-year-old man requires an extraction of an impacted wisdom tooth. He is not taking any prescription or over-the-counter drugs. He has no previous history of surgery. There is a history of bleeding problems in his mother's family, but he is not sure which individuals had the problems. Shortly after the tooth extraction, he rinses his mouth out with lukewarm water and develops severe bleeding from the tooth socket that cannot be controlled.

7. A 10-year-old boy presents with a nosebleed that is unresponsive to pinching of the nose and packing of the anterior nares. He is not taking any prescription or over-the-counter medications. Physical examination reveals scattered petechiae and ecchymoses over the anterior and posterior trunk and in the area where the blood pressure cuff was located. There is no lymphadenopathy or hepatosplenomegaly. A stool for occult blood is negative. A CBC shows a normal hemoglobin and WBC count. An abnormality is noted in the peripheral blood smear.

8. A 30-year-old woman presents with fever, headaches, and recurrent nosebleeds. Physical examination reveals retinal hemorrhages, widespread petechiae and ecchymoses, and a positive stool for occult blood. There is no lymphadenopathy or hepatosplenomegaly. Mental status examination is abnormal. The CBC shows a decreased hemoglobin and a normal WBC count and mean corpuscular volume. The corrected reticulocyte count is 10%. The peripheral smear shows numerous fragmented RBCs, polychromasia, and a platelet abnormality. There is a positive urine dipstick for blood. Renal tubular cell casts are present. The serum blood urea nitrogen is 60 mg/dL and the serum creatinine is 6 mg/dL.

9. A 55-year-old man has an anterior myocardial infarction. He is placed on aspirin, heparin, and warfarin.

10. An 18-year-old man presents with pain and swelling in the right calf. He states that his mother had numerous deep vein thromboses and pulmonary emboli and recently died from complications related to pulmonary embolization. He is concerned that he might have a similar problem. A Doppler ultrasound reveals a deep thrombosis in the right anterior tibial vein. He is placed on a standard dose of heparin and the PTT returns normal. A repeat test on a different sample also returns normal. The dose of heparin is then markedly increased and the PTT becomes prolonged. What is the most likely diagnosis?
A. Antiphospholipid syndrome
B. Antithrombin III deficiency
C. Factor V Leiden
D. Protein C or S deficiency

Answers

1. **G** is correct. Rat poison contains warfarin, which blocks epoxide reductase rendering vitamin K inactive. This prevents further γ-carboxylation of the vitamin K–dependent coagulation factors II (prothrombin), VII, IX, and X. Because factors X and II are in the final common pathway, both the PT and PTT are prolonged. The PT evaluates factors VII, X, V, II, and I (fibrinogen), and the PTT evaluates factors XII, XI, IX, VIII, X, V, II, and I. The platelet count and bleeding time are not affected by warfarin. Because the patient has serious bleeding, fresh frozen plasma is the treatment of choice.

2. **E** is correct. The patient has primary fibrinolysis due to release of urokinase from the transurethral resection of the prostate gland. Urokinase activates plasminogen to release plasmin. Plasmin degrades multiple coagulation factors (e.g., V, VIII, fibrinogen). This increases the PT and PTT. The degradation products of fibrinogen interfere with platelet aggregation causing an increase in the bleeding time. The platelet count is not affected. The test for fibrinogen degradation products is positive; however, D-dimers are negative because fibrin clots are not present in primary fibrinolysis.

3. **D** is correct. The patient has gram-negative sepsis due to *E. coli*. Endotoxins released from the pathogen damage endothelial cells causing the release of nitric oxide. Nitric oxide is a potent vasodilator. Vasodilation of the peripheral resistance arterioles produces warm skin, increases venous return to the heart, which, in turn, increases the cardiac output causing bounding pulses. Endotoxins also damage endothelial cells causing widespread release of tissue thromboplastin. Tissue thromboplastin activates the extrinsic coagulation system producing disseminated intravascular coagulation with the formation of fibrin thrombi within the microcirculation. Factors I, II, V, and VIII are consumed in the fibrin clots, which results in anticoagulation. Hence, the patient has a thrombohemorrhagic disorder leading to ischemia and excessive bleeding from all orifices, needle puncture sites, mucosa, and superficial scratches. Fibrin thrombi also trap platelets causing thrombocytopenia, which is responsible for producing petechiae and ecchymoses.

4. **F** is correct. Nonsteroidal anti-inflammatory drugs prevent platelet aggregation by preventing platelet synthesis of thromboxane A_2. This

prolongs the bleeding time, which is a test of platelet function up to the formation of a temporary platelet plug. The platelet count and PT and PTT are not affected.

5. **B** is correct. The history of menorrhagia, easy bruisability, bleeding from superficial scratches, and epistaxis all abating with oral contraceptives and recurring when off oral contraceptives is a classic scenario for von Willebrand disease. In this autosomal dominant disorder, there is a deficiency of von Willebrand factor (vWF), which is necessary for platelet adhesion to areas of endothelial injury. This prolongs the bleeding time without affecting the platelet count. vWF also complexes with factor VIII coagulant (VIII:C) in the circulation and prevents degradation of VIII:C. Therefore, deficiency of vWF automatically leads to decreased factor VIII:C activity and prolongation of the PTT. The PT is normal, because it does not evaluate VIII:C activity. The estrogen in oral contraceptives increases vWF and VIII:C activity which reverses the platelet and coagulation factor defects.

6. **C** is correct. The patient has mild hemophilia A, an X-linked recessive disorder with deficiency of VIII:C activity in the intrinsic coagulation system. Deficiency of VIII:C causes an increase in the PTT, but not the PT. The patient experienced bleeding from the extraction site, because the damaged small vessel lumens had only temporary platelet plugs held together by fibrinogen preventing the vessels from bleeding. The lack of thrombin from the VIII:C deficiency prevented conversion of the fibrinogen to fibrin producing a stable platelet thrombus held together by fibrin. When the patient rinsed his mouth out with lukewarm water, the temporary platelet plugs were dislodged causing serious bleeding.

7. **A** is correct. The patient has idiopathic thrombocytopenic purpura (ITP), the most common cause of thrombocytopenia in children. An IgG antibody is directed against platelet fibrinogen receptors causing macrophages in the spleen to phagocytose and destroy the sensitized platelets. Thrombocytopenia prolongs the bleeding time, because there are insufficient numbers of platelets to form platelet thrombi. The PT and PTT are normal, because coagulation factor synthesis is normal in ITP.

8. **A** is correct. The patient has thrombotic thrombocytopenic purpura (TTP). In this disorder, there is an acquired or genetic deficiency in vWF-cleaving metalloprotease in endothelial cells. Increase in circulating multimers of vWF increases platelet adhesion to areas of endothelial injury at arteriole-capillary junctions. Platelets are consumed owing to production of platelet thrombi in these areas of endothelial injury. TTP should not be confused with

disseminated intravascular coagulation, where activation of the coagulation system produces fibrin thrombi that consume factors I, II, V, and VIII and trap RBCs and platelets in the fibrin strands. The platelet thrombi in TTP damage RBCs producing fragmentation of RBCs in the blood. These fragmented cells are called schistocytes (see Chapter 6) and the anemia is microangiopathic hemolytic anemia. Hemoglobin is released into the blood and enters the urine producing hemoglobinuria. The patient demonstrates the clinical pentad of TTP: fever, thrombocytopenia, renal failure (BUN : creatinine ratio <15), microangiopathic hemolytic anemia with schistocytes, and central nervous system deficits.

9. **E is correct.** In an acute anterior myocardial infarction, aspirin is used to prevent thrombus formation either in the coronary arteries or the damaged endothelium in the left ventricle. Aspirin prevents platelet aggregation causing prolongation of the bleeding time without affecting the platelet count. Patients are also anticoagulated with heparin and warfarin. Heparin enhances antithrombin III activity leading to neutralization of many of the coagulation factors including thrombin and X in the final common pathway. This prolongs the PT and the PTT, although the latter test is a better test to follow heparin therapy. Warfarin inhibits further activation of the vitamin K–dependent coagulation factors (II, VII, IX, and X). Because factors II and X are in the final common pathway, the PT and PTT are both prolonged; however, the former test is a better test to follow warfarin therapy when it is converted into the international normalized ratio (INR).

10. **B (antithrombin III) is correct.** Heparin works by enhancing the activity of antithrombin III (ATIII); therefore, if the patient is deficient in ATIII, a standard dose of heparin is not sufficient to neutralize the clotting factors to prolong the PTT. However, using larger doses of heparin will enhance the activity of what little ATIII is present causing prolongation of the PTT.

A (antiphospholipid syndrome, APL) is incorrect. The APL syndrome is a thrombosis syndrome due to the presence of anticardiolipin antibodies and/or lupus anticoagulant. Standard doses of heparin will prolong the PTT in this condition.

C (factor V Leiden) is incorrect. Factor V Leiden is the most common hereditary thrombosis syndrome. Factor V Leiden is a mutant form of factor V that cannot be degraded by protein C and S. Standard doses of heparin will prolong the PTT.

D (protein C or S deficiency) is incorrect. Protein C and S normally inactivate factors V and VIII; therefore, deficiency of the proteins leads to an increase in these coagulation factors and tendency for developing thromboses. Standard doses of heparin will prolong the PTT.

CHAPTER 8

Immunohematology Disorders

I. **ABO Blood Group System**
   A. **ABO blood group antigens**
   1. Blood group O characteristics
      a. Most common blood group
         • No A or B antigens are present on the RBC membrane.
      b. Natural antibodies (isohemagglutinins) in serum
         (1) Anti-A IgM, anti-B IgM, anti-A and B IgG antibodies
         (2) Anti-A and B IgG antibodies (unlike IgM antibodies) are directed against a different antigen on group A and B RBCs.

   > Blood group antibodies are natural IgM antibodies. Natural antibodies develop against antigens that are *not* present on the RBC, which explains why blood group O patients have antibodies against both A and B antigens.

      c. Increased incidence of duodenal ulcers
   2. Blood group A characteristics
      a. Anti-B IgM antibodies
      b. Increased incidence of gastric carcinoma
   3. Blood group B characteristics
      • Anti-A IgM antibodies
   4. Blood group AB characteristics
      a. Least common blood group
      b. No natural antibodies

   B. **Newborns**
   1. Natural antibodies are *not* present at birth.
      • Synthesis of IgM begins shortly after birth.
   2. IgG antibodies are of maternal origin.
      a. Maternal IgG antibodies cross the placenta.
      b. Newborns begin synthesizing IgG shortly after birth.

   C. **Elderly people**
      • Frequently lose their natural IgM antibodies

   > Elderly patients may not have a hemolytic transfusion reaction if they are transfused with the wrong blood group because they frequently lose their natural antibodies. For example, if a patient is group B, he may not have anti-A IgM antibodies. Therefore, if he inadvertently

Group O: anti-A IgM, anti-B IgM, anti-A and B IgG
Group A: anti-B IgM
Group B: anti-A IgM
Group AB: no antibodies

Newborns: lack natural antibodies

Elderly people: frequently lose natural antibodies

	Forward Type		Back Type	
Blood group	Anti-A	Anti-B	A RBCs	B RBCs
O	–	–	+	+
A	+	–	–	+
B	–	+	+	–
AB	+	+	–	–

8-1: *Forward and back type to identify ABO blood groups. Forward type identifies the blood group antigen by reacting anti-A and anti-B against patient RBCs. Back type identifies the natural antibodies in the patient serum by reacting A RBCs and B RBCs against the patient serum. Refer to text for discussion. (From Goljan EF: Rapid Review Pathology, 2nd ed. St. Louis, Mosby, 2007, Fig. 15–01.)*

receives group A blood, there would *not* be a hemolytic transfusion reaction with destruction of the group A RBCs.

D. **Paternity issues**
   1. One or both parents are blood group AB.
      • Cannot have an O child
   2. Both parents are blood group O.
      • Cannot have an AB, A, or B child.
   3. One parent is group A and the other group B.
      • Can have an O children if both have AO and BO phenotypes
E. **Determining the ABO group** (Fig. 8-1)
   1. Forward type
      a. Identifies blood group antigen
         (1) Patient RBCs are added to test tube with anti-A test serum.
         (2) Patient RBCs are added to test tube with anti-B test serum.
      b. Blood group O does not react with anti-A or anti-B test serum.
      c. Blood group A reacts with anti-A test serum.
      d. Blood group B reacts with anti-B test serum.
      e. Blood group AB reacts with both anti-A and anti-B test serum.
   2. Back type
      a. Identifies the natural IgM antibodies
         (1) Patient serum is added to test tube with A test RBCs.
         (2) Patient serum is added to test tube with B test RBCs.
      b. Blood group O serum reacts with both A and B test RBCs.
         • Serum contains anti-A IgM and anti-B IgM.
      c. Blood group A serum reacts with B test RBCs.
         • Serum contains anti-B IgM.
      d. Blood group B serum reacts with A test RBCs.
         • Serum contains anti-A IgM.
      e. Blood group AB serum does *not* react with A or B test RBCs.
         • Serum does *not* contain any natural antibodies.

II. **Rh and Non-Rh Antigen Systems**
   A. **Rh antigen system**
      1. System has three closely located gene loci.

Forward typing: identifies blood group antigen

Back typing: identifies natural antibodies

a. Locus coding for D antigen
   (1) There is no D antigen.
      • Used in antigen profiles to indicate the absence of D antigen
   (2) Presence of D antigen is considered Rh positive.
      • 85% of the population
   (3) Absence of D antigen is considered Rh negative.
      • 15% of the population
   (4) D antigen has the greatest antigenicity of all the Rh antigens.

Five Rh antigens: D, C, c, E, e

b. Locus coding for C or c antigen
c. Locus coding for E or e antigen

2. Autosomal codominant inheritance
   a. Each antigen expresses itself when present.
   b. Child receives one set of three Rh antigens from each parent.
      (1) Example—child with CDe from the father and cde from the mother
      (2) Note that the child lacks E antigen.
   c. Possible Rh antigen profiles
      (1) DD, Dd, or dd
      (2) CC, Cc, or cc

Rh positive: D antigen positive

      (3) EE, Ee, or ee
3. Rh phenotype of an individual
   a. Patient RBCs are reacted with test antisera against each Rh antigen.
   b. Example—Rh phenotype positive for C, c, D, E antigens but negative for e antigen; phenotype is CcDE

B. **Alloimmunization**

Alloimmunization: antibodies develop against foreign antigens

1. Antibodies develop against antigens *not* present on an individual's RBCs.
   a. Patient exposure to Rh antigen they are lacking
      • Rh negative individual develops anti-D antibodies if exposed to D antigen.
   b. Patient exposure to non-Rh antigen they are lacking
      • Individual who is Kell antigen negative develops anti-Kell antibodies if exposed to Kell antigen.
   c. These Rh or non-Rh antibodies are called atypical antibodies.
      • The individual is considered sensitized if atypical antibodies are present.
2. Significance of atypical antibodies
   a. May produce a hemolytic transfusion reaction (HTR), as in the following examples
      (1) Individual with anti-D antibodies receives D antigen positive blood.
      (2) Anti-D IgG antibodies will attach to D antigen positive RBCs.
      (3) Splenic macrophages with receptors for IgG will phagocytose and destroy the D antigen positive RBCs.
      (4) Direct and indirect Coombs' test results are positive (see Chapter 5).

Individual with an atypical antibody must receive blood lacking the antigen.

   b. Transfusion requirements for sensitized individuals
      (1) Individual must receive blood that does *not* have the foreign antigen(s).

  (2) Example—individual with anti-D antibodies must receive D
    antigen negative blood.
C. **Clinically important non-Rh antigens**
 1. Duffy (Fy) antigens
  a. Binding site for infestation of RBCs by *Plasmodium vivax*
  b. Majority of black Americans lack the Fy antigen.
   • Offers protection against contracting *P. vivax* malaria
 2. I and i antigen systems
  a. IgM antibodies (cold agglutinins) may develop against I or i antigen.
  b. Increased risk for developing a cold immune hemolytic anemia (see
   Chapter 5)
   (1) Anti-i hemolytic anemia may occur in infectious mononucleosis.
   (2) Anti-I hemolytic anemia may occur in *Mycoplasma pneumoniae*
    infections.

> Fy antigen negative
> RBCs: protection against
> *P. vivax* malaria

III. **Blood Transfusion Therapy**
 A. **Blood donors**
  1. Autologous transfusion
   a. Process of collection, storage, and reinfusion of the individual's own
    blood
   b. Safest form of transfusion
  2. Tests performed on donor blood
   a. Group (ABO) and type (Rh)
   b. Antibody screen (indirect Coombs' test)
    • Detects atypical antibodies (e.g., anti-D, anti-Kell)
   c. Screening tests for infectious disease
    • Examples—syphilis, hepatitis B and C, HIV-1 and 2, HTLV-1

> Autologous transfusion:
> safest transfusion

> There is a risk for transmitting infection when transfusing blood.
> The most common infectious agent transmitted by blood
> transfusion is cytomegalovirus (CMV), which is present in donor
> lymphocytes. Risk for infection is virtually eliminated by
> transfusion of leukocyte-free blood.

> CMV: most common
> pathogen transmitted by
> transfusion

 B. **Patient crossmatch**
  1. Components of a standard crossmatch
   a. ABO group and Rh type
   b. Antibody screen for atypical antibodies
   c. Direct Coombs' test
    • Identifies atypical IgG antibodies on patient RBCs
   d. Major crossmatch
  2. Major crossmatch
   a. Purpose of a major crossmatch
    • Detect atypical antibodies directed against foreign antigens on donor
    RBCs
   b. Patient serum is mixed with a sample of RBCs from a donor unit.
    (1) Each unit of donor blood must have a separate crossmatch.

> A negative antibody
> screen ensures that a
> major crossmatch will be
> compatible.

(2) Lack of RBC agglutination or hemolysis indicates a compatible crossmatch.

> Patients with a negative antibody screen should have a compatible crossmatch, because no atypical antibodies are present. However, a compatible crossmatch does *not* guarantee that the recipient will not develop atypical antibodies against foreign antigens on donor RBCs, a transfusion reaction, or an infection.

3. Type and screen
   a. Purpose
      • For surgeries that generally do not require transfusion, but the possibility exists
   b. Testing
      (1) ABO and Rh typing
      (2) Antibody screen
      (3) Crossmatch with donor units is *not* performed.
   c. Advantages
      (1) Does not tie up donor blood
      (2) Reduces patient cost for transfusion
      (3) Easy to have blood available if transfusion is required
4. Use of blood group O packed RBCs for transfusion
   a. Can be transfused into any patient, regardless of the blood group
      (1) Blood group O RBCs lack A and B antigens.
      (2) Blood group O individuals are considered universal donors.
   b. Blood group O individuals can only receive O blood.
      • Anti-A IgM and anti-B IgM will hemolyze transfused A, B, or AB RBCs.
5. Transfusion of blood group AB individuals
   a. Can be transfused with blood from any blood group
      • They lack natural IgM antibodies.
   b. AB individuals are considered universal recipients.

> Before blood is transfused into newborns or patients with T-cell deficiencies, it must be irradiated to kill donor lymphocytes. This prevents the patient from developing a graft-versus-host reaction or a CMV infection.

C. **Blood component therapy** (Table 8-1)
D. **Transfusion reactions**
   1. Allergic reactions
      a. Most common transfusion reaction
      b. Type I IgE-mediated hypersensitivity reaction against proteins in donor blood
      c. Clinical findings
         (1) Urticaria with pruritus
         (2) Fever, tachycardia, wheezing

Blood group O individuals: universal donor

Blood group AB individuals: universal recipients

Allergic transfusion reaction: IgE mediated

TABLE 8-1
Blood Components

Component	Discussion
Packed RBCs	Purpose: increase O_2 transport to tissues Packed RBCs (1 unit) have less volume (300 mL) and a higher hematocrit than a unit of whole blood; does contain some leukocytes and platelets Each unit of packed RBCs should raise the Hb by 1 g/dL and the Hct by 3%. Lack of an incremental rise implies a hemolytic transfusion reaction or blood loss in the patient *Yersinia enterocolitica*, a pathogen that thrives on iron, is the most common contaminant of stored blood
Platelets	Purpose: stop medically significant bleeding related to thrombocytopenia (usually <30,000/mm³) or qualitative platelet defects (e.g., aspirin) Platelets have HLA antigens and ABO antigens on their surface; however, they lack Rh antigens Each unit of platelets should raise the platelet count by 5000–10,000/mm³
Fresh frozen plasma	Purpose: treatment of multiple coagulation deficiencies (e.g., DIC; cirrhosis) or treatment of warfarin over-anticoagulation if bleeding is life-threatening Contains no platelets, leukocytes, or RBCs Should be ABO compatible with the patient
Cryoprecipitate	Purpose: treatment of coagulation factor deficiencies involving fibrinogen and factor VIII (e.g., DIC) Cryoprecipitate contains fibrinogen, factor VIII, and factor XIII Desmopressin acetate stimulates production of all factor VIII components and is used instead of cryoprecipitate in treating mild hemophilia A and von Willebrand disease

DIC, disseminated intravascular coagulation; Hct, hematocrit; Hb, hemoglobin.

(3) Potential for anaphylactic shock
(4) Mild cases are treated with antihistamines.

> In IgA deficiency, patients may have antibodies directed against IgA from previous exposure to a blood product. Reexposure to IgA in a blood product may result in a severe anaphylactic reaction. Therefore, IgA-deficient individuals must receive blood or blood products that lack IgA.

2. Febrile reaction
   a. Pathogenesis
      (1) Recipient has anti-human leukocyte antigen (HLA) antibodies directed against foreign HLA antigens on donor leukocytes.
         • RBCs do *not* have HLA antigens.
      (2) Type II hypersensitivity reaction
   b. Clinical findings
      (1) Fever, chills, headache, and flushing
         • Fever due to cytokines released by leukocytes
      (2) Treated with antipyretics

Febrile transfusion reaction: anti-HLA antibodies against donor leukocytes (*not* RBCs)

> Anti-HLA antibodies develop when individuals are exposed to foreign HLA antigens (e.g., previous blood transfusion or organ transplant). Women commonly have these reactions owing to pregnancy, when there is an increased risk for exposure to fetal blood during delivery or after a spontaneous abortion.

3. Acute hemolytic transfusion reaction (HTR)
   a. May be intravascular or extravascular hemolytic reactions (see Chapter 5)
   b. Intravascular hemolysis
      (1) ABO blood group incompatibility
      (2) Example—group B patient receives group A donor blood.
         • Anti-A IgM attaches to A positive donor RBCs, producing intravascular hemolysis.
      (3) Type II hypersensitivity reaction
   c. Extravascular hemolysis
      (1) An atypical antibody reacts with a foreign antigen on donor RBCs.
         • Splenic macrophage phagocytosis and destruction of donor RBCs coated by the atypical antibody
      (2) Jaundice commonly occurs.
         • Unconjugated bilirubin (UCB) is the end product of macrophage degradation of hemoglobin (Hb).
      (3) Type II hypersensitivity reaction

Acute HTRs are due to blood group incompatibility or presence of an atypical antibody.

> Individuals who have been infused with blood in the past may have been exposed to a foreign blood group antigen and developed atypical antibodies that are no longer circulating; therefore, the pretransfusion antibody screen is negative. However, memory B cells are present and reexposure to the foreign antigen incites the formation of antibodies, resulting in an extravascular hemolytic anemia. This reaction may occur within hours to 3 to 10 days after the transfusion.

   d. Clinical findings
      (1) Fever, back pain, hypotension
      (2) Disseminated intravascular coagulation, oliguria (renal failure)
   e. Laboratory findings
      (1) Positive direct Coombs' test
         • IgG antibody or C3b is coating donor RBCs.
      (2) Positive indirect Coombs' test
         • Atypical antibody is present in serum.
      (3) *No* increase in Hb over pretransfusion levels.
      (4) Hemoglobinuria
         • Sign of intravascular hemolysis
      (5) Jaundice
         • Sign of extravascular hemolysis

IV. **Hemolytic Disease of the Newborn (HDN)**
  A. **General**
    1. Hemolysis in the fetus is due to transplacental transfer of maternal IgG.
    2. Also called erythroblastosis fetalis
       a. Erythroblastosis means presence of nucleated RBCs in peripheral blood.
       b. Indicates severe hemolytic anemia
    3. Alloimmune hemolytic anemia (see Chapter 5)
       a. Mother and fetus have different antigens on their RBCs.
       b. Example—mother is negative for D antigen and fetus is positive for D antigen.
       c. Example—mother is blood group O and fetus is blood group A.
    4. Types of HDN
       a. ABO HDN
       b. Rh HDN
  B. **ABO HDN**
    1. Epidemiology
       a. Most common HDN
          • Occurs in 20% to 25% of all pregnancies
       b. Mothers are blood group O.
       c. Fetus is either blood group A or B.
    2. Pathogenesis
       a. Blood group O individuals have anti-A and B IgG antibodies.
          (1) IgG antibodies cross the placenta and attach to fetal A or B RBCs.
          (2) Fetal splenic macrophages phagocytose sensitized RBCs.
             • Produces a mild anemia and unconjugated hyperbilirubinemia
          (3) UCB is disposed of in the mother's liver.
       b. May affect the firstborn or any future pregnancy
    3. Clinical and laboratory findings
       a. Jaundice develops within the first 24 hours after birth.
          (1) Most common cause of jaundice in this time period.
             • Fetal liver cannot handle the excess bilirubin load.
          (2) Risk for kernicterus is very small (see IV.C).
       b. Anemia
          (1) Mild normocytic anemia or no anemia at all
          (2) Exchange transfusions are rarely indicated.
       c. Positive direct Coombs' on fetal cord blood RBCs
          • Due to anti-A and B IgG antibodies coating fetal A or B RBCs
       d. Spherocytes are present in the cord blood peripheral smear.
          • Due to macrophage removal of a portion of the RBC membrane
  C. **Rh HDN**
    1. Pathogenesis
       a. Mother is Rh (D antigen) negative; fetus is Rh positive.
       b. Mother is exposed to fetal Rh positive blood (fetomaternal bleed).
          (1) Occurs during the last trimester or during childbirth itself

ABO HDN: most common HDN

ABO HDN: mother group O, fetus blood group A or B

ABO HDN: positive direct Coombs' on fetal RBCs

Rh HDN: mother Rh negative, fetus Rh positive

(2) Cytotrophoblast lining the chorionic villus is absent during the last trimester.
- Increased risk for a fetomaternal bleed

c. Mother develops anti-D IgG antibodies when exposed to fetal Rh positive cells.
- First Rh incompatible pregnancy does *not* affect the firstborn.

d. Subsequent Rh incompatible pregnancies produce anemia in the fetus.
(1) Anti-D IgG antibodies cross the placenta and attach to fetal Rh positive RBCs.
(2) Fetal splenic macrophages phagocytose RBCs, causing anemia.
(3) Severe anemia may result in high output cardiac failure (hydrops fetalis) and death.
  (a) Combined left- and right-sided heart failure with ascites and edema.
  (b) Extramedullary hematopoiesis is present in the liver and spleen.

2. Procedures used to follow sensitized women
a. Titration studies of anti-D at regular intervals
- Semiquantitative indicator and not adequate to estimate severity of hemolysis

b. Amniocentesis with measurement of bilirubin pigment
(1) Bilirubin has an optical density (OD) of 450-nm wavelength.
(2) The greater the increase of bilirubin in repeat amniocenteses, the greater the severity of hemolysis.

3. Clinical and laboratory findings
a. Degree of anemia is more severe than with ABO HDN.
- Increased numbers of nucleated RBCs in the peripheral blood

b. Jaundice develops shortly after birth.
(1) Level of UCB is much higher than with ABO HDN.
- Most of the UCB is *not* bound by albumin and circulates free in the blood.
(2) Increased risk for kernicterus
- Free, unbound lipid-soluble UCB poses the greatest risk for bilirubin entry into the brain (Fig. 8-2).

Kernicterus: free unconjugated bilirubin deposits in basal ganglia

> Kernicterus is the deposition of free (not bound to albumin) lipid-soluble UCB in the basal ganglia. Free bilirubin has access to the brain owing to an incompletely formed blood-brain barrier. Bilirubin damages neurons in the brain, causing severe dysfunction.

c. Positive direct and indirect Coombs' tests on fetal cord blood
d. Spherocytes are *not* present in cord blood.
- Macrophages phagocytose and destroy the entire RBC.

e. Exchange transfusions are required.
(1) Newborn's blood is removed and replaced with fresh blood.
(2) Corrects anemia and removes antibodies and unconjugated bilirubin.

ABO incompatibility: protects mother from Rh sensitization

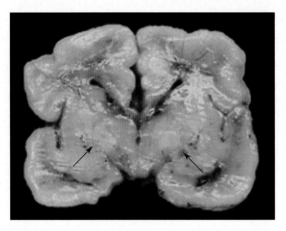

8-2: *Cross section of the brain of a newborn with kernicterus. The arrows depict yellow bilirubin pigment deposited in the basal ganglia. Bilirubin is toxic to neurons and produces long-term neurologic sequelae. (From Kumar V, Fausto N, Abbas A: Robbins and Cotran's Pathologic Basis of Disease, 7th ed. Philadelphia, WB Saunders, 2004, Fig. 10-16.)*

> ABO incompatibility protects the mother from developing Rh sensitization. For example, in a mother who is O negative and carrying a fetus who is B positive, B positive fetal RBCs entering her circulation are destroyed by maternal anti-B IgM antibodies, thereby preventing sensitization.

4. Prevention of Rh HDN in Rh negative mothers without anti-D
   a. Receive injection of anti-D globulin (Rh immune globulin) during the 28th week of pregnancy.
   b. Anti-D globulin does *not* cross the placenta.
      • Binds to and destroys fetal Rh positive RBCs if they enter her circulation
   c. Anti-D globulin lasts ~3 months in the mother's blood.
   d. Additional anti-D globulin is given after delivery if the baby is Rh positive.

Prevention of Rh HDN: Rh immune globulin (anti-D globulin)

> Special tests are performed on the mother's blood (e.g., Kleihauer-Betke or flow cytometry) that detect fetal RBCs in her blood. The amount of fetal blood is quantified and an appropriate amount of anti-D globulin is given to the mother within 72 hours. Anti-D globulin masks the antigenic sites on the fetal RBCs or destroys the fetal RBCs so that the mother does not host an antibody response against the D antigen. If the patient already has anti-D antibodies, there is no indication for giving the globulin either during or after delivery, because its main purpose is to prevent sensitization.

D. **Use of blue fluorescent light**
   1. Used as a treatment of jaundice in the newborn
   2. UCB in the skin absorbs light energy from blue fluorescent light.
      a. Photoisomerization converts UCB to a nontoxic water-soluble dipyrrole (called lumirubin).
      b. Lumirubin is excreted in bile or urine.

Blue fluorescent light: converts bilirubin in skin to water-soluble dipyrrole

Questions

1. An afebrile blood group O, Rh negative (O⁻) 75-year-old man has a massive lower gastrointestinal bleed from sigmoid diverticulosis. He has to be transfused with blood group O, Rh positive (O⁺) blood, because no group O, Rh negative (O⁻) blood is currently available in the blood banks in the area. He states that he has been transfused once in the past without any problems. In the pretransfusion workup, the patient has a negative antibody screen and a compatible major crossmatch with 4 units of group O, Rh positive (O⁺) blood. Midway through infusion of the third unit of blood he develops fever, headache, and tachycardia. The transfusion is stopped and a transfusion workup in the blood bank exhibits the following on a posttransfusion specimen of patient blood:

Patient temperature:	103°F (39.4°C)
Patient blood pressure:	130/86 mm Hg
Patient pulse:	130 beats/minute
Patient plasma:	clear
Patient antibody screen:	negative
Patient direct Coombs':	negative
Patient urine:	negative dipstick for blood

Which of the following best explains the mechanism for the transfusion reaction?
A. Delayed hemolytic transfusion reaction
B. Error in the major crossmatch
C. Hemolytic transfusion reaction related to receiving Rh positive blood
D. Histamine-related transfusion reaction
E. Patient anti-HLA antibodies directed against donor leukocytes

2. Which of the following is a characteristic of ABO hemolytic disease of the newborn (HDN) rather than Rh HDN due to anti-D?
A. Age-adjusted normocytic anemia
B. Newborn may develop anemia and jaundice in the first pregnancy
C. Positive direct Coombs' on umbilical cord RBCs
D. Severe anemia requiring an exchange transfusion
E. Unconjugated hyperbilirubinemia

3. Which of the following best characterizes a major crossmatch?
A. Guarantees survival of infused donor RBCs
B. Negative patient antibody screen usually correlates with a compatible crossmatch

  C. Prevents febrile transfusion reactions
  D. Prevents formation of antibodies against donor blood group antigens
  E. Prevents transmission of infectious diseases

4. A blood group O, Rh negative (O⁻) woman, during her first pregnancy, has a negative antibody screen. She delivers a blood group B, Rh positive (B⁺) baby. The baby develops unconjugated hyperbilirubinemia 8 hours after birth. Which of the following applies to this case?
  A. ABO incompatibility protects against Rh sensitization.
  B. Anti-D antibody caused destruction of fetal cells.
  C. Newborn has physiologic jaundice.
  D. She is not a candidate for Rh immune globulin.
  E. She is Rh compatible but ABO incompatible with her baby.

5. A 90-year-old woman who is blood group A, Rh negative (A⁻), inadvertently receives blood group B blood, Rh positive blood (B⁺). She does not develop a hemolytic transfusion reaction. Which of the following best describes why the patient has not hosted an immune response to the incompatible unit of blood?
  A. Absence of isohemagglutinins associated with old age
  B. Decreased anti-A IgM titers in the donor unit
  C. Defect in cellular immunity
  D. Patient has a genetic defect in converting pre-B cells into B cells
  E. Patient received packed RBCs rather than whole blood

6. A 32-year-old woman who is 5 days postpartum develops fever, low back pain, and a yellow discoloration in her eyes. Immediately after her delivery she had massive hemorrhage due to a retained placenta, for which she received 3 units of packed RBCs. Her pretransfusion antibody screen was negative, and all units of blood were compatible. A similar obstetric mishap occurred during her first pregnancy 14 years ago, which required 3 units of packed RBCs to normalize her blood loss. Her current CBC demonstrates a 2 g/dL drop in Hb concentration when compared to the posttransfusion level prior to discharge from the hospital. Both direct and indirect Coombs' test results are positive. A pink discoloration is noted in the serum. The total bilirubin is 3.5 mg/dL with predominantly unconjugated bilirubin present on fractionation. The serum alanine aminotransferase (ALT) concentration is 20 U/L. Which of the following best describes the mechanism for jaundice?
  A. Donor IgG antibodies are destroying patient RBCs
  B. Patient anti-HLA antibodies are destroying patient leukocytes
  C. Patient IgG antibodies are destroying transfused donor RBCs
  D. Posttransfusion fever due to cytomegalovirus
  E. Posttransfusion hepatitis due to hepatitis C

Answers

1. **E** (patient anti-HLA antibodies are directed against donor leukocytes) is correct. The patient has a febrile transfusion reaction. In these reactions, the recipient has anti-human leukocyte antigen (HLA) antibodies directed against foreign HLA antigens on donor leukocytes. Destruction of the donor leukocytes releases pyrogens causing fever as well as other findings such as chills, headache, and flushing.

   A (delayed hemolytic transfusion reaction) is incorrect. The antibody screen and direct Coombs' test are both negative. This excludes the presence of IgG antibodies in the serum attaching to foreign antigens on donor RBCs. This would lead to phagocytosis and destruction of the RBCs by splenic macrophages (extravascular hemolysis) and unconjugated hyperbilirubinemia. There is no mention made of jaundice in the patient.

   B (error in the major crossmatch) is incorrect. Although errors in crossmatching blood do occur, they are extremely rare. Furthermore, an error would not explain the correlation of fever and no evidence of hemolysis with infusion of the blood.

   C (hemolytic transfusion reaction related to receiving Rh positive blood) is incorrect. The patient had a negative antibody screen prior to his transfusions, which excludes the presence of pre-existing anti-D antibodies. Receiving D antigen positive blood would not result in the immediate development of antibodies leading to a hemolytic anemia. However, it is likely that in the future he would have to receive D antigen negative blood because of anti-D antibodies from D antigen positive transfusions.

   D (histamine-related transfusion reaction) is incorrect. The patient does not have an allergic type of transfusion reaction, which involves the release of histamine from mast cells leading to itching, flushing, and hives.

2. **B** (newborn may develop anemia and jaundice in the first pregnancy) is correct. In ABO HDN, O mothers already have anti-A and B IgG natural antibodies that react with different antigens in blood group A and B RBCs. Because IgG crosses the placenta, if the fetus is blood group A or B, the antibody will attach to the RBC and be removed by fetal splenic macrophages leading to a mild extravascular hemolytic anemia. In Rh HDN due to anti-D, the mother must first be sensitized by an Rh positive fetus before antibodies can cross the placenta and hemolyze fetal Rh positive cells in future pregnancies.

A (age-adjusted normocytic anemia) is incorrect. Both ABO and Rh HDN have a normocytic anemia; however, the former type is mild and the latter type is frequently severe.

C (positive direct Coombs' on umbilical cord RBCs) is incorrect. Both ABO and Rh HDN have a positive direct Coombs' test on cord blood RBCs, because both types have IgG antibodies coating the fetal RBCs. In ABO HDN the antibody is anti-A and B IgG, but in Rh HDN it is anti-D IgG.

D (severe anemia requiring an exchange transfusion) is incorrect. Only Rh HDN is associated with a severe anemia requiring transfusion to prevent hydrops fetalis (left- and right-sided heart failure).

E (unconjugated hyperbilirubinemia) is incorrect. Both ABO and Rh HDN have macrophage destruction of sensitized fetal RBCs leading to an unconjugated hyperbilirubinemia.

3. **B** (negative patient antibody screen usually correlates with a compatible crossmatch) is correct. An antibody screen (indirect Coombs' test) detects atypical antibodies that could potentially attack donor RBC antigens. If the antibody screen is negative, then the major crossmatch (recipient serum + donor RBCs) should be compatible.

A (guarantees survival of infused donor RBCs) is incorrect. All packed RBC transfusions contain a small amount of plasma containing the natural antibodies of the recipient. Therefore, if packed O RBCs are given to an A, B, or AB blood group patient, donor anti-A IgM, anti-B IgM, and anti-A and B IgG antibodies can attach to recipient RBCs, leading to a minimal degree of macrophage destruction of the recipient RBCs.

C (prevents febrile transfusion reactions) is incorrect. Febrile transfusion reactions are due to recipient anti-HLA antibodies against donor leukocytes. The antibody screen does *not* detect these antibodies; therefore, febrile transfusion reactions cannot be prevented.

D (prevents formation of antibodies against donor blood group antigens) is incorrect. With the possible exception of identical twins, no two individuals have exactly the same RBC antigen profile. Therefore, a recipient is exposed to foreign antigens from donor RBCs and can develop antibodies against them.

E (prevents transmission of infectious diseases) is incorrect. Although donor blood is screened for most of the important infectious diseases, some donors may be in the incubation phase of an infection and not have antibodies present in the blood.

4. **A** (ABO incompatibility protects against Rh sensitization) is correct. The newborn is both ABO and Rh incompatible with the mother. If a fetomaternal bleed occurred before or during delivery, the B⁺ fetal RBCs would have been destroyed by maternal anti-B IgM antibodies, significantly reducing the potential for sensitization against the fetal D antigen positive RBCs.

B (anti-D antibody caused destruction of fetal cells) is incorrect. The mother has a negative antibody screen, which rules out the possibility of Rh hemolytic disease of the newborn (HDN).

C (newborn has physiologic jaundice) is incorrect. The newborn has ABO HDN, which is the most common cause of jaundice in the first 24 hours after birth. Physiologic jaundice usually begins on day 3 of life. It is caused by normal macrophage destruction of fetal RBCs.

D (she is not a candidate for Rh immune globulin) is incorrect. The mother is Rh negative and has a negative antibody screen. Because the fetus is Rh positive, she is a candidate for receiving Rh immune globulin even though ABO HDN is protective against Rh sensitization.

E (she is Rh compatible but ABO incompatible with her baby) is incorrect. The mother is both ABO and Rh incompatible with the baby.

5. **A** (absence of isohemagglutinins associated with old age) is correct. As people age, their isohemagglutinins (natural antibodies) diminish in concentration or are entirely absent, which is most likely the case in this 90-year-old woman. Because she does not have any anti-B IgM antibodies in her serum, the donor B RBCs were not destroyed.

B (decreased anti-A IgM titers in the donor unit) is incorrect. Donor anti-A IgM antibodies are likely present; however, they would not likely produce significant destruction of the recipient's A RBCs.

C (defect in cellular immunity) is incorrect. There is a slight decrease in cellular immunity with old age; however, cellular immunity defects are not involved in any of the transfusion reactions (i.e., allergic, febrile, hemolytic).

D (patient has a genetic defect in converting pre-B cells into B cells) is incorrect. This type of defect occurs in Bruton's agammaglobulinemia, which is an X-linked recessive disorder. Because the patient is a woman, this diagnosis is excluded.

E (patient received packed RBCs rather than whole blood) is incorrect. Receiving packed RBCs does not have any effect on preventing hemolytic transfusion reactions.

6. **C** (patient IgG antibodies are destroying transfused donor RBCs) is correct. The patient has a delayed hemolytic transfusion reaction. She has a positive direct and indirect Coombs' test, free Hb in her serum, and a significant drop in her posttransfusion Hb concentration after leaving the hospital. It is likely that she was sensitized during her first pregnancy, but the antibody titers were too low to detect in the antibody screen she had prior to transfusion during her recent hospitalization.

A (donor IgG antibodies are destroying patient RBCs) is incorrect. Although donor packed RBCs do contain small amounts of plasma containing natural antibodies, they are not responsible for producing hemolytic transfusion reactions.

B (patient anti-HLA antibodies are destroying patient leukocytes) is incorrect. This describes a febrile type of hemolytic transfusion reaction, which is not present in this patient.

D (posttransfusion fever due to cytomegalovirus) is incorrect. Cytomegalovirus is the most common pathogen transmitted by blood transfusion; however, this patient's fever is related to a hemolytic transfusion reaction.

E (posttransfusion hepatitis due to hepatitis C) is incorrect. The time interval from her transfusion is too short to develop signs of hepatitis. A hemolytic transfusion reaction is responsible for her jaundice and fever.

9

Clinical Chemistry

I. Total Serum Protein

A. Components

1. Sum total of globulins (α_1-, α_2-, β-, γ-globulins) + albumin
2. Serum protein electrophoresis (SPE; Fig. 9-1A)
   a. Protein fractions separate on the basis of size and charge
   b. Albumin
      (1) Protein with the most negative charges
         • Contains the most acidic amino acids with COO^- groups
      (2) Migrates furthest to the anode (positive pole)
   c. Globulin fractions
      (1) α_1 Fraction
         • Contains α_1-antitrypsin
      (2) α_2 Fraction
         • Contains haptoglobin
      (3) β Fraction
         • Contains transferrin and complement
      (4) γ Fraction
         (a) Contains most of the immunoglobulins (Igs)
         (b) Contains proteins with the most positive charges
            • Remain close to the point of application, which is near the cathode (negative pole)
         (c) IgG is responsible for the normal size of the γ-globulin curve.
            • Most abundant immunoglobulin (IgG > IgA > IgM)

B. Increased total serum protein (hyperproteinemia)

1. Etiology
   a. Most commonly due to an increase in γ-globulins
   b. Examples—chronic inflammation, malignant plasma cell disorders
2. Chronic inflammation
   a. Increase in the synthesis of IgG antibodies
   b. Causes a diffuse enlargement of γ-globulin curve (Fig. 9-1B)
      (1) Many clones of plasma cells are synthesizing IgG.
         • Called a polyclonal gammopathy
      (2) Albumin is slightly decreased
         • Catabolic effect of inflammation
   c. Examples—tuberculosis, rheumatoid arthritis, cirrhosis, AIDS

> In AIDS, nonspecific polyclonal stimulation of B cells by Epstein-Barr virus and cytomegalovirus causes increased synthesis of IgG.

Total serum protein: globulins + albumin

γ-Globulin fraction: contains immuno-globulins; IgG most abundant

Hyperproteinemia: chronic inflammation most common cause

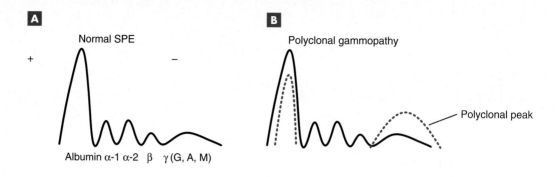

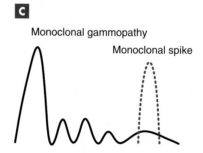

9-1: *Serum protein electrophoresis (SPE) with normal SPE (**A**), polyclonal gammopathy (**B**), and monoclonal gammopathy (**C**).*

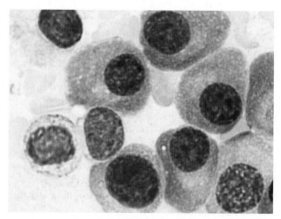

9-2: *Malignant plasma cells in multiple myeloma. The majority of malignant plasma cells show a gray-blue cytoplasm, peripherally located nuclei, and perinuclear clearing. (From Hoffbrand AV: Color Atlas: Clinical Hematology, 3rd ed. St. Louis, Mosby, 2000, Fig. 12.4B.)*

3. Malignant plasma cell disorders (Table 9-1, Fig. 9-2)
    a. Monoclonal B-cell disorders
        (1) Increase in a single immunoglobulin
        (2) Increase in corresponding light chain
    b. Ig detected as a monoclonal spike (M component) on SPE (see Fig. 9-1C)

Plasma cell dyscrasia:
monoclonal spike

TABLE 9-1
Selected Plasma
Cell Disorders

Disorder	Comments
MGUS	Most common monoclonal gammopathy Small IgG M spike in elderly patients Plasma cells <3% in bone marrow No BJ protein

Multiple myeloma	Epidemiology: rare under 40 years of age
	M spike occurs in 80–90% of cases
	   Usually IgG kappa
	   Urine BJ protein positive in 60–80% of cases
	Pathologic findings
	   Sheets of malignant plasma cells in bone marrow aspirate
	     (see Fig. 9-2)
	   Plasma cells >10% of cells in aspirate
	Bone pain: due to "punched out" lytic lesions (vertebra, skull, ribs)
	Hypercalcemia in 25% of cases
	Renal failure in 30–50% of cases, due to:
	   Proteinaceous tubular casts (contain BJ protein) damage tubular
	     epithelium
	   Nephrocalcinosis: calcification tubular basement membranes in
	     collecting ducts
	   Primary amyloidosis: light chains converted into amyloid
	Normocytic anemia with rouleaux
	Prolonged bleeding time: defect in platelet aggregation
	Recurrent infections: most common cause of death
	Median survival 6 months without treatment

Lymphoplasmacytic lymphoma (Waldenström's macroglobulinemia)	Neoplastic lymphoplasmacytoid B cells
	Elderly male-dominant disease
	M spike with IgM
	BJ protein is present
	Generalized lymphadenopathy (*not* present in myeloma)
	Anemia and bone marrow (*no* lytic lesions like myeloma), liver,
	   and spleen involvement
	Hyperviscosity syndrome due to increased IgM: retinal
	   hemorrhages, strokes, platelet aggregation defects
	Median survival 5 years

BJ, Bence-Jones; MGUS, monoclonal gammopathy of undetermined significance.

   c. Most commonly due to an increase in IgG.
     • Other plasma cell clones are suppressed
   d. Bence Jones (BJ) protein
     • Excess κ or λ light chains excreted in urine
   e. Immunoelectrophoresis or immunofixation
     • Identify Ig and light chain in serum and light chains in
      urine
C. **Decreased total serum protein (hypoproteinemia)**
   1. Etiology
     a. Decrease in albumin (hypoalbuminemia)
     b. Decrease in γ-globulin (hypogammaglobulinemia)

Bence Jones protein: light chains in the urine

Hypoproteinemia: hypoalbuminemia most common cause

    2. Hypoalbuminemia
      a. Decreased intake of protein
        • Example—kwashiorkor
      b. Decreased synthesis of albumin
        • Examples—cirrhosis, chronic inflammation
      c. Nephrotic syndrome (see Chapter 4)
        (1) Protein loss > 3.5 g protein/24 hours
        (2) Lipoid nephrosis most common cause in children
        (3) Membranous glomerulopathy most common cause in adults
      d. Gastrointestinal loss
        (1) Celiac disease
          • Loss of villi reduces absorptive surface
        (2) Chronic pancreatitis
          • Loss of enzymes interferes with protein degradation
        (3) Large villous adenoma
          • Loss of protein in mucus
      e. Third-degree burns
        • Loss of plasma in burns
    3. Hypogammaglobulinemia
      a. Bruton's agammaglobulinemia
        • Pure B-cell deficiency (children)
      b. Common variable immune deficiency
        • Pure B-cell deficiency (adults)
      c. Chronic lymphocytic leukemia
        • Neoplastic B cells cannot transform into plasma cells.
      d. Nephrotic syndrome
        • Globulins lost in the urine

II. **Serum Calcium and Phosphorus**
  A. **Overview**
    1. Superior and inferior parathyroid glands
      • Derive from fourth pharyngeal pouch and third pharyngeal pouch, respectively
    2. Parathyroid hormone (PTH)
      a. Increases calcium reabsorption in early distal tubule
      b. Decreases bicarbonate reclamation in proximal tubule
      c. Decreases phosphorus reabsorption in proximal tubule
      d. Maintains ionized calcium level in blood
        (1) Increases bone resorption and renal reabsorption of calcium
        (2) Vitamin D also involved in calcium maintenance
      e. Stimulated by hypocalcemia and hyperphosphatemia
      f. Suppressed by hypercalcemia and hypophosphatemia
    3. Total serum calcium
      a. Components of the total serum calcium (Fig. 9-3A)
        (1) Calcium bound to albumin (40%) and phosphorus and citrate (13%)

Total serum calcium: calcium bound + calcium free (ionized)

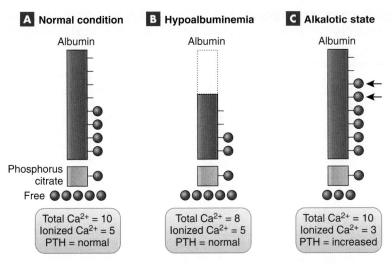

9-3: *Total serum calcium in a normal individual (**A**), individual with hypoalbuminemia (**B**), and individual with alkalosis (**C**). Refer to text for discussion. PTH, parathyroid hormone. (From Goljan EF: Rapid Review Pathology, 2nd ed. St. Louis, Mosby, 2007, Fig. 22-06.)*

    (2) Free, ionized calcium (47%)
        • Metabolically active fraction has a negative feedback with PTH
  b. Hypoalbuminemia (see Fig. 9-3B)
    (1) Decreased total serum calcium
        • Due to a decrease in calcium bound to albumin
    (2) Correction for decreased albumin
        • Corrected calcium = serum calcium − serum albumin + 4
    (3) Normal free ionized level, normal PTH
    (4) *No* evidence of tetany
  c. Effect of respiratory or metabolic alkalosis (Fig. 9-3C)
    (1) Increases negative charges on albumin
      (a) Less hydrogen ions on the COOH groups of acidic amino acids
        • Change of COOH groups to COO⁻
      (b) Extra negative charges bind some of the ionized calcium (arrows in schematic).
    (2) Total serum calcium remains normal.
    (3) Decreased ionized calcium, increased PTH
    (4) Patient develops tetany.

> Tetany is due to a decreased ionized calcium level. It causes partial depolarization of nerves and muscle, which lowers the threshold potential (E_t) causing it to come closer to the resting membrane potential (E_m). A smaller stimulus is required to initiate an action potential. Clinical findings of tetany include carpopedal spasm (thumb flexes into the palm) and Chvostek's sign (facial twitch after tapping the facial nerve).

Hypoalbuminemia: ↓ total serum calcium, normal ionized calcium

Alkalosis: normal total serum calcium, decreased ionized calcium

TABLE 9-2
Selected Causes of
Hypercalcemia

Disorder	Comments

Primary hyperparathyroidism	Epidemiology: most common nonmalignant cause of hypercalcemia
	  Female dominant (>50 yr old).
	  Association with MEN I and MEN IIa
	  Causes: adenoma (85% of cases), primary hyperplasia, carcinoma
	Laboratory findings
	  Increased serum PTH, increased calcium, decreased phosphorus
	  Normal anion gap metabolic acidosis: decreased proximal tubule reclamation of bicarbonate (proximal RTA)
	  Chloride/phosphorus ratio >33: ratio of <29/1 excludes primary HPTH
	Diagnosis: technetium-99m-sestamibi radionuclide scan
	Treatment: surgical removal of the adenoma

Malignancy-induced	Mechanisms: bone metastasis with activation of osteoclasts (most common), ectopic secretion of a PTH-related protein (e.g., squamous cell carcinoma of lung, renal cell carcinoma) Multiple myeloma: increased secretion of osteoclast-activating factor (IL-1) by malignant plasma cells Laboratory findings: hypercalcemia with decreased serum PTH
Sarcoidosis	Mechanism: macrophages in granulomas synthesize 1-α-hydroxylase, causing hypervitaminosis D
Hypervitaminosis D Thiazides	Increased calcium reabsorption in the jejunum and kidneys Mechanism: block in Na^+-Ca^- cotransporter increases Ca^+ reabsorption

HPTH, hyperparathyroidism; IL, interleukin; MEN, multiple endocrine neoplasia syndrome; PTH, parathyroid hormone; RTA, renal tubular acidosis.

Hypercalcemia: primary hyperparathyroidism, malignancy-induced most common causes

B. **Increased serum calcium (hypercalcemia)**
  1. Etiology (Table 9-2)
  2. Clinical findings
    a. Calcium renal stones
    b. Nephrocalcinosis
      (1) Metastatic calcification of collecting duct basement membrane
      (2) Produces nephrogenic diabetes insipidus with polyuria and renal failure
    c. Peptic ulcer disease
      • Calcium stimulates gastrin, which increases gastric acid.
    d. Acute pancreatitis
      • Calcium activates phospholipase.
    e. Osteitis fibrosa cystica
      (1) Occurs in primary hyperparathyroidism
      (2) Cystic and hemorrhagic bone lesion
        • Commonly occurs in the jaw
      (3) Caused by increased osteoclastic activity
    f. Subperiosteal bone resorption of phalanges and tooth sockets
      • Common finding in primary hyperparathyroidism

Hypocalcemia: most common cause previous thyroid surgery

C. **Decreased serum calcium (hypocalcemia)**
  1. Etiology (Table 9-3)

TABLE 9-3
Selected Causes of Hypocalcemia

Disorder	Comments

Hypoparathyroidism	Etiology
	    Previous thyroid surgery (most common cause)
	    Autoimmune hypoparathyroidism
	    DiGeorge syndrome: failure of descent of 3rd and 4th pharyngeal
	        pouches, absence of parathyroid glands, absent thymus (pure
	        T cell deficiency)
	    Hypomagnesemia: magnesium is a cofactor for adenylate cyclase;
	        cAMP is required for PTH activation
	        Causes of hypomagnesemia: diarrhea, aminoglycosides,
	            diuretics, alcoholism
	Laboratory findings
	    Hypocalcemia, hyperphosphatemia, decreased PTH

Hypovitaminosis D	Etiology
	    Lack of sunlight: decreased photoconversion of cholesterol to
	        vitamin D in the skin
	    Malabsorption (e.g., celiac disease): decreased reabsorption of
	        fat-soluble vitamin D
	    Cirrhosis: decreased synthesis of 25-hydroxyvitamin D (decreased
	        25-hydroxylation)
	    Drugs enhancing cytochrome system (e.g., alcohol, phenytoin):
	        increased metabolism of 25-hydroxyvitamin D
	    Chronic renal failure: decreased synthesis of
	        1,25-hydroxyvitamin D (decreased 1-α-hydroxylation)

Acute pancreatitis	Calcium is bound to fatty acids in enzymatic fat necrosis Poor prognostic sign
Pseudohypoparathyroidism	Autosomal dominant disease End-organ resistance to PTH Mental retardation, basal ganglia calcification, short 4th and 5th metacarpals ("knuckle-knuckle-dimple-dimple" sign) Hypocalcemia, normal to increased PTH

cAMP, cyclic adenosine monophosphate; PTH, parathyroid hormone.

2. Clinical findings
   a. Tetany (see II.A)
   b. Osteomalacia
      (1) Decreased mineralization of bone
         • Excess osteoid in bone
      (2) Pathologic fractures, bow legs
      (3) Called rickets in children
         (a) Pathologic fractures, bow legs
         (b) Craniotabes (soft skull bones)
         (c) Rachitic rosary
            • Defective mineralization and overgrowth of epiphyseal
              cartilage in ribs
   c. Secondary hyperparathyroidism
      (1) Hyperplasia of all four parathyroid glands
         • Compensation for hypocalcemia (e.g., hypovitaminosis D)
      (2) Decreased calcium, increased PTH

TABLE 9-4
Selected Causes of
Hyperphosphatemia

Condition	Comments
Chronic renal failure	Decreased excretion of phosphorus as titratable acid
Normal child	Children require increased serum phosphorus to drive calcium into bone for mineralization
Primary hypoparathyroidism	Decreased excretion of phosphorus as titratable acid
Increased phosphorus load	Newborn drinking undiluted cow milk
	Rhabdomyolysis: rupture of muscle
	Tumor lysis syndrome: treatment of cancer releases phosphorus from killed tumor cells

(3) May develop tertiary hyperparathyroidism (HPTH)
    (a) Glands become resistant to the hypercalcemic stimulus

Secondary HPTH: compensation for hypocalcemia

    (b) May bring serum calcium into a normal or increased range
  d. Calcification of basal ganglia
    (1) Occurs in autoimmune hypoparathyroidism
    (2) Due to metastatic calcification
      • Increased phosphorous drives calcium into the brain tissue

  D. Increased serum phosphorus

Hyperphosphatemia: renal failure most common cause

    1. Etiology (Table 9-4)
    2. Clinical findings
      a. Metastatic calcification
        • Excess phosphorus drives calcium into normal tissue
      b. Hypovitaminosis D
        • Hyperphosphatemia inhibits the synthesis of 1-α-hydroxylase.

  E. Decreased serum phosphorus

Hypophosphatemia: alkalosis most common cause

    1. Etiology (Table 9-5)
    2. Clinical findings
      a. Muscle weakness
        (1) Decreased synthesis of ATP causes muscle weakness.
        (2) Muscle paralysis and rhabdomyolysis may occur.
      b. RBC hemolysis

Insulin therapy: danger of developing hypophosphatemia

        • RBCs require ATP to maintain pumps and membrane integrity.
  F. Summary of laboratory findings in calcium and phosphorus disorders
  (Table 9-6)

III. **Serum Uric Acid**
    • End product of purine metabolism
  A. Increased serum uric acid (hyperuricemia)
    • Etiology (Table 9-7)

Hyperuricemia: gout most common cause

  B. Decreased serum uric acid (hypouricemia)
    • Etiology (Table 9-8)

IV. **Serum Iron**
    • See Chapter 5.

TABLE 9-5
Selected Causes of
Hypophosphatemia

Disorder	Comments
Hypovitaminosis D (extrarenal causes)	Decreased reabsorption of phosphorus from small intestine and kidneys
Insulin Rx in DKA	Increased cell uptake of glucose requires phosphorus for phosphorylation
Primary HPTH	Increased PTH decreases phosphorus reabsorption in the proximal tubules
Proximal tubule dysfunction	Phosphorus is normally reabsorbed in proximal tubule Nephrotoxic acute tubular necrosis: aminoglycosides (most common cause), heavy metals (lead, mercury) Fanconi syndrome: generalized proximal tubular dysfunction leading to glucosuria, phosphaturia, aminoaciduria, loss of bicarbonate, loss of uric acid
Respiratory/metabolic alkalosis	Alkalosis activates phosphofructokinase causing increased phosphorylation of glucose
Intravenous infusion of fructose	Fructose uses up phosphorus for phosphorylation (fructose 1-phosphate)
Vitamin D–resistant rickets	X-linked dominant disorder Defect in renal and gastrointestinal reabsorption of phosphorus

DKA, diabetic ketoacidosis; HPTH, hyperparathyroidism; PTH, parathyroid hormone; Rx, treatment.

TABLE 9-6
Summary of
Selected Calcium
and Phosphorus
Disorders

Disorder	Serum Calcium	Serum Phosphorus	Serum PTH
Primary hypoparathyroidism	↓	↑	↓
Vitamin D deficiency: e.g., renal failure	↓	↑	↑
Vitamin D deficiency: e.g., malabsorption	↓	↓	↑
Primary HPTH	↑	↓	↑
Malignancy-induced hypercalcemia	↑	↑	↓

HPTH, hyperparathyroidism; PTH, parathyroid hormone.

V. **Serum Glucose**
  A. **Overview**
    1. Metabolic fuel
      a. Muscle (initial stage of exercise), RBC, brain
      b. Glucose in fed state
        (1) Derives from metabolism of lactose, sucrose, maltose
        (2) Complete oxidation yields 36 to 38 ATP
      c. Glucose in fasting state
        (1) Liver glycogenolysis
          • Main supplier for 16 hours
        (2) Gluconeogenesis
          • Primary source of glucose

TABLE 9-7
Selected Causes of Hyperuricemia

Disorder	Comments

Gout	Pathogenesis
	  Decreased renal excretion (most common cause; 90% of cases)
	  Overproduction (10% of cases)
	Recurrent acute arthritis
	  Commonly involves the first metatarsophalangeal joint
	  Fever, pain, and neutrophilic leukocytosis
	  MSU phagocytosed by neutrophils in SF
	Chronic gout
	  Tophi are produced: deposits of MSU in soft tissue around joints

Diuretic therapy	Volume contraction increases proximal tubule reabsorption Decreased secretion in proximal tubule
Massive cell destruction	Increased release of purines leads to increased synthesis of uric acid Commonly occurs in the treatment of leukemias and lymphomas Allopurinol, an xanthine oxidase inhibitor, should be started *before* chemotherapy Polycythemia vera: increased number of hematopoietic cells with increased release of purines Urate nephropathy can cause acute renal failure
Metabolic acidosis	Uric acid competes with anions from other acids for excretion in the proximal tubule (e.g., ketoacids, lactic acid)
Lead poisoning	Decreases excretion of uric acid in the proximal tubules

MSU, monosodium urate; SF, synovial fluid.

TABLE 9-8
Selected Causes of Hypouricemia

Disorder	Comments
SIADH	Increased plasma volume from excessive renal reabsorption of water increases glomerular filtration rate: uric acid is lost in the urine Dilutional effect in plasma from excess water
Normal pregnancy	Normal increase in plasma volume increases glomerular filtration rate: uric acid is lost in urine Dilutional effect of increased plasma volume

SIADH, syndrome of inappropriate secretion of antidiuretic hormone.

Hyperglycemia: diabetes mellitus most common cause

Diabetes mellitus: type 2 most common type

2. Serum glucose is 15% higher than whole blood glucose.
   • Whole blood glucose × 1.15 equals serum glucose.
B. **Increased serum glucose (hyperglycemia)**
   1. Etiology (Table 9-9)
   2. Diabetes mellitus
      a. Classification
         (1) Type 1 and type 2 diabetes mellitus (Table 9-10)
         (2) Secondary causes
            • Examples—chronic pancreatitis, glucocorticoids, Cushing syndrome
         (3) Impaired glucose tolerance (IGT)
         (4) Gestational diabetes mellitus (GDM)

Disorder	Comments
Diabetes mellitus	Refer to text (V.B)
Endocrine hyperfunction	Acromegaly, hyperthyroidism, Cushing's syndrome, pheochromocytoma, glucagonoma
Acute myocardial infarction	Due to release of catecholamines from the CNS which increases glycogenolysis
Stroke	Due to release of catecholamines from the CNS which increases glycogenolysis
Metabolic acidosis	Inhibits glycolysis

CNS, central nervous system.

TABLE 9-9
Selected Causes of Hyperglycemia

Characteristic	Type 1	Type 2
Prevalence	5–10%	90–95%
Age of onset	<20 years	>30 years
Speed of onset	Rapid	Insidious
Body habitus	Usually thin	Usually obese (80% of cases)
Genetics	Family history uncommon HLA-DR3 and HLA-DR4 association	Family history common No HLA association
Pathogenesis	Lack of insulin Pancreas devoid of β-islet cells Insulitis: T cell cytokine destruction and autoantibodies against β-islet cells and insulin Triggers for destruction—viruses, drugs	Insulin resistance Decreased insulin receptors: down-regulation by increased adipose Postreceptor defects: most important factor. Examples—tyrosine kinase defects, GLUT-4 abnormalities
Clinical findings	Polyuria, polydipsia, polyphagia, weight loss	Insidious onset of symptoms Recurrent blurry vision: alteration in lens refraction from increased water via sorbitol (osmotically active) Recurrent infections: bacterial, *Candida* Target organ disease: nephropathy, retinopathy, neuropathy, CAD Reactive hypoglycemia: too much insulin is released for a glucose load (early finding)
	Ketoacidosis (hyperglycemia, coma; production of ketone bodies)	HNKC: enough insulin to prevent ketoacidosis but not enough to prevent hyperglycemia Lactic acidosis may occur due to shock
Treatment	Insulin	Weight loss: up-regulates insulin receptor synthesis Oral hypoglycemic agents; may require insulin

CAD, coronary artery disease; GLUT, glucose transport unit; HLA, human leukocyte antigen; HNKC, hyperosmolar nonketotic coma.

TABLE 9-10
Comparison Between Types 1 and 2 Diabetes Mellitus

(5) Maturity-onset diabetes of the young (MODY)
  (a) Autosomal dominant inheritance
  (b) Patients are younger than 25 years old.
  (c) Mild hyperglycemia
    • Impaired glucose-induced secretion of insulin release
  (d) Resistance to ketosis
  (e) May progress into type 2 diabetes mellitus
(6) Syndrome X (metabolic syndrome)
  (a) Genetic defect causes insulin resistance
    • Exacerbated by obesity
  (b) Hyperinsulinemia
    • Contributes to hypertriglyceridemia, hypertension, coronary artery disease
  (c) Obesity exacerbates insulin resistance
    • Increased adipose down-regulates insulin receptor synthesis

> Defining levels of the metabolic syndrome (syndrome X) include waist circumference > 102 cm (>40 in) in men and > 88 cm (>35 in) in women; serum triglyceride ≥150 mg/dL; HDL < 40 mg/dL in men and < 50 mg/dL in women; blood pressure ≥130/85 mm Hg; and a fasting glucose ≥110 mg/dL.

b. Pathologic processes in diabetes mellitus
  (1) Poor glycemic control
    • Key factor that produces organ damage
  (2) Nonenzymatic glycosylation (NEG)
    (a) Glucose combines with amino groups in proteins.
    (b) Produces advanced glycosylation products
      • Causing increased vessel permeability to protein, increased atherogenesis
    (c) Production of glycosylated HbA_{1c}
    (d) Pathologic effects
      • Renal failure, stroke
  (3) Osmotic damage
    (a) Aldose reductase converts glucose to sorbitol
      • Sorbitol draws water into tissue causing damage.
    (b) Pathologic effects
      • Cataracts, peripheral neuropathy, retinopathy
c. Insulin-induced hypoglycemia (see V.C)
d. Diabetic ketoacidosis (DKA, Fig. 9-4)
  (1) Complication of type 1 diabetes
  (2) Produces severe volume depletion and coma
    • Volume depletion due to loss of sodium and water with osmotic diuresis

Margin notes:

Syndrome X: insulin resistance syndrome

Good glycemic control prevents complications of diabetes.

Aldose reductase: converts glucose to sorbitol; osmotic damage

Insulin-induced hypoglycemia: most common complication of diabetes

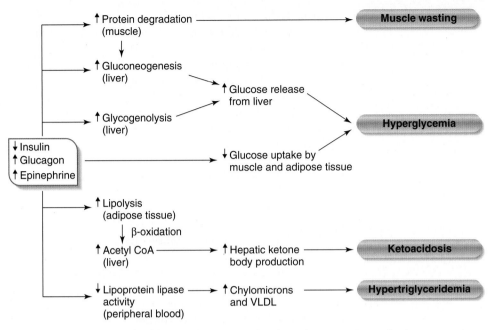

9-4: *Laboratory findings in diabetic ketoacidosis. VLDL, very low density lipoprotein. See text for discussion. (From Pelley JW, Goljan EF: Rapid Review Biochemistry, 2nd ed. St. Louis, Mosby, 2007, Fig. 9-5.)*

(3) Mechanisms for hyperglycemia
    (a) Increased gluconeogenesis
        • Due to increase in glucagon and epinephrine
    (b) Increased glycogenolysis in the liver
(4) Mechanism for ketone body synthesis
    (a) Increased lipolysis with release of fatty acids
    (b) Increased β-oxidation of fatty acids
        • Increases production of acetyl CoA
    (c) Acetyl CoA is converted by the liver to ketone bodies.
        • Acetone (fruity odor), acetoacetic and β-hydroxybutyric acid
(5) Mechanism for hypertriglyceridemia
    (a) Lack of hydrolysis of chylomicrons
        • Chylomicrons contain diet-derived triglyceride.
    (b) Lack of hydrolysis of very low density lipoprotein (VLDL)
        • VLDL contains liver-derived triglyceride.
(6) Laboratory findings in DKA
    (a) Hyperglycemia
        • Glucose ranges from 250 to 1000 mg/dL
    (b) Dilutional hyponatremia (see Chapter 2)
        • Glucose causes water to shift out of the intracellular fluid compartment into the extracellular fluid compartment.

Gluconeogenesis: most important mechanism of hyperglycemia in DKA

Ketone bodies: acetone, acetoacetic and β-hydroxybutyric acid

    (c) Hyperkalemia (see Chapter 2)
- Transcellular shift as excess H^+ ions enter cells in exchange for potassium.

    (d) Increased anion gap metabolic acidosis (see Chapter 2)
- Due to ketoacidosis and lactic acidosis

    (e) Prerenal azotemia (see Chapter 4)
- Due to volume depletion

e. Hyperosmolar nonketotic coma

    (1) Complication of type 2 diabetes

    (2) Increased mortality rate (20–50%)
- Patients are older and usually have underlying cardiac and renal problems.

f. Laboratory diagnosis

    (1) Criteria

        (a) Two fasting plasma glucose values ≥126 mg/dL
- Set for high sensitivity

        (b) Two-hour glucose evaluation after 75 g glucose challenge > 200 mg/dL (normal < 140 mg/dL)

    (2) Glycosylated hemoglobin (HbA_{1c})

        (a) Evaluates long-term glycemic control

        (b) Mean glucose value for the preceding 8 to 12 weeks

        (c) Test is *not* used to diagnose diabetes.

        (d) HbA_{1c} < 7% reduces microvascular complications.

    (3) Fructosamine
- Reflects glycemic control for the preceding 2 weeks

> HbA_{1c}: evaluates long-term glycemic control

g. Impaired glucose tolerance

    (1) Hyperglycemia that is nondiagnostic of diabetes

        (a) Fasting glucose 100 to 125 mg/dL

        (b) Two-hour glucose test after 75 g glucose challenge 140 to 200 mg/dL

    (2) Increased risk for macrovascular disease and neuropathy

    (3) Approximately 30% develop diabetes within 10 years.

h. Gestational diabetes mellitus

    (1) Glucose intolerance develops during pregnancy due to

        (a) Increased placental size

        (b) Anti-insulin effect of human placental lactogen

    (2) Screening

        (a) All pregnant women screened between 24 and 28 weeks' gestation

        (b) 50 g glucose challenge followed by 1-hour glucose level
- ≥140 mg/dL is a positive screen (normal < 140 mg/dL)

        (c) Positive screen is confirmed with a 3-hour oral (100 g) glucose tolerance test
- Fasting ≥ 95 mg/dL, 1 hour ≥ 180 mg/dL, 2 hour ≥ 155 mg/dL, 3 hour ≥ 140 mg/dL (GDM diagnosed if two or more values are above the criteria.)

(3) Neonatal risks if GDM poorly controlled

    (a) Neonatal hypoglycemia

      • High insulin levels at birth drives glucose into the hypoglycemic range.

    (b) Respiratory distress syndrome

      • High fetal insulin levels inhibit surfactant synthesis.

(4) Maternal risk

    • More than 50% develop type 2 diabetes at a later date.

C. Decreased serum glucose (hypoglycemia)

  1. Etiology (Table 9-11)

  2. Clinical findings in reactive hypoglycemia

    a. Fed-state hypoglycemia

    b. Sweating, trembling, palpitations, anxiety

      • Adrenergic findings

  3. Clinical findings in fasting hypoglycemia

    a. Neuroglycopenic symptoms

    b. Confusion, hallucinations, blurred vision, seizures, coma

  4. Laboratory diagnosis; Whipple triad:

    a. Serum glucose < 40 mg/dL

    b. Symptoms of hypoglycemia

    c. Reversal of symptoms when serum glucose returned to normal

VI. Serum Blood Urea Nitrogen (BUN) and Creatinine

  • See Chapter 4

VII. Serum Sodium, Chloride, Potassium, Bicarbonate

  • See Chapter 2

VIII. Serum Cholesterol and Triglyceride

  A. Lipoprotein fractions

    1. Chylomicron

      a. Synthesized in intestinal epithelium

      b. Transports diet-derived triglyceride in the blood

      c. Absent during fasting

      d. Increased chylomicrons produce turbidity in plasma.

        • Chylomicrons float on top of plasma (supranate) when a test tube is refrigerated upright overnight.

      e. Hydrolyzed by capillary lipoprotein lipase (CLP)

        (1) Becomes a chylomicron remnant

        (2) Remnant is metabolized by the liver.

    2. Very low density lipoprotein (VLDL)

      a. Transports liver-synthesized triglyceride in the blood

      b. Increased VLDL produces turbidity in plasma.

        • Produces a turbid infranate when a test tube is refrigerated upright overnight

      c. Hydrolyzed by CLP

        (1) Produces intermediate density lipoprotein (IDL)

Neonatal hypoglycemia: high insulin drives glucose into hypoglycemic range

Hypoglycemia: insulin excess in type 1 diabetic most common cause

Chylomicron: diet-derived triglyceride

Increased plasma turbidity: due to hypertriglyceridemia

VLDL: liver-derived triglyceride

TABLE 9-11
Selected Causes of Hypoglycemia

Disorder	Comments
Excess insulin	Reactive type of hypoglycemia May also occur with sulfonylurea drugs Increased serum insulin, decreased serum C-peptide (marker of endogenous insulin synthesis; suppressed by taking insulin)
IGT, type 2 diabetes	Reactive type of hypoglycemia Excessive amount of insulin is released for the glucose absorbed (early finding)
Idiopathic postprandial syndrome	Lack of energy, mental dullness, chronic anxiety Symptoms are *rarely* accompanied by hypoglycemia Treatment is frequent high-protein meals
Addison's disease	Fasting type of hypoglycemia Decreased gluconeogenesis due to hypocortisolism (gluconeogenic hormone)
Insulinoma	Fasting type of hypoglycemia Benign β-islet cell tumor Hypoglycemia, increased serum insulin, increased C-peptide
Alcohol excess	Fasting type of hypoglycemia Decreased gluconeogenesis: pyruvate is converted to lactate by increased NADH in alcohol metabolism Decreased glycogen stores
Hypopituitarism	Fasting type of hypoglycemia Deficiency of growth hormone and cortisol: both are gluconeogenic hormones
Chronic renal failure	Fasting type of hypoglycemia Kidney is a site for gluconeogenesis
Starvation	Fasting type of hypoglycemia Decrease in gluconeogenesis
Pediatric hypoglycemias	Fasting type of hypoglycemia Von Gierke's glycogenosis: deficient glucose 6-phosphatase (gluconeogenic enzyme) Carnitine deficiency: decreased β-oxidation of fatty acids for fuel All tissues are glucose dependent Leucine sensitivity: leucine directly stimulates insulin release Prematurity: diminished glycogen stores and decreased gluconeogenic enzymes Galactosemia: deficient GALT; decreased substrates for gluconeogenesis Hereditary fructose intolerance: deficient aldolase B decreased substrates for gluconeogenesis Maple syrup urine disease: deficiency branched chain α-keto acid dehydrogenase; decreased substrates for gluconeogenesis

GALT, galactose 1-phosphate uridyltransferase; IGT, impaired glucose tolerance.

  (2) IDL produces low-density lipoprotein (LDL).
 d. IDL remnant is metabolized by the liver
 3. Low-density lipoprotein (LDL)
  a. Transports cholesterol in the blood

LDL: transports cholesterol

   (1) Derived from hydrolysis of VLDL
   (2) Serum cholesterol < 200 mg/dL is considered normal for any age bracket.

b. Calculated LDL = cholesterol − high density lipoprotein − triglyceride/5
  (1) Formula should *not* be used if triglyceride is >400 mg/dL.
    • Must directly measure LDL
  (2) Triglyceride divided by 5 equals VLDL.
  (3) Chylomicrons falsely lower the calculated LDL.
    (a) Increased triglyceride increases VLDL.
    (b) Fasting is necessary to obtain an accurate triglyceride and calculated LDL.
c. Functions of cholesterol
  (1) Component of the cell membrane
  (2) Synthesis of vitamin D, adrenal cortex hormones, bile salts and acids
d. Ranges of LDL
  (1) <100 mg/dL: optimal
    • Risk for coronary heart disease (CHD) markedly reduced
  (2) 100–129 mg/dL: near optimal
  (3) 130–159 mg/dL: borderline high level
  (4) 160–189 mg/dL: high level
  (5) >190 mg/dL: very high level
    • Highest risk for CHD

> The intensity of treatment to lower cholesterol is directly related to the degree of risk for CHD. The LDL cholesterol goal is <100 mg/dL if the patient has known coronary heart disease. For persons without CHD, the LDL cholesterol goal is subdivided into those with a 0–1 risk factor (goal < 160 mg/dL) or those with multiple (2+) risk factors (goal < 130 mg/dL). The risk factors include age (male ≥ 45 years, female ≥ 55 years); family history of premature CHD (e.g., family member with myocardial infarction before 55 years of age); current cigarette smoking; blood pressure ≥140/90 mg/dL (or on antihypertensive medicine); and HDL < 40 mg/dL (if ≥60 mg/dL, subtract 1).

4. High-density lipoprotein (HDL)
  a. "Good cholesterol"
    (1) Should be >40 mg/dL
      • Values < 40 mg/dL increase risk for coronary heart disease.
    (2) Increased by exercise, wine, estrogen
    (3) Inverse relationship of HDL with VLDL
      • Example—increased VLDL automatically decreases HDL.
  b. Synthesized by the liver and small intestine
  c. Functions of HDL
    (1) Source of apolipoproteins for other lipoprotein fractions
    (2) Removes cholesterol from atherosclerotic plaques
      • Reverse cholesterol transport

HDL: removes cholesterol from plaques for disposal in the liver

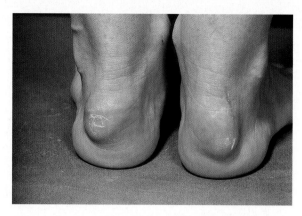

9-5: *Achilles tendon xanthoma. Note the slightly yellow-colored nodules on the heels. These lesions are pathognomonic for familial hypercholesterolemia. (From McKee PH, Colonje JE, Granter SR: Pathology of the Skin, 3rd ed. St. Louis, Mosby, 2005, Fig. 12.8.)*

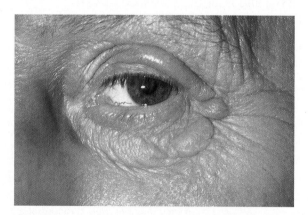

9-6: *Xanthelasma. Note the yellow, periorbital plaques. These are a common manifestation of hypercholesterolemia. (From McKee PH, Colonje JE, Granter SR: Pathology of the Skin, 3rd edition. St. Louis, Mosby, 2005, Fig. 12.18.)*

B. **Lipoprotein disorders with increased cholesterol and/or triglyceride** (Table 9-12, Figs. 9-5 through 9-8)

C. **Decreased serum cholesterol or triglyceride** (Table 9-13)

IX. **Bilirubin**

A. **Bilirubin metabolism** (Fig. 9-9)

1. Unconjugated bilirubin (UCB)

a. Senescent RBCs are phagocytosed by splenic macrophages.

b. UCB (indirect bilirubin) is the end product of heme degradation.

• UCB is lipid-soluble.

UCB: end product of heme degradation in splenic macrophages

TABLE 9-12

Lipoprotein Disorders

Type	Comments

Type I	AR inheritance: childhood disease
	Pathogenesis: deficiency of CLP or apo-C-II (normally activates CLP)
	  Chylomicrons are primarily increased in early childhood and VLDL also increases later in life
	Presents with acute pancreatitis: pancreatic vessels with chylomicrons rupture
	Increase in serum TG (>1000 mg/dL; primarily due to chylomicrons); turbid supranate (chylomicrons) and
	  clear infranate with refrigeration; normal (usual case) to moderately increased serum CH

Type II	Type IIa: increase in serum CH (>260 mg/dL) and LDL (>190 mg/dL); serum TG < 300 mg/dL
	Type IIb: increase in serum CH (>260 mg/dL) and LDL (>190 mg/dL); serum TG > 300 mg/dL
	Genetic causes
	  Polygenic hypercholesterolemia (type IIa): most common type (85% of cases). Multifactorial (polygenic)
	    inheritance; alteration in regulation of LDL levels with primary increase in serum LDL and normal TG
	  Familial combined hypercholesterolemia (type IIb): AD inheritance; CH and TG begin to increase around
	    puberty; associated with syndrome X (insulin resistance syndrome). Increase in CH and TG; decrease in
	    HDL
	  Familial hypercholesterolemia (type IIa): AD inheritance; absent or defective LDL receptors; lipid deposits—
	    Achilles tendon xanthoma (diagnostic; Fig. 9-5), xanthelasma (yellow plaques on eyelid; Fig. 9-6).
	    Premature CAD; increase in serum CH and LDL; serum TG < 300 mg/dL; decrease in HDL
	Acquired causes
	  Primary hypothyroidism: decreased synthesis of LDL receptors
	  Blockage of bile flow: bile contains CH
	  Nephrotic syndrome: increased liver synthesis of CH

Type III	Familial dysbetalipoproteinemia or "remnant disease": AR inheritance Pathogenesis: defective apo E; decreased liver uptake of IDL and chylomicron remnants Palmar xanthomas in flexor creases (Fig. 9-7); increased risk for CAD Both serum CH and TG > 300 mg/dL; LDL < 190 mg/dL; confirm diagnosis with ultracentrifugation to identify remnants, lipoprotein electrophoresis, identify apo E gene defect

Type IV	Familial hypertriglyceridemia: AD inheritance; most common hyperlipoproteinemia
	  Pathogenesis: increased production of VLDL
	  Eruptive xanthomas (yellow, papular lesions; Fig. 9-8)
	  Increased risk for CAD and peripheral vascular disease
	  Increase in TG (>300 mg/dL); serum CH normal to moderately increased (250–500 mg/dL); serum
	    LDL < 190 mg/dL; decrease in HDL (inverse relationship with VLDL); turbid infranate after refrigeration
	Acquired causes
	  Excess alcohol intake: most common cause; increased production of VLDL, decreased activity of CLP
	  Oral contraceptives: estrogen increases production of VLDL
	  Diabetes mellitus: decreased adipose and muscle CLP (decreased VLDL clearance). Increased LDL; decreased
	    HDL
	  Chronic renal failure: increased production of VLDL and decreased clearance of VLDL
	  Thiazide diuretics, β-blockers: ? increase production or decrease clearance of VLDL

Type V	Most commonly familial hypertriglyceridemia + an exacerbating disorder: e.g., diabetic ketoacidosis, alcoholism
	Pathogenesis: increase in chylomicrons and VLDL due to decreased activation and release of CLP
	Hyperchylomicronemia syndrome
	  Eruptive xanthomas
	  Increased incidence of acute pancreatitis
	  Lipemia retinalis: retinal vessels look like milk, blurry vision
	  Dyspnea and hypoxemia: impaired gas exchange in pulmonary capillaries
	  Hepatosplenomegaly
	  Increase in serum TG (usually >1000 mg/dL); normal serum CH and LDL
	  Turbid supranate and infranate after refrigeration

AD, autosomal dominant; AR, autosomal recessive; CAD, coronary artery disease; CH, cholesterol; CLP, capillary lipoprotein lipase; TG, triglyceride.

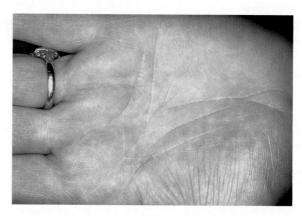

9-7: *Palmar xanthomas. Note the yellow, macules on the palm that are accentuated in the creases. These are characteristic lesions in type III hyperlipoproteinemia. (From McKee PH, Colonje JE, Granter SR: Pathology of the Skin, 3rd ed. St. Louis, Mosby, 2005, Fig. 12.20.)*

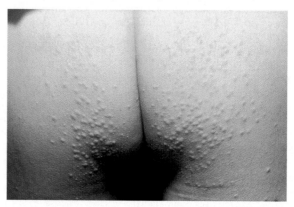

9-8: *Eruptive xanthomas. Note the numerous small, yellow papules on the buttocks. These lesions occur with any marked increase in triglyceride (i.e., type 1, IV, and V hyperlipoproteinemias). (From McKee PH, Colonje JE, Granter SR: Pathology of the Skin, 3rd edition. St. Louis, Mosby, 2005, Fig. 12.3.)*

TABLE 9-13
Causes of Decreased Serum Cholesterol and/or Triglyceride

Disorder	Comments
Apolipoprotein B deficiency	AR disorder Pathogenesis: deficiency of apolipoprotein B-48 and B-100 Malabsorption: chylomicrons accumulate in villi and prevent reabsorption of micelles Marked decrease in vitamin E (fat soluble vitamin) Ataxia, hemolytic anemia with thorny erythrocytes (acanthocytes) Deficiency of chylomicrons, VLDL, LDL, and HDL with concomitant decrease in CH and TG
Low carbohydrate diet Malnutrition	Decrease in TG Decrease in CH and TG
Statin drug therapy	Statin drugs block HMG CoA reductase Decreases CH and LDL
Acute myocardial infarction	Significant decrease in CH (40%–50% decrease) after 48 hr

AR, autosomal recessive; CH, cholesterol; HMG CoA, hydroxymethylglutaryl coenzyme A; TG, triglyceride.

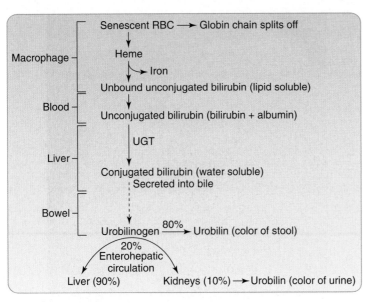

9-9: *Bilirubin metabolism. Refer to text for discussion. UGT, uridyl transferase. (From Goljan EF: Rapid Review Pathology, 2nd ed. St. Louis, Mosby, 2007, Fig. 18-01.)*

2. UCB combines with albumin in the blood.
    a. UCB is taken up by hepatocytes.
    b. UCB is conjugated to produce conjugated bilirubin (CB).
        • CB (direct bilirubin) is water soluble.
3. CB is secreted into the intrahepatic bile ducts.
    a. Temporarily stored in the gallbladder
    b. Enters the duodenum via the common bile duct
    c. CB is never normally found in the blood or urine.
4. Intestinal bacteria convert CB to urobilinogen (UBG)
    a. UBG is spontaneously oxidized to urobilin.
    b. Urobilin produces the brown color of stool.
5. A small amount of UBG is recycled to the liver and kidneys.
    • Color of urine is due to urobilin.
B. **Jaundice**
    1. Jaundice is due to an increase in UCB and/or CB.
        • Jaundice is first noticed in the sclerae (Fig. 9-10).
    2. Classification of causes of jaundice is based on the percentage of CB (Table 9-14).
        • Percent CB = CB/total bilirubin
    3. Schematics showing common causes of jaundice (Box 9-1)

X. **Alkaline Phosphatase (ALP)**
    A. **Overview**
        1. ALP is present in many tissues

CB: water soluble

Urobilin: color of stool and urine

Viral hepatitis: most common cause of jaundice

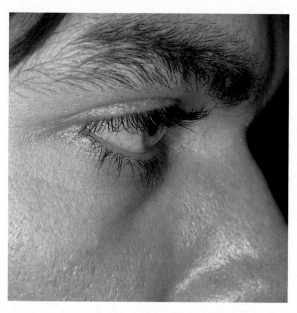

9-10: *Jaundice. Note the yellow discoloration of the sclera. (From Savin J, Hunter JA, Hepburn NC: Diagnosis in Color: Skin Signs in Clinical Medicine. London, Mosby-Wolfe, 1997, Fig. 6.28.)*

    2. Examples—bone (in osteoblasts), liver (synthesized in bile ducts), placenta

    3. Function in osteoblasts
- Dephosphorylates pyrophosphate, which normally inhibits bone mineralization

B. Increased serum ALP
- Etiology (Table 9-15)

C. Decreased serum ALP

    1. Decreased serum ALP has no clinical significance.

    2. Decreased leukocyte ALP occurs in chronic myelogenous leukemia (see Chapter 6).

XI. **Gamma Glutamyltransferase (GGT)**

  A. Overview

    1. GGT is located in the smooth endoplasmic reticulum in hepatocytes.
- Same location as cytochrome P-450 system in the liver (see Chapter 1)

    2. Enzyme is increased with drug "induction" of the cytochrome P-450 system

    3. Examples of inducing drugs and chemicals
- Alcohol, barbiturates, phenytoin, polycyclic hydrocarbons (cigarette smoke)

  B. Increased serum GGT

    1. Etiology

      a. Obstructive jaundice (intra- and extrahepatic types)
- Excellent marker of obstruction similar to ALP

Serum ALP and GGT: markers of liver cholestasis

TABLE 9-14
Causes of
Jaundice

Classification	UB	Urine UBG	Examples of Disorders
Unconjugated CB < 20%			
Increased production of UCB	Absent	↑	Extravascular hemolytic anemias: e.g., hereditary spherocytosis, Rh and ABO HDN

Decreased uptake and/or conjugation of UCB	Absent	Normal	Gilbert's syndrome: AD disorder
			  Common genetic defect in uptake/conjugation of UCB
			  Jaundice occurs with fasting
			  No histologic changes in the liver
			Crigler-Najjar syndromes: genetic disorders with decreased to absent conjugating enzymes
			Physiologic jaundice of newborn: begins on day 3 of life; caused by normal macrophage destruction of fetal RBCs

Mixed CB 20–50%	↑	↑	Viral hepatitis: defect in uptake, conjugation of UCB and secretion of CB

Obstructive
CB > 50%
	↑	Absent	Obstruction to intrahepatic bile flow
			  Drug-induced (e.g., OCP)
			  Primary biliary cirrhosis
			  Dubin-Johnson syndrome: genetic defect in secretion into intrahepatic bile ducts; black pigment in hepatocytes
			  Rotor's syndrome: similar to Dubin-Johnson syndrome but *without* black pigment in hepatocytes
			Obstruction to extrahepatic bile flow
			  Gallstone in common bile duct
			  Carcinoma of head of pancreas

CB, conjugated bilirubin; HDN, hemolytic disease of newborn; OCP, oral contraceptive pill; UB, urine bilirubin; UBG, urobilinogen; UCB, unconjugated bilirubin.

TABLE 9-15
Causes of
Increased Serum
Alkaline
Phosphatase

Causes	Discussion
Normal child	Due to bone growth and increased osteoblastic activity (see Chapter 1)
Pregnancy	Derived from the placenta
Elderly	Due to reactive bone formation at the margin of weight-bearing joints in osteoarthritis (degenerative arthritis)
Obstructive jaundice	Excellent marker of intrahepatic and extrahepatic jaundice Increased pressure on bile duct epithelium leads to increased synthesis of ALP (not released from damaged tissue)
Bone fracture	Due to increased osteoblastic activity
Osteoblastic metastasis	Tumors secrete factors that enhance osteoblastic activity leading to increased density in bone Occurs with prostate cancer (most common) and breast cancer

ALP, alkaline phosphatase.

BOX 9-1

SCHEMATICS SHOWING COMMON CAUSES OF JAUNDICE

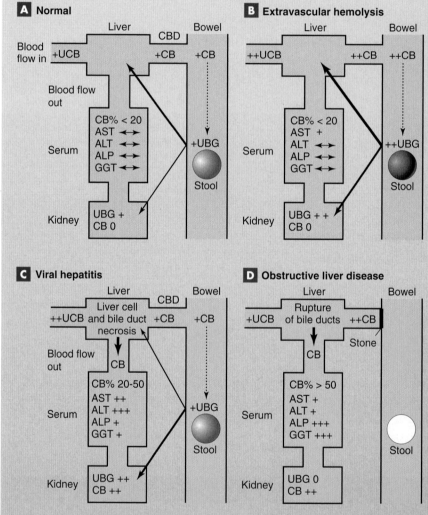

AST > ALT in alcoholic hepatitis

In this discussion, the symbol (+) is used to indicate degrees of magnitude. Normal bilirubin metabolism (**A**) shows liver uptake of lipid-soluble unconjugated bilirubin (+UCB) and its conjugation to water-soluble conjugated bilirubin (+CB). CB is secreted into the common bile duct (CBD) and is emptied into the bowel. Intestinal bacteria convert CB to urobilinogen (+UBG), which spontaneously oxidizes to the pigment urobilin. Urobilin is responsible for the

BOX 9-1—cont'd

color of stool. A small percentage of UBG is reabsorbed into the blood. Most of it enters the liver (*large diameter arrow*) and a small percentage (*small diameter arrow*) enters the urine (UBG+). Urobilin is responsible for the color of urine. All of the normal bilirubin in blood is UCB (CB% < 20%) derived from macrophage destruction of senescent RBCs. UCB cannot enter urine, because it is attached to albumin in the blood and is lipid-soluble, *not* water-soluble. CB is never a normal finding in urine, because it does not have contact with blood in its metabolism.

B, In **extravascular hemolysis** (e.g., hereditary spherocytosis), there is increased macrophage production of UCB causing an increase in serum UCB (++; CB% < 20%). There is a corresponding increase in uptake and conjugation of UCB, conjugation to CB (++), and conversion of CB in the bowel to UBG (++). This causes darkening of the stool. There is a greater percentage of UBG recycled back to the liver (*wider arrow*) and urine (*other dark arrow*). The increase in urine UBG (++) darkens the color of urine. Because RBCs contain the enzyme aspartate aminotransferase (AST), hemolysis of RBCs causes an increase in serum AST (+). Alanine aminotransferase (ALT), alkaline phosphatase (ALP), and γ-glutamyltransferase (GGT) levels are normal.

In **viral hepatitis (C)**, there is generalized liver dysfunction involving uptake and conjugation of UCB, secretion of CB into bile ducts, and recycling of UBG. Serum UCB is increased (++) owing to a decrease in uptake and conjugation. Serum and urine CB are increased (++) because of liver cell necrosis and disruption of bile ductules between hepatocytes. Urine UBG is increased (++), because UBG is redirected from the liver (*smaller diameter arrow*) to the kidneys (*larger diameter arrow*). Because there is an increase in serum UCB and CB, there is a mixed hyperbilirubinemia with a CB% of 20–50. In viral hepatitis, ALT is higher (+++) than AST (++) and there is a slight increase in ALP and GGT (+). In alcoholic hepatitis, AST is greater than ALT, because alcohol damages mitochondria, which is where AST is normally located.

In **obstructive liver disease (D)**, there is an increase in serum and urine CB (++) due to obstruction of intrahepatic or extrahepatic bile flow (stone in the CBD in this case). This causes increased pressure in the intrahepatic bile ductules leading to rupture and egress of CB into sinusoidal blood. There is absence of UBG in the stool (light-colored) and urine. %CB is >50% and there is a marked increase in serum ALP and GGT (+++) and only a slight increase in serum AST and ALT (+).

TABLE 9-16
Causes of
Increased Serum
Transaminases

Causes	Discussion
Viral hepatitis	Highest transaminase levels of all liver diseases
	ALT > AST: ALT is the last enzyme to return to normal
	Greater increase in acute hepatitis than chronic hepatitis
Alcoholic hepatitis	AST > ALT: AST is primarily located in the mitochondria and alcohol damages mitochondria; ALT is frequently normal
Reye's syndrome	Primarily occurs in children with viral infection (e.g., varicella, flu) and exposure to salicylates
	Salicylates damage hepatocytes: produces diffuse fatty change (increases transaminases) and disrupts the urea cycle (increases serum ammonia)
HELLP syndrome	Occurs in association with preeclampsia/eclampsia
	H = hemolytic anemia with schistocytes (due to fibrin clots in DIC, see Chapter 5)
	EL = elevated transaminases due to hepatic necrosis around the triads
	LP = low platelets due to DIC
Drug-induced hepatitis	Examples—isoniazid (caused by toxic metabolite), halothane, acetaminophen, methyldopa

ALT, alanine aminotransferase; AST, aspartate aminotransferase; DIC, disseminated intravascular hemolysis.

b. Drug ("induction") of the cytochrome P-450 system
  • Excellent marker of alcohol ingestion
2. Useful in differentiating source of increased ALP
  a. Both enzymes are increased in intrahepatic and extrahepatic obstruction.
  b. Normal GGT with increased ALP indicates that ALP is *not* of liver origin.

XII. **Aspartate Aminotransferase (AST), Alanine Aminotransferase (ALT)**

Transaminases: markers of diffuse liver cell necrosis

  A. **Overview**
    1. AST and ALT are the primary markers of diffuse liver cell necrosis.
      • Usually *not* increased with focal liver cell necrosis (e.g., metastasis, granulomas)
    2. ALT is more specific for liver than AST.
  B. **Increased serum transaminases**
    • Etiology (Table 9-16)
  C. **Decreased serum transaminases**
    1. Pyridoxine deficiency in pregnancy
    2. Fulminant hepatitis

Fulminant hepatitis: acute drop in transaminases, prolonged PT

      a. No more liver parenchyma is present to destroy.
      b. Classic laboratory findings in fulminant hepatitis
        (1) Sudden drop in transaminases
        (2) Prolongation of the prothrombin time
  D. **Summary of liver function tests** (Table 9-17)
  E. **Viral hepatitis**
    1. Summary table of viral hepatitis (Table 9-18)
    2. Hepatitis B serologic tests (Fig. 9-11)

TABLE 9-17
Summary of Liver Function Tests

Test	Significance
Liver cell necrosis	
Serum alanine aminotransferase (ALT)	Specific enzyme for liver cell necrosis
	Present in the cytosol
	ALT > AST: viral hepatitis
Serum aspartate aminotransferase (AST)	Present in mitochondria
	Alcohol damages mitochondria: AST > ALT indicates alcoholic hepatitis
Cholestasis	
Serum γ-glutamyltransferase (GGT)	Intra- or extrahepatic obstruction to bile flow
	Induction of cytochrome P-450 system (e.g., alcohol): increases GGT
Serum alkaline phosphatase (ALP)	Normal GGT and increased ALP: source of ALP other than liver (e.g., osteoblastic activity in bone)
	Increased GGT and ALP: liver cholestasis
Bilirubin excretion	
CB < 20%	Unconjugated hyperbilirubinemia: e.g., extravascular hemolytic anemias, Gilbert's syndrome
CB 20–50%	Mixed hyperbilirubinemia (e.g., viral hepatitis)
CB > 50%	Conjugated hyperbilirubinemia (e.g., liver cholestasis)
Urine bilirubin	Bilirubinuria: viral hepatitis, intra- or extrahepatic obstruction of bile ducts
Urine UBG	Increased urine UBG: extravascular hemolytic anemias, viral hepatitis
	Absent urine UBG: liver cholestasis
Hepatocyte function	
Serum albumin	Albumin is synthesized by the liver
	Hypoalbuminemia: severe liver disease (e.g., cirrhosis)
Prothrombin time (PT)	Majority of coagulation factors are synthesized in the liver
	Increased PT: severe liver disease
Blood urea nitrogen (BUN)	Urea cycle is present in the liver
	Decreased serum BUN: cirrhosis, fulminant liver failure
Serum ammonia	Ammonia is metabolized in the urea cycle
	Increased serum ammonia: cirrhosis, Reye's syndrome, fulminant liver failure
Immune function	
Serum IgM	Increased in primary biliary cirrhosis
Antimitochondrial antibody	Primary biliary cirrhosis
Anti–smooth muscle antibody	Autoimmune hepatitis
Antinuclear antibody	Autoimmune hepatitis
Tumor marker	
α-Fetoprotein (AFP)	Hepatocellular carcinoma

CB, conjugated bilirubin; UBG, urobilinogen; UCB, unconjugated bilirubin

a. Hepatitis B surface antigen (HBsAg)
  (1) Appears within 2 to 8 weeks after exposure
    • First marker of infection
  (2) Persists up to 4 months in acute hepatitis
    • HBsAg > 6 months defines chronic HBV.

HBsAg > 6 months defines chronic HBV

TABLE 9-18
Summary of Viral Hepatitis (Hepatitis A through E)

Virus	Transmission	Clinical Findings	Serology
HAV	Fecal–oral	No carrier state Does *not* lead to chronic hepatitis Occurs in day care centers, prisons, travelers to developing countries, and male homosexuals (anal intercourse)	Anti-HAV-IgM: active infection Anti-HAV-IgG: recovery or vaccination (protective antibody)
HBV	Parenteral, sexual, vertical (pregnancy, breast feeding)	Carrier state may occur Chronic hepatitis in 10% of immunocompetent patients Risk for hepatocellular carcinoma	See text (XII.E)
HCV	Parenteral, sexual	Carrier state may occur Mild hepatitis; jaundice uncommon Chronic hepatitis in >70% of cases Associated with posttransfusion hepatitis Risk for hepatocellular carcinoma	Screen: EIA Anti-HCV IgG: infection Confirmatory tests: RIBA, HCV RNA Positive RIBA + HCV RNA indicates infection Positive RIBA and negative HCV RNA indicates recent recovery
HDV	Parenteral, sexual	Carrier state may occur Requires HBsAg to replicate Coinfection: HBV and HDV exposure at same time Superinfection: HBV carrier exposed to blood containing HBV and HDV	Anti-HDV IgM or IgG: indicates active infection IgG is *not* a protective antibody
HEV	Fecal–oral (waterborne)	No carrier state or chronic infection Fulminant hepatitis may develop in pregnant women	Anti-HEV IgM: active Anti-HEV IgG: recovery (protective antibody)

EIA, enzyme immunoassay; HBsAg, hepatitis B surface antigen; RIBA, recombinant immunoblot assay.

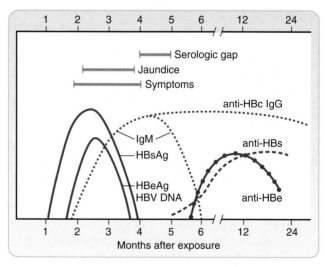

9-11: Schematic of hepatitis B serology tests. See text for discussion. (From Goljan: Rapid Review Pathology, 2nd ed. St. Louis, Mosby, 2007, Fig. 18.02, p 372.)

b. Hepatitis B e antigen (HBeAg) and HBV-DNA
   (1) Infective particles
   (2) Appear after HBsAg and disappear before HBsAg
c. Anti-HBV core antibody IgM (anti-HBc IgM)
   (1) Nonprotective antibody
       (a) Remains positive in acute infection
       (b) Disappears by 6 months
   (2) Persists during "window phase" or "serologic gap"
       • HBsAg, HBV DNA, and HBeAg are absent
   (3) Converts to anti-HBc IgG after 6 months
d. Anti-HBV surface antibody (anti-HBs)
   (1) Protective antibody
   (2) Marker of immunization after HBV vaccination
e. Chronic HBV
   (1) Persistence of HBsAg >6 months
   (2) "Healthy" chronic carrier
       (a) Presence of HBsAg
       (b) Presence of anti-HBc IgG
       (c) Absence of DNA and e antigen
   (3) Infective chronic carrier
       (a) Presence of HBsAg
       (b) Presence of infective particles (DNA and e antigen)
       (c) Presence of anti-HBc IgG
       (d) Increased risk for postnecrotic cirrhosis and hepatocellular carcinoma
f. Summary of HBV serology tests (Table 9-19)

F. **Summary chart of laboratory findings in selected liver disorders** (Table 9-20)

> Anti-HBc IgM: only marker present during window phase
>
> Anti-HBs: protective antibody; immunization or recovery from past infection
>
> Chronic carriers: HBsAg > 6 months, anti-HBc IgG

XIII. **Lactate Dehydrogenase (LDH)**
   A. **Overview**
      1. LDH is widespread in tissue
      2. LDH isoenzymes
         a. Five LDH isoenzymes
            • $LDH_2 > LDH_1$, $LDH_1 > LDH_3$, $LDH_4 \sim LDH_5$
         b. $LDH_1 > LDH_2$ (flip)
            (1) Acute myocardial infarction
                (a) LDH_1 is present in cardiac muscle.
                (b) Appears within 10 hours; peaks 2 to 3 days; disappears within 7 days
            (2) RBC hemolysis
                (a) LDH_1 is present in RBCs.
                (b) Occurs with iatrogenic hemolysis of blood sample or intravascular hemolytic anemia
   B. **Increased serum LDH**
      • Etiology (Table 9-21)
   C. **Decreased serum LDH**
      • No clinical significance

TABLE 9-19
Serologic Studies in Hepatitis B

HBsAg	HBeAg HBV DNA	Anti-HBc IgM	Anti-HBc IgG	Anti-HBs	Interpretation
+	–	–	–	–	Earliest phase of acute HBV
+	+	+	–	–	Acute infection
–	–	+	–	–	Window phase, or serologic gap
–	–	–	+	+	Recovered from HBV
–	–	–	–	+	Immunized
+	–	–	+	–	"Healthy" carrier
+	+	–	+	–	Infective carrier

Anti-HBc, core antibody; anti-HBs, surface antibody; HBeAg, e antigen; HBsAg, surface antigen.

TABLE 9-20
Summary Chart of Laboratory Findings in Selected Liver Disorders

Disease	%CB	AST	ALT	ALP	GGT	UB	Urine UBG
Normal						Absent	↑
Viral hepatitis	20–50%	↑↑↑	↑↑↑↑	↑	↑	↑↑	↑↑
Alcoholic hepatitis	20–50%	↑↑	↑	↑	↑↑↑	↑↑	↑↑
Cholestasis	>50%	↑	↑↑	↑↑↑	↑↑↑	↑↑↑	Absent
Extravascular hemolysis	<20%	↑↑ RBC	N	N	N	Absent	↑↑

Arrows represent degree of magnitude
ALP, alkaline phosphatase; ALT, alanine aminotransferase; AST, aspartate aminotransferase; CB, conjugated bilirubin; UB, urine bilirubin; UBG, urobilinogen.

TABLE 9-21
Causes of Increased Serum Lactate Dehydrogenase (LDH)

Disorder	Comments
Acute myocardial infarction	LDH isoenzymes more useful than total LDH. LDH isoenzymes have now been replaced by troponins I and T to detect infarctions after 3 days
Diffuse liver cell necrosis	Not as good an indicator as the serum transaminases
Disseminated malignancy	Nonspecific marker of disseminated malignancy
RBC hemolysis	Falsely increased in a hemolyzed specimen Excellent marker for intravascular hemolysis Excellent marker for megaloblastic anemias (i.e., folate and vitamin B_{12} deficiency); increased destruction of hematopoietic cells outside of the bone marrow sinusoids releases large quantities of LDH
Dysgerminoma	Malignant ovarian tumor: only germ cell tumor of the ovary to have an increase in serum LDH

XIV. **Creatine Kinase**
   A. **Overview**
      1. Primarily located in muscle
      2. CK isoenzymes
         a. Three isoenzymes

Disorder	Comments
Acute myocardial infarction (CK:MB)	CK isoenzymes are more useful than total CK CK-MB: begins to increase within 4–8 hr; peaks at 24 hr; disappears within 1.5 to 3 days Reappearance after day 3 is a reinfarction CK-MB also increased in cardiac contusion, Duchenne muscular dystrophy, myocarditis
Skeletal muscle injury (CK-MM)	Trauma to muscle: e.g., car accident, severe exercise Myositis: inflammation of muscle (e.g., polymyositis) Myopathy: primary hypothyroidism, Duchenne muscular dystrophy Rhabdomyolysis: rupture of muscle (e.g., hypophosphatemia, hypokalemia, heat stroke)
Miscellaneous causes of increased CK-BB	Some cases of head injury Anterior chest wall injury Cancers involving prostate, colon, lung, esophagus

(1) CK-MM
   (a) Accounts for >95% of skeletal muscle CK
   (b) Accounts for 70% to 75% of cardiac muscle CK
(2) CK-MB
   (a) Primarily in cardiac muscle
   (b) Very small percentage in skeletal muscle
(3) CK-BB
   • Found predominantly in brain and lung

B. **Increased serum CK**
   • Etiology (Table 9-22)

CK-MB is predominantly in cardiac muscle

C. **Decreased serum CK**
   • No clinical significance

D. **Serum troponin I (cTnI) and T (cTnT)**
  1. Normally regulate calcium-mediated contraction
    a. Appear within 3 to 6 hours; peak in 24 hours; disappear within 7 to 10 days
    b. Troponins are the gold standard for diagnosis of acute MI
      • More specific for myocardial tissue than CK-MB and last longer
    c. Cannot diagnose reinfarction
      • Underscores why CK-MB is still utilized
  2. Schematic of cardiac enzymes used in the diagnosis of myocardial infarction (Fig. 9-12)

cTnI, cTnT: gold standard for diagnosis of acute MI

XV. **Porphyria**
  A. **Overview**
    1. Porphyrins are compounds that bind to iron
      a. Precursors for heme synthesis in the bone marrow and liver
      b. Heme is found in Hb, myoglobin, and cytochromes.
      c. Porphyrinogen compounds
        (1) Colorless and nonfluorescent in the reduced state

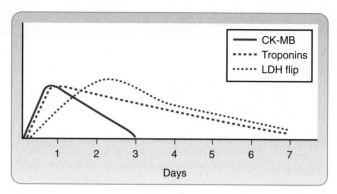

9-12: *Schematic of cardiac enzymes used in the diagnosis of an acute myocardial infarction. See text for discussion. (From Goljan EF: Rapid Review Pathology, 2nd ed. St. Louis, Mosby, 2007, Fig. 10.04.)*

(2) Wine-red color in urine and fluoresce under ultraviolet light when oxidized

(3) Absorb ultraviolet light in blood vessels near the skin surface
  • Photosensitizing agents that produce vesicles and bullae

B. **Acute intermittent porphyria (AIP)**
  1. Autosomal dominant disorder
  2. Defect in porphyrin metabolism (Fig. 9-13)
    a. Deficiency of uroporphyrinogen synthase (step 3)
      • Alias porphobilinogen deaminase
    b. Proximal increase in porphobilinogen (PBG) and δ-aminolevulinic acid (ALA)
    c. Urine is colorless when first voided.
      (1) Exposure to light
        • Causes oxidation of PBG to porphobilin producing port-wine color
      (2) Classic "window-sill test"
    d. Heme has a negative feedback relationship with ALA synthase.
    e. Decreasing heme precipitates porphyric attacks by increasing porphyrin synthesis.
      • Example—drugs enhancing liver cytochrome P-450 system (e.g., alcohol)
  3. Clinical findings
    a. Neurologic dysfunction
      (1) Recurrent bouts of severe abdominal pain simulating acute abdomen
      (2) Often mistaken for a surgical abdomen
        • Patient has "bellyful of scars."
    b. Psychosis, peripheral neuropathy, dementia
C. **Porphyria cutanea tarda (PCT)**
  1. Genetic or acquired disease involving porphyrin metabolism
    • Associated with hepatitis C and excessive alcohol intake
  2. Deficiency of uroporphyrinogen decarboxylase (step 5)

AIP: deficiency of uroporphyrinogen synthase (porphobilinogen deaminase)

AIP: "bellyful of scars"

PCT: deficiency of uroporphyrinogen decarboxylase

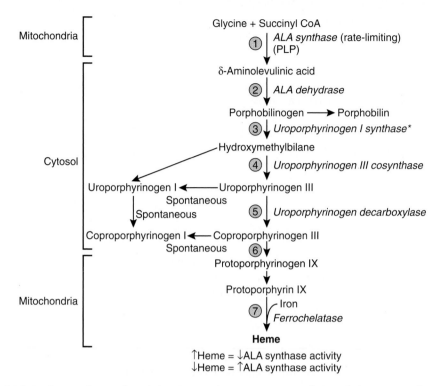

9-13: *Porphyrin synthesis and metabolism. Heme is the most important porphyrin and plays a minor role in oxygen transfer reactions. Enzyme deficiencies in porphyrin synthesis result in various types of porphyria. *Alias porphobilinogen deaminase. ALA, δ-aminolevulinic acid; PLP, pyridoxal phosphate. (From Pelley JW, Goljan EF: Rapid Review Biochemistry, 2nd ed. St. Louis, Mosby, 2007, Fig. 8-7.)*

     a. Urine is wine-red color on voiding.
     b. Uroporphyrin I is increased in urine.
   3. Clinical findings
     a. Photosensitive bullous skin lesions
        (1) Caused by porphyrin metabolites deposited in the skin
        (2) Patients avoid light
     b. Hyperpigmentation, fragile skin
     c. Increased amounts of lanugo (fine, downy hair)

XVI. **Miscellaneous Tests**
  A. **Amniotic fluid (AF) testing**
    1. Composition
     a. Fetal contributions
       (1) Urine (primary component)
       (2) Gastrointestinal tract
       (3) Amniotic membranes
     b. High salt content causes ferning when dried on a slide.
       • Excellent sign of premature rupture of the amniotic sac
    2. Swallowed and recycled by the fetus

Amniotic fluid: mainly composed of fetal urine

3. Polyhydramnios
   a. Excessive amniotic fluid
   b. Causes
      (1) Tracheoesophageal (TE) fistula
         • Proximal esophagus ends blindly; AF is not reabsorbed.
      (2) Duodenal atresia
         • Duodenum distal to entry of common bile duct is atretic; AF is not reabsorbed.
4. Oligohydramnios
   a. Decreased amount of AF
      • Produces fetal deformations
   b. Etiology
      (1) Juvenile polycystic kidney disease
         • Decreased production of urine
      (2) Renal agenesis
         • Decreased production of urine
      (3) May also be due to leaking amniotic sac.

B. **α-Fetoprotein (AFP) in pregnancy**
   1. Increased maternal AFP
      a. Open neural tube defect
         (1) Anencephaly, myelomeningocele
         (2) Related to folate deficiency
         (3) Folate stores should be adequate *before* pregnancy.
            • Neural tube development is complete by the end of the first month of gestation.
      b. Other causes
         (1) Omphalocele
         (2) TE fistula
         (3) Placental disease
            • Infarctions, thrombosis, large placentas (e.g., Rh hemolytic disease of newborn)
      c. Management of increased maternal AFP
         (1) Ultrasound
         (2) Measure AF AFP levels
         (3) Measure AF acetylcholinesterase levels
            • Increased in open neural tube defects
   2. Decreased maternal AFP
      a. Down syndrome
      b. Other causes
         • Fetal death, hydatidiform mole, maternal diabetes mellitus
      c. Management of decreased serum maternal AFP
         • Ultrasound

C. **Fetal lung maturity (FLM) testing**
   1. Measurement of surfactant
      • Most sensitive indicator of FLM
   2. Surfactant
      a. Components of surfactant

Polyhydramnios: TE fistula, duodenal atresia

Oligohydramnios: primarily due to renal problems

Increased AFP in pregnancy: open neural tube defect

Decreased maternal serum AFP: possible Down syndrome

(1) Lecithin (phosphatidyl choline)

(2) Phosphatidyl glycerol

b. Synthesized by type II pneumocytes during 34th to 36th weeks

c. Decreases alveolar surface tension to prevent atelectasis

• Atelectasis refers to collapse of the small airways in the lungs.

d. Cortisol and thyroxine increase surfactant synthesis.

• Maternal administration of glucocorticoids increases surfactant synthesis if babies must be delivered before term.

e. Insulin inhibits surfactant synthesis.

(1) Poor maternal glycemic control increases fetal insulin.

• Decreases fetal surfactant synthesis

(2) Increased fetal risk for respiratory distress syndrome

3. Measurement of surfactant in AF

a. Many techniques available

• Examples—thin layer chromatography, fluorescence polarization, agglutination ("shake test")

b. Lecithin/sphingomyelin (L:S) ratio

• L:S ratio > 2 indicates adequate surfactant.

L:S ratio > 2: adequate surfactant

D. **Tumor markers**

1. Clinical usefulness

a. Screen for cancer

b. Determine degree of tumor burden

c. Detect recurrent cancer

d. Direct or monitor therapy

e. Establish prognosis

2. Types of tumor markers

a. Ectopic hormone production

• Calcitonin, erythropoietin (EPO), antidiuretic hormone (ADH)

b. Tumor-associated antigens

• Carcinoembryonic antigen (CEA), AFP

c. Enzymes

• Acid phosphatase, prostate-specific antigen (PSA)

d. Immunoglobulin (Ig)

• Bence Jones protein (light chains), monoclonal Ig

e. Molecular markers

• Gene mutations—amplification, translocations

f. Receptor assays

• Estrogen and progesterone receptor assays in breast cancer

3. Summary of important tumor markers (Table 9-23)

E. **Antistreptococcal testing**

1. Used to evaluate *Streptococcus pyogenes* infections

a. Tests are *not* specific for a certain type of *Streptococcus* infection.

b. Rising titers indicate a recent infection.

2. Antistreptolysin O (ASO) titer; increased in:

a. Rheumatic fever

• Usually follows previous *Streptococcal* pharyngitis

**TABLE 9-23
Clinically
Important Tumor
Markers**

Marker	Associated Cancer and Discussion
AFP	Liver (hepatocellular), testis/ovary (yolk sac tumor)
Calcitonin	Thyroid (medullary carcinoma)
	May produce hypocalcemia
CEA	Colon, breast, lung (small cell carcinoma)
PSA	Prostate: sensitive but not specific for cancer (increased in BPH)
	Other more sensitive ways of reporting PSA: rate of change of PSA values with time (PSA velocity); ratio between serum PSA and volume of prostate gland (prostate density); measurement of free versus bound forms of circulating PSA
BJ protein	Multiple myeloma, Waldenström's macroglobulinemia
CA15-3	Breast
CA19-9	Pancreas
CA125	Surface-derived ovarian cancer (e.g., serous cystadenocarcinoma)
ACTH	Lung (small cell carcinoma), thyroid (medullary carcinoma); ectopic type of Cushing's syndrome
ADH	Lung (small cell carcinoma); produces hyponatremia
EPO	Kidney, liver; secondary polycythemia
hCG	Testis (choriocarcinoma), molar pregnancy (choriocarcinoma); gynecomastia in males
Insulin-like factor	Liver (hepatocellular); produces hypoglycemia
PTH-related protein	Kidney, lung (squamous carcinoma); produces hypercalcemia
*ERB (HER)*B2 oncogene	Breast; receptor amplification type of mutation in breast cancer is a poor prognostic sign
t(9;22) translocation	Chronic myelogenous leukemia; translocation involves *ABL* oncogen; *BCR*-fusion gene more specific for CML than Philadelphia chromosome
t(8;14) translocation	Burkitt's lymphoma; translocation involve *MYC* oncogene. EBV important in pathogenesis
t(14;18) translocation	B cell follicular lymphoma; overexpression type of mutation involving *BCL2* antiapoptosis gene
t(15;17) translocation	Acute promyelocytic leukemia (M3); translocation produces abnormality in retinoic acid metabolism
ERA/PRA receptors	Breast; increased activity of receptor in breast cancer tissue indicates tumor is estrogen stimulated; patient is candidate for antiestrogen therapy

ACTH, adrenocorticotropic hormone; ADH, antidiuretic hormone; AFP, α-fetoprotein; BPH, benign prostatic hyperplasia; BJ, Bence Jones; CA, cancer antigen; CEA, carcinoembryonic antigen; EBV, Epstein-Barr virus; EPO, erythropoietin; ERA, estrogen receptor assay; hCG, human chorionic gonadotrophin; PRA, progesterone receptor assay; PSA, prostate-specific antigen; PTH, parathyroid hormone.

    b. Poststreptococcal glomerulonephritis
       • Usually follows previous *Streptococcal* pharyngitis or skin infection
    c. Scarlet fever
       • Erythrogenic strain of *Streptococcus* produces erythematous rash.
    d. Bacterial endocarditis
    e. Tonsillitis/pharyngitis
  3. Anti-DNAase B titer; increased in:
    • Streptoccal pyoderma and poststreptococcal glomerulonephritis
  4. Streptozyme
    • Screening test that detects antibodies to several streptococcal antigens
 F. **Cystic fibrosis (CF)**
  1. Autosomal recessive disease

2. Pathogenesis
   a. Three nucleotide deletion on chromosome 7 (most common mutation)
      (1) Nucleotides normally code for phenylalanine
      (2) Mutations can be identified
   b. Production of a defective CF transmembrane conductance regulator (CFTR) for chloride ions
   c. CFTR Cl^- is degraded in the Golgi apparatus.
      • Due to defective protein folding
   d. Loss of CFTR Cl^- causes decreased Na^+ and Cl^- reabsorption in sweat glands.
      • Basis of the sweat test
   e. Effect of loss of CFTR Cl^- in other secretions
      (1) Increased Na^+ and water reabsorption from luminal secretions
      (2) Decreased Cl^- secretion out of epithelial cells into luminal secretions
      (3) Net effect is dehydration of body secretions due to lack of NaCl.
         • Secretions are dehydrated in bronchioles, pancreatic ducts, bile ducts, meconium, and seminal fluid.
3. Clinical findings
   a. Nasal polyps (25% of cases)
   b. Respiratory infections/failure
   c. Malabsorption
      • Pancreatic exocrine deficiency
   d. Type 1 diabetes mellitus
      • Due to chronic pancreatitis
   e. Infertility in males
      • Atresia of vas deferens
4. Sweat chloride test
   a. Pilocarpine iontophoresis initiates localized skin sweating.
   b. Sweat chloride >60 mEq/L is consistent with CF.

G. *Helicobacter pylori* testing
1. Gram-negative curved bacillus
   • Urease producer
2. Disease associations with *H. pylori*
   a. Duodenal and gastric ulcers
   b. Type B antral chronic atrophic gastritis
   c. Gastric adenocarcinoma
   d. Low-grade B-cell malignant lymphoma
3. Tests to identify *H. pylori*
   a. Endoscopic biopsy
      • Identify organisms
   b. Urease tests
      (1) Detect urease in a gastric biopsy
      (2) Sensitivity 90%, specificity 99% to 100%
   c. Serologic test
      (1) Does *not* differentiate current or past infection
      (2) Does *not* determine whether treatment has worked
      (3) Sensitivity 50% and specificity 85%

Cystic fibrosis: defective CFTR Cl^- is degraded in Golgi apparatus

Cystic fibrosis: loss NaCl in sweat, loss of NaCl in luminal secretions (dehydrated)

Respiratory infections: most common cause of death in CF

H. pylori: urease producer

    d. Radiolabeled urea breath test
      (1) *H. pylori* converts orally administered labeled urea to labeled CO_2.
      (2) Labeled CO_2 is detected in the breath.
      (3) Sensitivity >97% and specificity >90%
    e. Stool antigen test
      (1) Detects pyloroantigens
      (2) Least expensive test
      (3) Helps support a diagnosis of infection
      (4) Useful in determining whether treatment is effective
      (5) Sensitivity 92%, specificity 90% to 100%

H. Carcinoid syndrome (carcinoid tumors)
  1. Most common small bowel malignancy
  2. Neuroendocrine tumor
    a. Contain neurosecretory granules visible on electron microscopy
    b. Carcinoid tumors are malignant.
  3. Locations
    a. Tip of the vermiform appendix
      (1) Most common site
      (2) Usually remains localized
    b. Terminal ileum
      (1) Commonly metastasize to liver
      (2) Tumor produces bioactive compounds (e.g., serotonin).
        • Compounds are delivered to the liver by the portal vein.
      (3) Serotonin is metabolized to 5-hydroxyindoleacetic acid (5-HIAA).
        • 5-HIAA is excreted in the urine.
      (4) Serotonin is completely metabolized.
        • It does *not* enter the systemic circulation.
    c. Bronchus
      (1) Serotonin can directly enter the circulation.
      (2) Rarely produces carcinoid syndrome
  4. Clinical features
    a. Liver metastasis must occur to produce the syndrome.
      (1) Serotonin is secreted by metastatic tumor nodules.
      (2) Serotonin enters hepatic vein tributaries.
        • Gains access to the systemic circulation
    b. Findings due to serotonin
      (1) Flushing of the skin
        • Due to vasodilation
      (2) Diarrhea
        • Due to increased bowel motility
      (3) Increase in urine 5-HIAA

I. Wilson's disease
  1. Epidemiology
    • Autosomal recessive disorder
  2. Pathogenesis

Carcinoid tumors: malignant neuroendocrine tumors

Carcinoid tumor terminal ileum: metastasis to liver causes carcinoid syndrome

Carcinoid syndrome: flushing and diarrhea

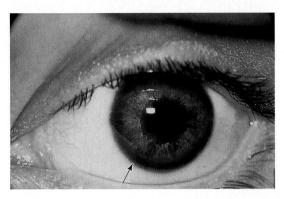

9-14: *Kayser-Fleischer ring. The arrow depicts deposition of a copper-colored pigment in Descemet's membrane in the cornea. (From Perkin GD: Mosby's Color Atlas and Text of Neurology. St. Louis, Mosby, 2002, Fig. 8-15.)*

    a. Gene mutation results in:
       (1) Defective hepatocyte transport of copper into bile for excretion
       (2) Decreased synthesis of ceruloplasmin
         • Binding protein for copper in blood
    b. Unbound copper eventually accumulates in blood.

> Ceruloplasmin is the binding protein for copper that is reabsorbed from the intestinal tract into the blood. It is synthesized in the liver and secreted into the plasma where it represents 90% to 95% of the total serum copper concentration. The remaining 5% to 10% of copper is free copper that is loosely bound to albumin. When ceruloplasmin is eventually metabolized in the liver, the copper is normally excreted into the bile. The gene defect in Wilson's disease affects a copper transport system that produces a dual defect: decreased synthesis of ceruloplasmin in the liver and decreased excretion of copper into bile. Accumulation of copper in the liver causes damage to hepatocytes leading to chronic hepatitis and cirrhosis. In a few years, unbound copper is released from the liver into the circulation (increased in blood and urine) where it can cause hemolysis or damage to the brain, kidneys, cornea, and other tissues.

Wilson's disease: ↓ synthesis ceruloplasmin, ↓ excretion of copper in bile

   3. Clinical and laboratory findings
    a. Kayser-Fleischer ring (Fig. 9-14)
      • Due to free copper deposits in Descemet's membrane in the cornea
    b. Central nervous system disease
      • Produces a movement disorder and dementia
    c. Decreased total serum copper
      • Due to decreased ceruloplasmin
    d. Decreased serum ceruloplasmin
      • Useful in diagnosing Wilson's disease in early stages of the disease
    e. Increased serum and urine free copper
      • Useful in diagnosing Wilson's disease in later stages of the disease

Kayser-Fleischer ring: excess copper in Descemet's membrane of cornea

Questions

Refer to the following choices in answering questions 1 through 4:

A. Type I hyperlipoproteinemia
B. Type II hyperlipoproteinemia
C. Type III hyperlipoproteinemia
D. Type IV hyperlipoproteinemia
E. Type V hyperlipoproteinemia

Each lettered option designates a lipid disorder. For questions 1 through 4, select the *one* lettered option that is most closely associated with it. In answering these questions, each lettered option may be selected once, more than once, or not at all.

1. A 28-year-old man has bilateral Achilles tendon xanthomas.

2. A 42-year-old man has yellow papular lesions on his buttocks and trunk. After refrigeration of a turbid blood sample, there is a turbid infranate without any supranate.

3. A 35-year-old man has yellow lesions on his palms and within the palmar creases. Serum cholesterol and triglyceride are both elevated.

4. A 25-year-old woman is a type 1 diabetic in ketoacidosis. She has yellow papular lesions on her buttocks and trunk. After refrigeration of a turbid blood sample, there is a turbid supranate and infranate.

5. A 65-year-old man on the fifth day of hospitalization for an acute anterior myocardial infarction has recurrence of chest pain and an increase in both CK-MB and troponins I and T. Examination of the heart and lungs is normal. Which of the following is most likely responsible for the laboratory test abnormalities?
A. Myocardial rupture
B. Papillary muscle dysfunction
C. Reinfarction
D. Right ventricular infarction
E. Ventricular aneurysm

6. A 42-year-old woman complains of diarrhea and episodic flushing of the skin. She does not smoke cigarettes. Physical examination demonstrates a nodular liver. A pelvic examination is normal. A barium study reveals a constricting mass in the terminal ileum. Which of the following laboratory findings is most likely present?

A. Increased serum α-fetoprotein
B. Increased serum antistreptolysin O
C. Increased serum CA 125
D. Increased serum CA-19–9
E. Increased urinary 5-hydroxyindoleacetic acid

Refer to the following list for questions 7 through 11:
A. Kidney
B. Placenta
C. Liver
D. Lung
E. Testicle
F. Thyroid

For questions 7 through 11, select the *one* lettered option that is most closely associated with it. Each lettered option may be selected once, more than once, or not at all.

7. Site for a tumor that could potentially produce Cushing's syndrome and hyponatremia

8. Site for a tumor that could potentially produce hypercalcemia and secondary polycythemia

9. Site for a tumor that could potentially produce hypoglycemia and secondary polycythemia

10. Site for a tumor that produces an increase of both α-fetoprotein (AFP) and human chorionic gonadotropin (hCG)

11. Site for a tumor that can produce hypocalcemia

Refer to the following chart for questions 12 through 17:

	HBsAg	HBeAg HBV DNA	Anti-HBc IgM	Anti-HBc IgG	Anti-HBs
A.	–	–	+	–	–
B.	+	+	+	–	–
C.	–	–	–	+	+
D.	–	–	–	–	+
E.	+	–	–	+	–
F.	+	+	–	+	–

Each letter aligns with a set of options relating to hepatitis B serology test results. For questions 12 through 17, select the *one* lettered option that is most closely associated with it. Each lettered option may be selected once, more than once, or not at all.

12. Patient with hepatitis B who is noninfective and in the serologic gap

13. Patient who has recovered from hepatitis B

14. Patient who has been vaccinated against hepatitis B

15. Patient with symptomatic acute hepatitis B

16. Patient with infective chronic hepatitis B

17. Patient who is a "healthy" carrier for hepatitis B

Refer to the following table for questions 18 through 21:

% CB	Urine Bilirubin	Urine UBG	AST	ALT	ALP	GGT
	*negative	*↑	*normal	*normal	*normal	*normal
A. <20	negative	↑↑	↑	normal	normal	normal
B. >50	↑↑	negative	↑	↑	↑↑↑	↑↑↑
C. 20–50	↑	↑↑	↑↑	↑	↑↑	↑↑↑
D. 20–50	↑	↑↑	↑↑	↑↑↑	↑	↑
E. <20	negative	normal	normal	normal	normal	normal

*Values in top row are normal values. Number of arrows relates to the degree of elevation.
ALP, alkaline phosphatase; ALT, alanine aminotransferase; AST, aspartate aminotransferase; CB, conjugated bilirubin; GGT, gamma glutamyltransferase; UBG, urobilinogen.

Each letter entry designates a set of options relating to liver function test results. For questions 18 through 21, select the *one* lettered option that is most closely associated with it. Each lettered option may be selected once, more than once, or not at all.

18. A 24-year-old woman has hereditary spherocytosis and jaundice.

19. A 25-year-old medical student returns from a trip to Mexico on spring break. Three weeks later, he develops low-grade fever and jaundice. Physical examination shows painful hepatomegaly. The urine is dark yellow and the stool is light-colored.

20. A 32-year-old alcoholic has fever, jaundice, and tender hepatomegaly. A liver biopsy exhibits fatty change, Mallory's bodies, and a neutrophilic infiltrate.

21. A 22-year-old medical student develops jaundice only when he stays up all night studying. His physical examination is normal. All hepatitis serologic tests are negative.

22. A 30-year-old man with acute myelogenous leukemia is going to be placed on remission chemotherapy. Which of the following drugs should be used to prevent urate nephropathy?
A. Allopurinol
B. Aspirin
C. Probenecid
D. Sulfinpyrazone
E. Thiazides

23. A 75-year-old man with point tenderness in the lower vertebral column has an increased serum alkaline phosphatase. He does not smoke cigarettes. His stool guaiac is negative. Which of the following tests or procedures would be the most cost effective step in the initial evaluation of this patient?
A. Colonoscopy
B. Digital rectal examination
C. Prostate-specific antigen
D. Radionuclide bone scan
E. Serum gamma glutamyltransferase

24. A 35-year-old has a 3-month history of epigastric pain without radiation into the back. The stool is black and is positive for blood. He has a past history of gastric ulcer disease due to *Helicobacter pylori.* Which of the following tests would be the most cost effective and will identify the cause of his pain and provide an indicator on whether treatment is effective?
A. Radiolabeled urea breath test
B. Serologic test
C. Stool antigen test
D. Urease test on a gastric biopsy

25. A newborn child has a seizure within 1 hour after birth. The serum glucose is 20 mg/dL. The mother had gestational diabetes mellitus and was in poor glycemic control throughout the pregnancy. Which of the following hormones is most likely responsible for the hypoglycemia?
A. Cortisol
B. Glucagon
C. Insulin
D. Prolactin
E. Thyroxine

26. A 33-year-old man has a history of chronic liver disease and a movement disorder. Physical examination also reveals a discoloration in Descemet's membrane in the cornea. Which of the following laboratory findings would most likely be reported?
A. Decreased serum ceruloplasmin
B. Increased iron saturation
C. Increased serum iron
D. Increased total serum copper
E. Normal serum prothrombin time

27. A 45-year-old woman with rheumatoid arthritis has a increased serum total protein. The hyperproteinemia is most likely due to an increase in which of the following protein fractions?
A. Albumin
B. Immunoglobulin A
C. Immunoglobulin G
D. Immunoglobulin M

28. A 62-year-old man, who lives alone, has pitting edema of his lower legs. The serum total protein concentration is decreased. He subsists primarily on bread and diet cola. A urinalysis is negative for protein. Which of the following best explains the pathogenesis of the hypoproteinemia?
A. Acquired hypogammaglobulinemia
B. Decreased intake of protein
C. Malignant plasma cell disorder
D. Nephrotic syndrome

29. In a 24-year-old man with a healing bone fracture, which of the following laboratory test results are expected?

	Serum ALP	Serum GGT
A.	Increased	Increased
B.	Increased	Normal
C.	Normal	Increased
D.	Normal	Normal

ALP, alkaline phosphatase; GGT, γ-glutamyltransferase.

30. Which of the following occur in both type 1 and type 2 diabetes mellitus?
A. Antibodies against islet cells
B. Association with HLA-Dr3/Dr4
C. Down-regulation of insulin receptor synthesis
D. Ketoacidosis
E. Osmotic damage

31. A 45-year-old intensive care nurse complains of recurrent episodes of forgetfulness and tiredness. Laboratory studies show a serum glucose level of 25 mg/dL, an increase in serum insulin, and absent serum C-peptide. Which of the following is the most likely cause of her hypoglycemia?
A. Benign tumor of β-islet cells
B. Ectopic secretion of an insulin-like factor
C. Malignant tumor of α-islet cells
D. Patient injection of human insulin

Refer to Figure 9-15 for questions 32 through 35:

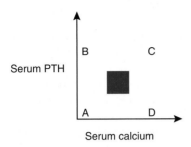

9-15: *Refer to questions 32 to 35.*

Each lettered set of options relates to serum parathyroid hormone (PTH) and serum calcium disorders. For questions 32 through 35, select the *one* lettered option that is most closely associated with it. Each lettered option may be selected once, more than once, or not at all. The square represents the normal reference interval for serum PTH and serum calcium.

32. A 45-year-old has end-stage diabetic nephropathy. When a blood pressure is taken, his thumb adducts into his palm.

33. A 52-year-old man is taking an aminoglycoside for an infection. He develops tetany. A serum magnesium level is decreased.

34. A 58-year-old woman has a recurrent history of calcium oxalate stones, hypercalciuria, peptic ulcer disease, constipation, and diastolic hypertension.

35. A 49-year-old woman with a previous history of a radical mastectomy 7 years ago complains of bone pain. A bone scan is reported as abnormal. The QT interval is shortened on an ECG.

Refer to Figure 9-16 for questions 36 and 37:

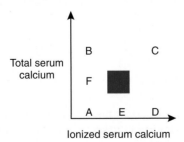

9-16: *Refer to questions 36 and 37.*

Each letter describes a set of options comparing total serum calcium to ionized serum calcium levels. For questions 36 and 37, select the *one* lettered option that is most closely associated with it. Each lettered option may be selected once, more than once, or not at all. The square represents the normal reference interval for total serum calcium and ionized serum calcium.

36. The patient is an 8-year old boy generalized pitting edema and effusion due to lipoid nephrosis. There is no evidence of tetany.

37. The patient is a 22-year-old woman who is having an hysterical reaction after seeing a mouse running under her desk. Her thumbs are flexed into the palms.

38. A 58-year-old man has pain in the lower lumbar spine and pelvis. Initial laboratory studies show a normocytic anemia and marked rouleaux of red blood cells. Serum blood urea nitrogen (BUN) is 70 mg/dL, and serum creatinine is 7 mg/dL. A bone marrow aspirate is performed and reveals sheets of malignant plasma cells. Which of the following additional laboratory findings is most likely to be reported?
A. Decreased erythrocyte sedimentation rate
B. Decreased serum calcium level
C. Increased prothrombin time
D. Monoclonal protein spike on serum protein electrophoresis
E. Normal bleeding time

39. Which of the following is most responsible for the hyperglycemia in diabetic ketoacidosis?
A. Anaerobic glycolysis
B. Decreased uptake of glucose in tissue
C. Gluconeogenesis
D. Glycogenolysis

40. A 22-year-old woman has a history of intermittent, abdominal pain that occurs after she has a glass of wine. Recently, after collecting a urine specimen for culture, she notices that the urine color has changed from a yellow to a wine-red color after sitting on the window sill in her kitchen. Which of the following compounds is most likely responsible for the color change in the urine?
A. Hemoglobin
B. Myoglobin
C. Porphobilin
D. Urobilin
E. Uroporphyrin I

41. A 3-year-old child has a recurrent history of fatty stools and respiratory infections. Physical examination reveals a polyp in the right nasal cavity. Which of the following tests should be ordered?
A. Chromosome analysis
B. Stool culture
C. Sweat chloride
D. Total serum immunoglobulin

Answers

1. **B** (type II hyperlipoproteinemia) is correct. The patient has familial hypercholesterolemia, which is an autosomal dominant disorder with absent or defective low density lipoprotein (LDL) receptors. Achilles tendon xanthomas are pathognomonic for the disease. Patients have an increase in serum cholesterol (>260 mg/dL) and LDL (>190 mg/dL) and a decrease in high-density lipoprotein (HDL).

2. **D** (type IV hyperlipoproteinemia) is correct. The patient most likely has familial hypertriglyceridemia, which has an autosomal dominant inheritance pattern. It is most often due to increased production of very low density lipoprotein (VLDL) by the liver. The yellow, papular skin lesions are called eruptive xanthomas. Patients have an increase in TG (>300 mg/dL) and LDL is usually <190 mg/dL. There is a decrease in serum HDL, due to an increase in VLDL. There is a turbid infranate after refrigeration.

3. **C** (type III hyperlipoproteinemia) is correct. The patient has familial dysbetalipoproteinemia or "remnant disease," which has an autosomal recessive inheritance pattern. It is due to defective apolipoprotein E, which leads to decreased liver uptake of intermediate density lipoprotein (IDL) and chylomicron remnants in the blood. Palmar xanthomas commonly occur in the flexor creases. Both serum CH and TG are >300 mg/dL.

4. **E** (type V hyperlipoproteinemia) is correct. This type of hyperlipoproteinemia is most often a combination of familial hypertriglyceridemia (type IV hyperlipoproteinemia) plus an exacerbating disorder where there is decreased activation and release of capillary lipoprotein lipase. This leads to an accumulation of both chylomicrons and VLDL resulting in a turbid supranate (chylomicrons) and infranate after refrigeration. Diabetic ketoacidosis with insulin deficiency is the most common setting for this hyperlipoproteinemia. Eruptive xanthomas commonly occur, as in this patient.

5. **C** (reinfarction) is correct. CK-MB isoenzymes, a marker for acute myocardial infarction, are usually gone by 3 days. Therefore, reappearance of CK-MB after 3 days indicates reinfarction or further extension of an existing myocardial infarction. Troponins I and T are the gold standard for diagnosing

an acute myocardial infarction. However, troponin I remains increased for a week, while troponin T remains increased for 10 to 14 days; therefore, they cannot be used to diagnose a reinfarction.

A (myocardial rupture) is incorrect. Rupture of the myocardium either produces a murmur (e.g., mitral regurgitation from posteromedial papillary muscle infarction) or cardiac tamponade with muffling of the heart sounds and jugular neck vein distention. These are not present in the patient.

B (papillary muscle dysfunction) is incorrect. The posteromedial papillary muscle is supplied by the right coronary artery. Dysfunction or infarction due to thrombosis of the artery should produce the pansystolic murmur of mitral valve regurgitation. Cardiac examination is normal in the patient.

D (right ventricular infarction) is incorrect. The right coronary artery supplies the right ventricle. Infarction of the right ventricle produces signs of right-sided heart failure, which include neck vein distention and the murmur of tricuspid valve regurgitation. These findings are not present in the patient.

E (ventricular aneurysm) is incorrect. Ventricular aneurysms are a late finding in an acute myocardial infarction. They do not produce reappearance of CK-MB.

6. **E** (increased urinary 5-hydroxyindoleacetic acid) is correct. The patient has carcinoid syndrome. In this patient, the primary site for the carcinoid tumor is the terminal ileum, where it has produced an obstructive lesion. When there is no liver metastasis, the serotonin produced by the tumor is drained by the portal vein to the liver where it is metabolized into 5-hydroxyindoleacetic acid (5-HIAA) and excreted in the urine. The syndrome is produced when there is metastasis to the liver, where serotonin may enter hepatic vein tributaries, hence gaining access to the systemic circulation. Serotonin is a vasodilator and produces flushing of the skin. It also increases colonic motility leading to diarrhea.

A (increased serum α-fetoprotein, AFP) is incorrect. Serum AFP is increased in hepatocellular carcinoma secondary to cirrhosis of the liver. It is not a marker of metastatic disease to the liver.

B (increased serum antistreptolysin O, ASO) is incorrect. Serum ASO titers are increased in group A streptococcal disease (*Streptococcus pyogenes*) involving the pharynx. It is not increased in the carcinoid syndrome.

C (increased serum CA 125) is incorrect. This tumor marker is increased in surface-derived ovarian tumors. The pelvic examination is normal in this patient.

D (increased serum CA-19–9) is incorrect. This tumor marker is increased in carcinoma of the pancreas. Cigarette smoking is the most common cause of this cancer, which usually involves the head of the pancreas producing obstructive jaundice. Jaundice is not present in this patient, and the barium study indicates a primary lesion in the terminal ileum.

7. **D** (lung) is correct. A small cell carcinoma of the lung can ectopically produce adrenocorticotropic hormone (ACTH) producing Cushing's syndrome and antidiuretic hormone producing hyponatremia.

8. **A** (kidney) is correct. A renal cell carcinoma can ectopically secrete parathyroid hormone-related protein producing hypercalcemia and erythropoietin (EPO) producing secondary polycythemia.

9. **C** (liver) is correct. A hepatocellular carcinoma can produce an insulin-like factor producing hypoglycemia or EPO producing secondary polycythemia.

10. **E** (testicle) is correct. A yolk sac tumor of the testicle can produce an increase in AFP and a choriocarcinoma of the testicle containing trophoblastic tissue can produce an increase in human chorionic gonadotropin.

11. **F** (thyroid) is correct. A medullary carcinoma of the thyroid derives from C cells that synthesize calcitonin. Calcitonin is a hormone that inhibits osteoclasts leading to hypocalcemia.

12. **A** is correct. The only marker for acute hepatitis B in the early recovery phase when all the tumor antigens have disappeared is anti-HBc IgM. It converts to anti-HBc IgG after 6 months.

13. **C** is correct. Markers for recovery are anti-HBc IgG and anti-HBs.

14. **D** is correct. Patients develop protective anti-HBs antibodies against HBsAg in the vaccine.

15. **B** is correct. Markers of acute, symptomatic hepatitis B include HBsAg, HBeAg and HBV DNA (infective particles), and anti-HBc IgM. With recovery, the infective particles leave first, followed by HBsAg.

16. **F** is correct. Chronic hepatitis B is defined as HBsAg present for over 6 months. Infective carriers have HBsAg, HBeAg and HBV DNA (infective particles), and anti-HBc IgG.

17. **E** is correct. Healthy chronic carriers have HBsAg and anti-HBc IgG. They lack HBeAg and HBV DNA (infective particles).

18. **A** is correct. In hereditary spherocytosis (see Chapter 5), spherocytes are removed extravascularly by macrophages leading to an increase in unconjugated bilirubin (UCB) and a CB < 20%. AST is present in RBCs; therefore, there is a slight increase in AST. Urine UBG is increased due to increased production of CB by the liver and increased conversion of CB to UBG in the colon.

19. **D** is correct. The student most likely has hepatitis A. Hepatitis produces a mixed jaundice (CB 20–50%). Urine UBG is increased, because UBG that is normally recycled back to the liver is redirected into the urine. Serum transaminases are markedly increased with serum ALT greater than AST. Serum ALP and GGT are only slightly increased.

20. **C** is correct. The patient has alcoholic hepatitis, which produces a mixed jaundice (CB 20–50%). Urine UBG is increased, because UBG that is normally recycled back to the liver is redirected into the urine. Serum transaminases are increased with serum AST (mitochondrial enzyme) greater than ALT (cytosol enzyme). Because AST is normally located in the mitochondria of hepatocytes, alcohol, a mitochondrial toxin, causes preferential release of AST into the blood. Serum ALP is slightly increased; however, serum GGT is markedly increased, because alcohol induces enzyme synthesis in the hepatocyte cytochrome P-450 system in the smooth endoplasmic reticulum. GGT is also located in the SER and is increased as well.

21. **E** is correct. The patient has Gilbert's disease, which is an autosomal dominant disease characterized by decreased uptake and conjugation of bilirubin particularly exacerbated by the fasting state. Baseline UCB levels are increased to over twice normal in the fasting state leading to visible evidence of jaundice (CB < 20%). Next to viral hepatitis, it is the second overall most common cause of jaundice in the United States. It has no clinical significance.

22.   **A** (allopurinol) is correct. Allopurinol is an xanthine oxidase inhibitor, which prevents the conversion of xanthine to uric acid. In treating cancers with a high tumor burden, patients must be placed on this drug to prevent excessive production of uric acid from purines released by the dying cancer cells. Excessive uric acid in the kidneys may result in acute renal failure due to blockage of the renal tubules by urate crystals.

B   (aspirin) is incorrect. Aspirin in low doses decreases uric acid in the urine and in high doses is uricosuric. In either situation, aspirin is not used to prevent urate nephropathy.

C   (probenecid) is incorrect. Probenecid is a uricosuric drug that is used in treating underexcretors with gout. It is not used to prevent urate nephropathy.

D   (sulfinpyrazone) is incorrect. Sulfinpyrazone is a uricosuric drug that is used in treating underexcretors with gout. It is not used to prevent urate nephropathy.

E   (thiazides) is incorrect. Thiazides can produce hyperuricemia by increasing proximal tubule reabsorption of uric acid (due to volume depletion) and decreasing proximal tubule secretion of uric acid. This would increase the risk for urate nephropathy.

23.   **B** (digital rectal examination) is correct. The patient most likely has metastatic prostate cancer to the lower vertebral column. Prostate cancer produces osteoblastic metastases (stimulates an increase in osteoblastic activity) leading to an increase in bone density and an increase in alkaline phosphatase originating from osteoblasts. With metastasis to bone, a digital rectal examination would very likely detect prostate cancer, because it originates in the periphery of the gland. It would be the least expensive initial step in evaluating this patient.

A   (colonoscopy) is incorrect. Prostate cancer is the most common cancer in men and the most common cause of osteoblastic metastases. The stool guaiac test is negative, and therefore, a colonoscopy to rule out colorectal cancer as a cause of the bone lesions would not be the initial step in evaluating the patient.

C   (prostate-specific antigen) is incorrect. Although this test is indicated and would be increased, a digital rectal examination will give more immediate information as to the cause of the patient's back pain and increased serum alkaline phosphatase.

D   (radionuclide bone scan) is incorrect, Although this test is indicated and would most likely show metastatic disease in the bone, a digital rectal examination will give more immediate information as to the cause of the patient's back pain and increased serum alkaline phosphatase.

E   (serum gamma glutamyltransferase) is incorrect. This test is excellent in helping to localize the source of an increased alkaline phosphatase. However, the presentation is very characteristic of prostate cancer and, though indicated, would not give immediate information regarding the cause of the patient's back pain.

24. **C** (stool antigen test) is correct. The stool antigen test detects pyloroantigens. It is the least expensive test and helps support a diagnosis of infection and determine whether treatment is effective. The sensitivity is 92% and specificity 90% to 100%.

A (radiolabeled urea breath test) is incorrect. *H. pylori* converts orally administered labeled urea to labeled CO_2, which is detected in the breath. It is an expensive test, when compared to the stool antigen test. It has a sensitivity >97% and a specificity >90%.

B (serologic test) is incorrect. This does *not* differentiate current or past infection. The patient has a history of *H. pylori*–induced peptic ulcer disease. The test also does *not* determine whether treatment has been effective.

D (urease test on a gastric biopsy) is incorrect. This is an expensive test that has excellent sensitivity (90%) and specificity 99% to 100%; however, it would have to be repeated to see if treatment was effective.

25. **C** (insulin) is correct. Due to the mother's poor glycemic control, the fetus also had hyperglycemia and an increase in insulin in response to the hyperglycemia. Insulin decreases surfactant synthesis, so an additional problem in the newborn could be respiratory distress syndrome. After delivery, the newborn child had a hyperglycemia and increased insulin, the latter driving the glucose down into hypoglycemic ranges prompting a seizure. This underscores the need to give these newborns glucose after birth to prevent hypoglycemia.

A (cortisol) is incorrect. Cortisol is a gluconeogenic hormone and would not be expected to produce hypoglycemia.

B (glucagon) is incorrect. Glucagon is a gluconeogenic hormone and would not be expected to produce hypoglycemia. Furthermore, it would likely be decreased due to the increased glucose levels.

D (prolactin) is incorrect. Prolactin has no effect on the blood glucose level.

E (thyroxine) is incorrect. Thyroxine has no significant effect on the blood glucose level.

26. **A** (decreased serum ceruloplasmin) is correct. A Kayser-Fleischer ring (rusty-colored pigment around the perimeter of the cornea), chronic liver disease, and a movement disorder are features of Wilson's disease, an autosomal recessive disease. Wilson's disease is due to a defect in the hepatocyte transport system for copper secretion into bile and a decrease in the synthesis of ceruloplasmin, which is the binding protein of copper. The total serum copper equals copper that is bound to ceruloplasmin (95% of the total) plus copper that is unbound (free). In Wilson's disease, the total serum copper level is decreased, because ceruloplasmin is decreased. However, the free copper level in the serum and urine is increased due to defective excretion in the bile and subsequent accumulation of copper in the serum.

B (increased iron saturation) is incorrect. Movement disorders and deposition of iron in the cornea are not associated with disorders of iron metabolism (e.g., hemochromatosis).

C (increased serum iron) is incorrect. Hemochromatosis (not Wilson's disease) is associated with an increase in the serum iron.

D (increased total serum copper) is incorrect. In Wilson's disease, the total serum copper level is decreased, because ceruloplasmin is decreased.

E (normal serum prothrombin time) is incorrect. The patient has chronic liver disease (chronic hepatitis or cirrhosis). Therefore, the prothrombin time is most likely increased due to decreased synthesis of coagulation factors in the liver.

27. **C** (immunoglobulin G) is correct. An increased serum total protein is most often due to an increase in immunoglobulins (Igs). Igs are primarily increased in chronic inflammation and malignant plasma cell disorders (e.g., multiple myeloma). Because the patient has rheumatoid arthritis, a chronic inflammatory disease, the immunoglobulins are increased. The primary Ig to increase in chronic inflammation is IgG. A serum protein electrophoresis would show a polyclonal gammopathy (diffuse increase in the γ-globulin curve).

A (albumin) is incorrect. An increase in albumin is uncommon and would most likely be present in a patient with volume depletion, which is not present in this patient.

B (immunoglobulin A) is incorrect. IgA is not the primary Ig that is increased in chronic inflammation. An exception to this rule is alcoholic cirrhosis, where it is often increased along with IgG.

D (immunoglobulin M) is incorrect. An increase in IgM is present in acute inflammation and in Waldenström's macroglobulinemia.

28. **B** (decreased intake of protein) is correct. The patient's diet is lacking protein leading to a decrease in albumin and a corresponding decrease in total protein. Albumin is primarily responsible for maintaining plasma oncotic pressure; therefore, hypoalbuminemia leads to leakage of protein-poor fluid into the interstitial space caused pitting edema.

A (acquired hypogammaglobulinemia) is incorrect. Hypogammaglobulinemia is an uncommon cause of a decrease in total serum protein. Furthermore, it would not explain the pitting edema in the patient.

C (malignant plasma cell disorder) is incorrect. A malignant plasma cell disorder (e.g., multiple myeloma) produces an increase in serum total protein, not a decrease.

D (nephrotic syndrome) is incorrect. The nephrotic syndrome is characterized by massive losses of protein in the urine (>3.5 g/24 hours) leading to hypoalbuminemia and a decrease in total serum protein. The patient does not have proteinuria.

29. **B** (increased serum ALP, normal serum GGT) is correct. In a healing fracture, there is increased osteoblastic activity. Because osteoblasts contain ALP, ALP is increased in serum. GGT is not present in osteoblasts; therefore, it remains normal

A (increased serum ALP, increased serum GGT) is incorrect. GGT is not present in osteoblasts; therefore, it is normal in a healing bone fracture. An increase in both ALP and GGT is present in intrahepatic and extrahepatic cholestasis. Increased pressure of bile on the bile duct epithelium causes increased synthesis of both enzymes.

C (normal serum ALP, increased serum GGT) is incorrect. A normal serum ALP and increased serum GGT is present in alcoholics. Alcohol induces synthesis of enzymes located in the smooth endoplasmic reticulum of the liver. These include enzymes in the cytochrome P-450 system and GGT.

D (normal serum ALP, normal serum GGT) is incorrect. In a healing bone fracture, serum ALP is increased and serum GGT is normal.

30. **E** (osmotic damage) is correct. Osmotic damage occurs in tissues with aldose reductase (e.g., lens, Schwann cells). Glucose is converted to sorbitol by aldose reductase. Sorbitol is osmotically active and draws water into the tissue leading to osmotic damage (e.g., cataracts, peripheral neuropathy). Osmotic damage primarily occurs with poor glycemic control, so both types of diabetes mellitus experience this mechanism of damage.

A (antibodies against islet cells) is incorrect. These antibodies occur in 80% to 90% of patients with type 1 diabetes within the first year of diagnosis. Type 2 diabetics do not have these antibodies.

B (association with HLA-Dr3/Dr4) is incorrect. These HLA types are seen in patients with type 1 diabetes mellitus. These HLA types place the patient at increased risk for eventual destruction of the islet cells by viruses (e.g., coxsackievirus) or other environmental factors.

C (down-regulation of insulin receptors) is incorrect. Type 2 diabetes mellitus is more often associated with obesity than type 1 diabetics. Increased adipose down-regulates insulin receptor synthesis. This underscores why weight reduction is important in type 2 diabetes, since loss of adipose upregulates insulin receptor synthesis. The hyperglycemia in type 2 diabetics is most directly related to postreceptor defects (e.g., defects in tyrosine kinase activity).

D (ketoacidosis) is incorrect. Ketoacidosis occurs in absolute insulin deficiency, which characterizes type 1 diabetes mellitus. In type 2 diabetes, there is enough insulin to prevent ketone body synthesis but not enough to keep blood glucose in the normal range. Patients with type 2 diabetes are prone to developing hyperosmolar nonketotic coma. The metabolic acidosis in these patients is due to lactic acidosis from volume depletion and hypovolemic shock, not ketoacidosis.

31. **D** (patient injection of human insulin) is correct. When preproinsulin in the β-islet cells is delivered to the Golgi apparatus, proteolytic reactions generate insulin and a cleavage peptide called C-peptide. Hence, C-peptide is a marker for endogenous synthesis of insulin. Injection of human insulin increases serum insulin and produces hypoglycemia. Hypoglycemia suppresses β-islet cells, causing a decrease in endogenous synthesis of insulin and a corresponding decrease or absence of C-peptide.

   A (benign tumor of β-islet cells) is incorrect. Benign tumors of the β-islet cells, or insulinomas, synthesize excess insulin, resulting in fasting hypoglycemia. Both serum insulin and serum C-peptide levels are increased in an insulinoma.

   C (ectopic secretion of an insulin-like factor) is incorrect. An insulin-like factor that causes hypoglycemia is most often produced by a hepatocellular carcinoma. Hypoglycemia suppresses β-islet cells, resulting in a decrease in serum insulin and C-peptide.

   D (malignant tumor of α-islet cells) is incorrect. Tumors of α-islet cells secrete glucagon, which produces hyperglycemia (not hypoglycemia) by stimulating gluconeogenesis.

32. **B** (increased serum PTH, decreased serum calcium) is correct. The patient has chronic renal failure and tetany (thumb adducts into palm) related to hypovitaminosis D. The second hydroxylation of vitamin D occurs in the proximal tubules of the kidneys where 1-α-hydroxylase is located. Decreased vitamin D results in decreased reabsorption of calcium from the small bowel leading to hypocalcemia. Hypocalcemia has a negative feedback with PTH causing an increase in PTH (secondary hyperparathyroidism). The increase in PTH enhances osteoclastic activity leading to an attempt to restore the serum calcium to normal.

33. **A** (decreased serum PTH, decreased serum calcium) is correct. Aminoglycosides are magnesium wasters and commonly lead to hypomagnesemia. Magnesium is a cofactor for adenylate cyclase. cAMP is required for PTH activation. Therefore, hypomagnesemia leads to hypoparathyroidism and a corresponding decreased in serum PTH and calcium, the latter resulting in tetany.

34. **C** (increased serum PTH, increased serum calcium) is correct. The patient has primary hyperparathyroidism, which is most often due to a benign parathyroid gland adenoma. The adenomas do not respond to the increase in serum calcium by decreasing the synthesis of PTH. All the clinical findings listed in the patient (renal stones, peptic ulcer disease, constipation, hypertension) are commonly present in primary hyperparathyroidism.

35. **D** (decreased serum PTH, increased serum calcium) is correct. The bone pain in the patient is due to breast cancer metastasis to the bone. In this case, it has produced hypercalcemia (short QT interval in an ECG) leading to suppression of PTH synthesis by the parathyroid glands. The metastatic lesions in the bone have activated osteoclasts leading to lytic lesions and an increase in serum calcium.

36. **E** (decreased total serum calcium, normal ionized serum calcium) is correct. The patient has nephrotic syndrome with a loss of albumin. The hypoalbuminemia should lower the total calcium without affecting the ionized calcium level.

37. **F** (normal total serum calcium, decreased ionized serum calcium) is correct. The patient has respiratory alkalosis due to hyperventilation. Alkalosis lowers the ionized calcium level (produces tetany) without affecting the total calcium, because albumin has more negative charges (more COOH groups on acidic amino acids are COO^-) and binds more ionized calcium.

38. **D** (monoclonal protein spike on serum protein electrophoresis) is correct. The patient has multiple myeloma complicated by renal failure (BUN:creatinine <15, see Chapter 4). A monoclonal spike in the γ-globulin region can be expected on serum protein electrophoresis. The spike is caused by a single immunoglobulin (usually IgG) and its corresponding light chain (usually κ), which are secreted by clones derived from a single neoplastic plasma cell. Renal failure is a common complication of multiple myeloma. Excess light chains, called Bence Jones protein, are usually present in the urine. In this case, renal failure is due to the formation of casts composed of Bence Jones protein blocking the tubular lumens and inciting a foreign body giant cell reaction.

A (decreased erythrocyte sedimentation rate, ESR) is incorrect. Rouleaux (RBCs stacked together like coins) is due to an increase in fibrinogen /or anemia, in this case, anemia. Rouleaux causes RBCs to settle faster in plasma and increases (not decreases) the erythrocyte sedimentation rate (ESR). The ESR is not a very specific test and is not a key test used to diagnose plasma cell malignancies.
B (decreased serum calcium level) is incorrect. The patient has multiple myeloma, which causes osteolytic lesions and the potential for hypercalcemia (not hypocalcemia).
C (increased prothrombin time) is incorrect. In multiple myeloma, coagulation studies, including prothrombin time, are normal.
E (normal bleeding time) is incorrect. In multiple myeloma, the bleeding time is usually prolonged, because rouleaux interferes with platelet aggregation.

39. **C** (gluconeogenesis) is correct. In diabetic ketoacidosis (DKA), complete deficiency of insulin causes the release of glucagon from α-islet cells (paracrine effect) in the pancreas. Glucagon is the main hormone that stimulates gluconeogenesis and maintains the hyperglycemia in DKA.

A (anaerobic glycolysis) is incorrect. Anaerobic glycolysis is the oxidation of glucose to lactate. This reaction uses glucose for energy rather than for maintaining glucose levels in the blood in DKA.

B (decreased uptake of glucose in tissue) is incorrect. Receptors for insulin are located on adipose cells and muscle cells. Insulin is not present in DKA; therefore, glucose cannot enter these cells to be metabolized. Although decreased uptake of glucose does contribute to hyperglycemia in DKA, it is not as important as gluconeogenesis.

D (glycogenolysis) is incorrect. Glycogenolysis is increased in DKA; however, glycogen stores are depleted within 36 hrs, which limits its role in maintaining hyperglycemia in DKA.

40. **C** (porphobilin) is correct. The patient has acute intermittent porphyria (AIP), which is an autosomal dominant disease due to a deficiency of uroporphyrinogen synthase (alias porphobilinogen deaminase). This enzyme converts porphobilinogen (PBG) to hydroxymethylbilane in heme synthesis. Deficiency of the enzyme causes a proximal accumulation of PBG and δ-aminolevulinic acid, which are excreted in the urine. PBG is colorless unless it is exposed to light and is oxidized to porphobilin, which has a wine-red color. A characteristic feature of the disease is recurrent neurologically induced abdominal pain precipitated by drugs that induce the liver cytochrome P-450 system (e.g., alcohol) or dietary restriction. Patients with abdominal pain frequently undergo surgical exploration ("bellyful of scars") only to find that no organic lesions are present. The confirmatory test is to document the enzyme deficiency in red blood cells.

A (hemoglobin) is incorrect. Hemoglobinuria occurs with intravascular hemolysis. Hemoglobin produces a red discoloration of urine that is present when voiding and does not require exposure to light to produce color.

B (myoglobin) is incorrect. Myoglobinuria occurs when there is massive damage to skeletal muscle (e.g., severe exercise, trauma). Myoglobin produces a red discoloration of urine when voided and does not change color after exposure to light.

D (urobilin) is incorrect. Urobilin is the oxidation product of urobilinogen, which is normally present in trace amounts in urine. Urobilin is the pigment that is responsible for the yellow color of urine. If urobilin is increased in the urine (e.g., extravascular hemolytic anemia, hepatitis), the urine is a dark yellow color and does not turn wine-red with exposure to light.

E (uroporphyrin I) is incorrect. Uroporphyrin I produces a wine-red color to urine when voided. It is increased in porphyria cutanea tarda (PCT). PCT is an acquired or hereditary disorder characterized by a deficiency of uroporphyrinogen decarboxylase, which converts uroporphyrinogen III to coproporphyrinogen III. The former compound spontaneously converts into uroporphyrinogen I and its colored oxidation product, uroporphyrin I. PCT is associated with photosensitive skin lesions consisting of vesicles and bullae. The skin is fragile and fine hair develops over the face. The patient does not have any of these physical findings.

41. C (sweat chloride) is correct. The child has cystic fibrosis (CF), which is an autosomal recessive disease. Owing to a three-nucleotide deletion on chromosome 7, a defective CF transmembrane conductance regulator (CFTR) for Cl⁻ ions is produced that is degraded in the Golgi apparatus. Loss of CFTR Cl⁻ causes decreased Na⁺ and Cl⁻ reabsorption in sweat glands which is the basis of the sweat test (sweat Cl⁻ > 60 mEq/L). In luminal secretions, there is lack of Na⁺ and Cl⁻ leading to thick, dehydrated secretions that block lumens producing respiratory infections (e.g., pneumonia) and pancreatic exocrine deficiency (produces malabsorption). Nasal polyps occur in 25% of children with CF and are highly predictive of CF.

A (chromosome analysis) is incorrect. A chromosome analysis is normal. Special studies are required to identify the three nucleotide deletion.

B (stool culture) is incorrect. The diarrhea is secondary to malabsorption of fat and is not related to a bacterial pathogen.

D (total serum immunoglobulin) is incorrect. Although certain types of immunodeficiency conditions can produce malabsorption and respiratory infections (i.e., common variable immunodeficiency), they are not associated with nasal polyps in children. Therefore, this test would not be useful in diagnosing CF.

10

Endocrine Disorders

I. Overview of Endocrine Testing

A. Tests to evaluate hypofunction and hyperfunction

1. Negative feedback loops
   a. Control an increase or decrease in hormone production
   b. Example—decreased calcium should increase parathyroid hormone (PTH)
2. Stimulation tests
   a. Evaluate hypofunctioning disorders
      - Example—adrenocorticotropic hormone (ACTH) stimulation test used in the workup of hypocortisolism
   b. Causes of hypofunction
      (1) Autoimmune destruction
         - Examples—Addison's disease, hypoparathyroidism
      (2) Infarction
         - Example—Sheehan's postpartum necrosis
      (3) Decreased hormone stimulation
         - Example—decreased thyroid-stimulating hormone (TSH) in hypopituitarism causes atrophy of thyroid gland
      (4) Enzyme deficiency, infection, neoplasia, congenital disorder
3. Suppression tests
   a. Evaluate hyperfunctioning disorders
      - Example—dexamethasone suppression test evaluates hypercortisolism
   b. Most hyperfunctioning disorders *cannot* be suppressed.
      - Notable *exceptions* are prolactinoma and pituitary Cushing's syndrome
   c. Causes of hyperfunction
      (1) Adenoma, hyperplasia, cancer
      (2) Inflammation causes increased release of stored hormone.
         - Examples—acute thyroiditis, early phase of Hashimoto's thyroiditis

> Endocrine gland hypofunction: most common cause is autoimmune disease

> Endocrine gland hyperfunction: most common cause is a benign adenoma

II. Hypothalamus Disorders

A. Hyperfunction disorders

1. Destructive lesion decreases synthesis of dopamine (prolactin inhibiting factor)
2. Examples
   a. Langerhans' histiocytosis
      - Malignant histiocytes destroy hypothalamus.

        b. Sarcoidosis (see Chapter 3)
- Granulomatous inflammation

    3. Produces galactorrhea

  B. **Hypofunction disorders**

    1. Destructive lesions

      a. Pituitary adenoma (see Table 10-1)
- Most common tumor affecting the hypothalamus

      b. Craniopharyngioma (see Table 10-1)

      c. Langerhans' histiocytosis

      d. Sarcoidosis

    2. Clinical disorders producing laboratory test abnormalities

      a. Secondary hypopituitarism
- No releasing hormones to stimulate the anterior pituitary

      b. Central diabetes inspidus
        (1) Antidiuretic hormone (ADH) is synthesized in the supraoptic and paraventricular nuclei.
        (2) Lack of ADH causes polyuria (urine output > 2.5–3 L/day) and polydipsia (increased thirst)

      c. Growth disorders
- Decreased growth hormone releasing hormone decreases growth hormone causing dwarfism in children

III. **Pituitary Gland Disorders**

  A. **Pituitary hyperfunction disorders**

    1. Prolactinoma

      a. Caused by a benign adenoma secreting prolactin
- Overall most common pituitary tumor

      b. Clinical and laboratory findings
        (1) Secondary amenorrhea
- Prolactin inhibits gonadotropin-releasing hormone (GnRH).
        (2) Galactorrhea
- Only occurs in women, *not* men
        (3) Impotence in men
- Loss of libido due to decrease in testosterone
        (4) Serum prolactin is usually >200 ng/mL.
        (5) Decreased FSH and LH
- Due to decreased GnRH

      c. Other causes of galactorrhea
        (1) Postpartum, stress, nipple stimulation
        (2) Primary hypothyroidism
- Decreased serum T_4 causes increase in thyrotropin-releasing hormone, which stimulates prolactin secretion.
        (3) Drugs: oral contraceptives, haloperidol, phenothiazines, methyldopa
        (4) Estrogen-producing tumors: granulosa cell tumor of ovary

      d. Treatment of prolactinoma
- Dopamine analogues (e.g., cabergoline) or surgery

Secondary amenorrhea + galactorrhea: prolactinoma

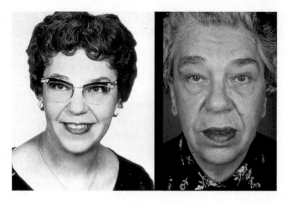

10-1: *Acromegaly showing the patient before development of the tumor (picture on the left) and after development of the tumor (picture on the right). Note the coarse facial features and enlargement of the jaw and lips. (From Damjanov I: Pathology for the Health-Related Professions, 2nd ed. Philadelphia, WB Saunders, 2000, p 407.)*

2. Growth hormone (GH) adenoma
   a. Functions of GH
      (1) Stimulates liver synthesis/release of insulin-like growth factor (IGF)-1
      (2) Stimulates gluconeogenesis and amino acid uptake in muscle
      (3) Negative feedback relationship with glucose and IGF-1
   b. Functions of IGF-1
      • Stimulates growth of bone (linear and lateral), cartilage, soft tissue
   c. Clinical findings
      (1) Children develop gigantism
         • Due to increased linear bone growth
      (2) Adults develop acromegaly (Fig. 10-1)
         (a) Increased lateral bone growth (e.g., hands, feet, jaw)
            • No linear growth because the epiphyses are fused
         (b) Prominent jaw
            • Spacing between the teeth
         (c) Frontal bossing
            • Enlarged frontal sinus increases the hat size.
         (d) Macroglossia, cardiomyopathy (cause of death)
   d. Laboratory findings
      (1) Increased GH and IGF-1 (better test)
         • Hormones are *not* suppressed by glucose administration.
      (2) Hyperglycemia
         • Due to increase in gluconeogenesis
B. **Anterior pituitary hypofunction**
   1. Etiology (Table 10-1)
   2. Clinical findings (Table 10-2)
C. **Posterior pituitary hypofunction; diabetes insipidus**
   1. Types
      a. Central diabetes insipidus (CDI)
         • Decreased amount of antidiuretic hormone (ADH)

> Acromegaly: increased lateral bone growth, organomegaly, hyperglycemia

> Hypopituitarism in adults: most common cause is nonfunctioning adenoma

TABLE 10-1
Causes of Anterior Pituitary Hypofunction

Disorder	Comments
Nonfunctioning pituitary adenoma	Association with multiple endocrine neoplasia (MEN) I syndrome: pituitary adenoma, hyperparathyroidism, pancreatic tumor (Zollinger-Ellison or insulinoma) Enlarged sella turcica with erosions of the clinoid processes Bitemporal hemianopsia, headache
Sheehan's postpartum necrosis	Pituitary gland doubles in size during pregnancy due to synthesis of prolactin; it is especially vulnerable to infarction if the patient develops hypovolemic shock (e.g., blood loss) Sudden cessation of lactation due to loss of prolactin Eventual development of hypopituitarism
Craniopharyngioma	Most common cause of hypopituitarism in children Benign pituitary tumor derived from Rathke's pouch remnants Rathke's pouch is an ectodermal derivative derived from the oral cavity. It develops into the anterior lobe of the pituitary gland; located above the sella turcica. Tumor extends into sella turcica and destroys the gland.
Pituitary apoplexy	Hemorrhage/infarction of a pituitary adenoma
Lymphocytic hypophysitis	Female dominant autoimmune destruction of the pituitary gland Occurs during or after pregnancy
Hypothalamic destruction	Decreased synthesis of releasing factors for anterior pituitary hormones

Water deprivation test: distinguishes CDI and NDI

    b. Nephrogenic diabetes insipidus (NDI)
      • Collecting tubules refractory to ADH
  2. Etiology and clinical findings (see Chapter 2)
  3. Water deprivation test
    a. Distinguishes CDI and NDI
    b. Normal findings in a normal individual after water deprivation
      (1) Increased plasma osmolality (POsm)
        • Stimulates release of ADH
      (2) Increased UOsm
        • Urine is concentrated by ADH reabsorption of free water.
    c. Findings in CDI and NDI after water restriction
      (1) Increased POsm (hypernatremia)
        • Loss of free water decreases total body water (TBW), which increases serum sodium and POsm.
      (2) Decreased UOsm
        • Decreased or absent concentration of urine
    d. Findings in CDI and NDI after injection of ADH
      (1) In CDI, UOsm increases >50% from the baseline
      (2) In NDI, UOsm increases <50% from the baseline

Psychogenic polydipsia (excessive water drinking) is another cause of polyuria. Before the water deprivation test, the POsm and serum Na+ are usually decreased, while in CDI and NDI, they are usually increased. After the water

TABLE 10-2
Clinical and Laboratory Findings in Hypopituitarism

Trophic Hormone Deficiency	Discussion
Gonadotropins (FSH, LH)	Children have delayed puberty Adult females have secondary amenorrhea Males have impotence: decreased libido due to decreased testosterone GnRH stimulation test: 　No significant increase of FSH/LH in hypopituitarism 　Eventual increase of FSH/LH in hypothalamic disease
Growth hormone (GH)	Decreased GH decreases synthesis and release of IGF-1: not very sensitive tests for screening due to their pulsatile release Children have growth delay: bone growth does *not* match the chronologic age of the child Adults have hypoglycemia: decreased gluconeogenesis Stimulation tests: clonidine, arginine-insulin, sleep: no increase in GH or IGF-1.
Thyroid-stimulating hormone (TSH)	Secondary hypothyroidism: decreased serum T_4 and TSH Cold intolerance, constipation, weakness No increase in TSH after TRF stimulation
Adrenocorticotropic hormone (ACTH)	Secondary hypocortisolism: decreased ACTH and cortisol Hypoglycemia: decreased gluconeogenesis Hyponatremia: mild SIADH due to loss of inhibitory effect of cortisol on ADH 　Metyrapone test: stimulation test of pituitary ACTH reserve. Metyrapone inhibits adrenal 11-hydroxylase, which causes a decrease in cortisol and a corresponding increase in plasma. ACTH (pituitary) and 11-deoxycortisol (adrenal), which is proximal to the enzyme block; in hypopituitarism, neither ACTH nor 11-deoxycortisol is increased. Short ACTH stimulation test: no increase in serum cortisol over decreased baseline levels Prolonged ACTH stimulation test: eventual increase in cortisol over the decreased baseline value once the adrenal gland is restimulated

GnRH, gonadotropin-releasing hormone; IGF, insulin-like growth factor; SIADH, syndrome of inappropriate secretion of antidiuretic hormone; TRF, thyrotropin-releasing factor.

deprivation test, the POsm and UOsm are similar to those of a normal individual.

IV. **Thyroid Gland Disorders**
   A. **Overview of thyroid hormone**
      1. Hormones are stored as colloid.
         • Activation of proteases releases hormones into peripheral blood.
      2. Free T_4 (FT_4) is peripherally converted to free T_3 (FT_3) by an outer ring deiodinase.

   > The euthyroid sick syndrome refers to alterations in thyroid hormones that are unrelated to intrinsic thyroid disease. The syndrome is

Serum reverse T_3: increased in euthyroid sick syndrome

associated with inhibition of the outer ring deiodinases in peripheral tissue that normally convert FT_4 to FT_3. Factors that inhibit the enzymes include severe systemic disease, psychiatric disturbances, and drugs (e.g., oral cholecystographic dyes, amiodarone, propanolol). If FT_4 is *not* converted to FT_3, the FT_3 concentration is always decreased. Some of the FT_4 is converted to reverse T_3, which is metabolically inactive. An increase in serum reverse T_3 is an excellent marker of thyroid hormone alterations associated with the euthyroid sick syndrome. The FT_4 levels are variable (normal, increased, decreased) depending on which one of the deiodinases is inhibited.

3. FT_3 is a metabolically active hormone.
4. FT_4 is a prohormone.

FT_4/FT_3: negative feedback with TSH

5. FT_4 and FT_3 have a negative feedback relationship with TSH.
   a. Increase in FT_4/FT_3 should produce a decrease in TSH.
   b. Decrease in FT_4/FT_3 should produce an increase in TSH.
6. T_4 and T_3 bind to thyroid-binding globulin (TBG).
   • One-third of TBG binding sites are normally occupied.

B. **Thyroid function tests**
   1. Total serum T_4 (Fig. 10-2A)
      a. Represents T_4 bound to TBG and free (unbound) T_4 (FT_4)

Total serum T_4: T_4 bound to TBG + FT_4

   (1) Figure 10-2A shows one third of TBG binding sites on two TBGs occupied by T_4.
      • Total of 6 T_4 bound to TBG.
   (2) There are 4 FT_4.
   (3) The total serum T_4 is 10.
   (4) Thyroid-stimulating hormone (TSH) is normal, because FT_4 is normal.
      b. Increase in TBG synthesis increases total serum T_4 (Fig. 10-2B).
   (1) Estrogen increases the synthesis of TBG.
      • Pregnancy, oral contraceptive pill, hormone replacement
   (2) Extra TBG automatically has one third of its binding sites occupied by T_4.
      • Total of 9 T_4 bound to TBG.
   (3) The 3 T_4 used to bind to the extra TBG are replaced by 3 T_4 released from the thyroid gland.
   (4) FT_4 remains normal (4).
   (5) Total serum T_4 is increased ($9 + 4 = 13$).
   (6) TSH is normal because FT_4 is normal.
   (7) No signs of thyrotoxicosis are present.
      c. Decrease in TBG synthesis decreases total serum T_4.
   (1) Causes of a decreased TBG
      • Anabolic steroids, nephrotic syndrome (urinary loss)

Alterations in TBG: alter total serum T_4; no effect on FT_4 and TSH

   (2) Total serum T_4 is decreased.
   (3) FT_4 and TSH remain normal.
   (4) No signs of hypothyroidism

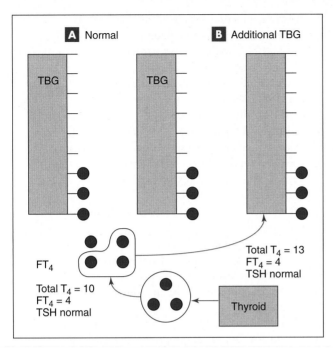

10-2: *Schematic of total serum thyroxine (T$_4$) in a normal individual (A) and in an individual with an increase in thyroid-binding globulin (TBG; B). The actual numbers do not represent the true concentration of T$_4$ and free T$_4$ (FT$_4$). The bars represent TBG and the circles are T$_4$ bound to TBG and T$_4$ that is free (FT$_4$). FT$_4$ normally has a negative feedback with thyroid-stimulating hormone (TSH). Refer to text for a complete discussion. (From Goljan EF: Rapid Review Pathology, 2nd ed. St. Louis, Mosby, 2007, Fig. 22-2.)*

    d. Normal TBG with increase or decrease in total serum T$_4$
       (1) Increased FT$_4$: Graves' disease, thyroiditis
       (2) Decreased FT$_4$: hypothyroidism
  2. Serum TSH
    a. Best overall screening test for thyroid function
    b. Increased TSH
      • Primary hypothyroidism
    c. Decreased TSH
       (1) Thyrotoxicosis (e.g., Graves' disease)
       (2) Hypopituitarism
         • Causes secondary hypothyroidism
  3. ^{131}I radioactive uptake
    a. Evaluates synthetic activity of the thyroid gland
      • Iodide is used to synthesize thyroid hormone.
    b. Increased uptake indicates increased synthesis of T$_4$.
      • Examples—Graves' disease, toxic nodular goiter
    c. Decreased uptake indicates
       (1) Inactivity of the gland
         • Example—patient taking thyroid hormone
       (2) Inflammation of the gland
         • Example—acute/subacute/chronic thyroiditis

Serum TSH: best screening test of thyroid function

Increased ^{131}I radioactive uptake: hyperfunctioning gland (e.g., Graves' disease)

Decreased ^{131}I radioactive uptake: hypofunctioning or inflamed gland

    d. Evaluates functional status of thyroid nodules
       (1) Decreased uptake in a nodule
         • "Cold" nodule—cyst, cancer
       (2) Increased uptake in a nodule
         • "Hot" nodule—toxic nodular goiter
  4. Serum thyroglobulin
    • Marker for thyroid cancer

C. Increased thyroid hormone
  1. Thyrotoxicosis: hormone excess regardless of cause
    a. Increased synthesis, e.g., Graves' disease
    b. Patient taking excess thyroid hormone
    c. Early phase of thyroiditis
       (1) Gland destruction releases excess hormones
       (2) Hashimoto's thyroiditis
       (3) Acute thyroiditis
         • Usually a viral or bacterial infection
       (4) Subacute painless thyroiditis
         • Autoimmune disease that develops postpartum
  2. Hyperthyroidism
    a. Thyroid hormone excess due to increased synthesis
    b. Examples—Graves' disease, toxic nodular goiter
  3. Graves' disease
    a. Epidemiology
       (1) Most common cause of hyperthyroidism and thyrotoxicosis
       (2) Female dominant autoimmune disease
    b. Pathogenesis
       (1) Thyroid-stimulating (IgG) antibodies against TSH receptor
       (2) Causes hyperthyroidism
         • Type II hypersensitivity reaction
       (3) Inciting events that may initiate onset of the disease
         • Infection, withdrawal of steroids, iodide excess, postpartum development
    c. Clinical features unique to Graves' disease
       (1) Infiltrative ophthalmopathy (exophthalmos)
         • Proptosis and muscle weakness of the eye (Fig. 10-3)
       (2) Pretibial myxedema
         • Due to excess glycosaminoglycans in the dermis
    d. Clinical findings in all causes of thyrotoxicosis
       (1) Weight loss, fine tremor, heat intolerance, diarrhea
       (2) Sinus tachycardia
         • Increased risk for atrial fibrillation
       (3) Brisk reflexes
    e. Laboratory findings
       (1) Increased serum T_4, decreased serum TSH
       (2) Increased ^{131}I uptake (Graves' disease)
       (3) Decreased ^{131}I uptake
         • Thyroiditis, patient taking excess thyroid hormone

---

Margin notes:

Graves' disease: anti-TSH receptor antibody, type II hypersensitivity

Exophthalmos: proptosis of eye; unique to Graves' disease

Graves' hyperthyroidism: ↑ serum T_4, ↑ ^{131}I uptake, ↓ serum TSH

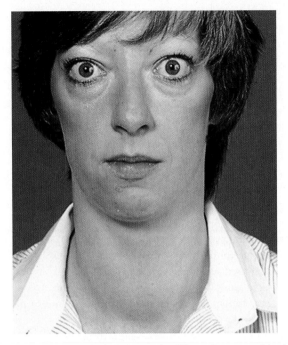

10-3: *Graves' disease. The patient has exophthalmos and a diffuse enlargement of the thyroid gland (goiter). (From Forbes C, Jackson W: Color Atlas and Text of Clinical Medicine, 2nd ed. St. Louis, Mosby, 2003, Fig. 7.61.)*

    (4) Hyperglycemia
      • Increased glycogenolysis
    (5) Hypocholesterolemia
      • Increased LDL receptor synthesis
    (6) Hypercalcemia
      • Increased bone turnover
    (7) Absolute lymphocytosis
  f. Treatment of Graves' disease
    (1) β-Blockers decrease adrenergic effects.
    (2) Thionamides decrease hormone synthesis.

Treatment Graves' disease: β-blockers, thionamides

D. **Decreased thyroid hormone (hypothyroidism)**
  1. Etiology
    a. Hashimoto's thyroiditis
    b. Subacute painless lymphocytic thyroiditis
    c. Hypopituitarism, iodine deficiency, enzyme deficiency
  2. Cretinism
    a. Hypothyroidism in infancy or early childhood
    b. Brain requires thyroxine for its maturation.
    c. Etiology
      (1) Maternal hypothyroidism
        • *Before* the fetal thyroid is developed
      (2) Enzyme or iodine deficiency

Cretinism: most often caused by maternal hypothyroidism

           d. Severe mental retardation

           e. Increased weight and short stature

              • Pituitary dwarfism: decreased weight and short stature

     3. Hashimoto's thyroiditis

           a. Epidemiology

              (1) Most common cause of hypothyroidism

              (2) Autoimmune thyroiditis

           b. Pathogenesis

              (1) Cytotoxic T cells destroy parenchyma

                 • Initial thyrotoxicosis, eventual hypothyroidism

              (2) Blocking IgG autoantibodies against the TSH receptor

                 • Decrease hormone synthesis

              (3) Antimicrosomal and thyroglobulin antibodies

                 • Develop as a result of gland injury

     4. Clinical findings

           a. Proximal muscle myopathy

              • Increased serum creatine kinase

           b. Weight gain

              • Due to hypometabolic state with retention of water and salt

           c. Dry and brittle hair, coarse yellow skin

           d. Periorbital puffiness, hoarse voice, myxedema (Fig. 10-4)

           e. Fatigue, cold intolerance, constipation

           f. Diastolic hypertension

              • Due to retention of sodium and water

           g. Delayed recovery of Achilles reflex, mental slowness, dementia

     5. Laboratory findings

           a. Primary type: decreased serum T_4, increased serum TSH

           b. Secondary type: decreased serum T_4, decreased serum TSH

           c. Antimicrosomal and antithyroglobulin antibodies

              • Present in Hashimoto's thyroiditis

           d. Hypercholesterolemia

              • Due to decreased synthesis of LDL receptors

     6. Treatment

           a. Thyroid hormone replacement

           b. Bring serum TSH into the normal range

   E. **Summary of laboratory findings in thyroid disorders** (Table 10-3)

V. **Parathyroid Gland Disorders**

   A. **Increased serum calcium** (see Chapter 9)

   B. **Decreased serum calcium** (see Chapter 9)

VI. **Adrenal Gland Disorders**

   A. **Overview of adrenal cortex hormones** (Fig. 10-5)

     1. Zona glomerulosa produces mineralocorticoids (e.g., aldosterone).

     2. Zona fasciculata produces glucocorticoids.

         • 11-Deoxycortisol and cortisol are 17-hydroxycorticoids (17-OH).

     3. Zona reticularis produces sex hormones.

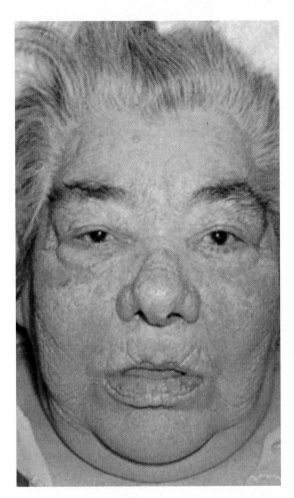

10-4: *Primary hypothyroidism in a patient with Hashimoto's thyroiditis. The patient has a puffy face, particularly around the eyes, and coarse hair. (From Forbes C, Jackson W: Color Atlas and Text of Clinical Medicine, 2nd ed. St. Louis, Mosby, 2003, Fig. 7.72.)*

TABLE 10-3 Laboratory Findings in Thyroid Disease

Disorder	Serum T$_4$	Free T$_4$	Serum TSH	^{131}I Uptake
Graves' disease	↑	↑	↓	↑
Patient taking excess hormone	↑	↑	↓	↓
Initial phase of thyroiditis	↑	↑	↓	↓
Primary hypothyroidism	↓	↓	↑	↔
Secondary hypothyroidism (e.g., hypopituitarism)	↓	↓	↓	↔
Increased TBG (e.g., excess estrogen)	↑	Normal	Normal	↔
Decreased TBG (e.g., anabolic steroids)	↓	Normal	Normal	↔

T$_4$, thyroxine; TBG, thyroid-binding globulin; TSH, thyroid-stimulating hormone; ↔, not indicated.

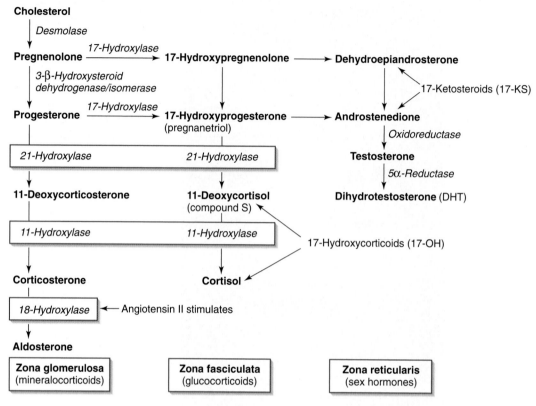

10-5: *Adrenocortical hormone synthesis. The zona glomerulosa produces mineralocorticoids (e.g., aldosterone), the zona fasciculata produces glucocorticoids (e.g., cortisol), and the zona reticularis produces sex hormones (e.g., testosterone). The 17-hydroxycorticoids (17-OH) are 11-deoxycortisol and cortisol. The 17-ketosteroids (17-KS, weak androgens) are dehydroepiandrosterone and androstenedione. Testosterone is converted to dihydrotestosterone (DHT) by 5α-reductase. (From Goljan EF: Rapid Review Pathology, 2nd ed. St. Louis, Mosby, 2007, Fig. 22-7.)*

      a. 17-Ketosteroids (17-KS)
        • Dehydroepiandrosterone (DHEA) and androstenedione
      b. Testosterone
        • Converted to dihydrotestosterone (DHT) by 5-α-reductase

B. **Overview of adrenal medulla hormones**
    1. Neural crest origin
    2. Produces catecholamines
      • Epinephrine (EPI) and norepinephrine (NOR)
    3. Metabolic products of EPI and NOR
      • Metanephrine and vanillylmandelic acid (VMA)
    4. Metabolic product of dopamine is homovanillic acid (HVA).

C. **Adrenocortical hyperfunction; Cushing's syndrome**
    1. Etiology
      a. Prolonged corticosteroid therapy
        • Most common cause

Cushing's syndrome:
most common cause
corticosteroid therapy

b. Pituitary Cushing's disease
  (1) 60% of cases
  (2) Due to a pituitary adenoma
  (3) Increased ACTH and cortisol
c. Adrenal Cushing's disease
  (1) 25% of cases
  (2) Most often due to an adenoma
    • Also primary hyperplasia, carcinoma
  (3) Decreased ACTH and increased cortisol
d. Ectopic Cushing's disease
  (1) 15% of cases
  (2) Usually small cell carcinoma of lung
    • Ectopic ACTH production
  (3) Markedly increased ACTH and cortisol

2. Clinical findings
  a. Weight gain
    (1) Due to hyperinsulinism from hyperglycemia
      • Insulin increases storage of fat (triglyceride) in adipose
    (2) Fat deposition in face ("moon facies"), upper back ("buffalo hump"), and trunk (truncal obesity) (Fig. 10-6)
  b. Purple striae
    (1) Stretch marks with hemorrhage into subcutaneous tissue
    (2) Hypercortisolism weakens collagen causing rupture of vessels
  c. Muscle weakness, hirsutism, hypertension

3. Laboratory findings
  a. Increased urine for free cortisol
    (1) Very high positive and negative predictive value
    (2) Excellent screening test
  b. Low-dose dexamethasone (cortisol analogue) suppression test
    (1) Cannot suppress cortisol in all types
    (2) Good screening test
  c. High-dose dexamethasone suppression test
    • Can suppress cortisol in pituitary Cushing's disease but *not* the other types
  d. Hyperglycemia
    • Cortisol enhances gluconeogenesis.
  e. Hypokalemic metabolic alkalosis
    • Due to increased weak mineralocorticoids

4. Summary of Cushing's syndromes (Table 10-4)

D. **Adrenocortical hyperfunction; hyperaldosteronism**
  • See Chapter 2

E. **Adrenal medulla hyperfunction; pheochromocytoma**
  1. Epidemiology
    a. Unilateral (~90% of cases)
    b. Benign adenoma (~90% of cases)
    c. Arises in the adrenal medulla (~90% of cases)

Cushing's syndrome: truncal obesity, thin extremities, purple stria

Pituitary Cushing's syndrome: suppression of cortisol by high-dose dexamethasone

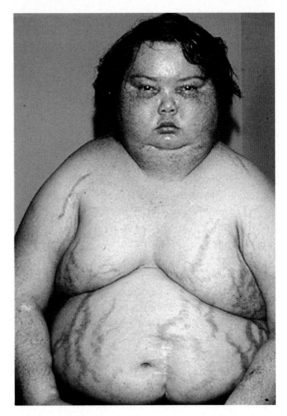

10-6: *Patient with Cushing's syndrome, showing "moon facies," truncal obesity, and purple abdominal striae. (From Damjanov I: Pathology for the Health-Related Professions, 2nd ed. Philadelphia, WB Saunders, 2000, p 426.)*

TABLE 10-4
Summary of Pituitary, Adrenal, and Ectopic Cushing's Syndromes

Laboratory Test	Pituitary Cushing	Adrenal Cushing	Ectopic Cushing
Serum cortisol	↑	↑	↑
Urine free cortisol	↑	↑	↑
Low dose dexamethasone	Cortisol *not* suppressed	Cortisol *not* suppressed	Cortisol *not* suppressed
High-dose dexamethasone	Cortisol suppressed	Cortisol *not* suppressed	Cortisol *not* suppressed
Plasma ACTH	Normal* to ↑	↓	Markedly ↑

*Normal: a plasma ACTH in the normal range is *not* normal in the presence of an increase in serum cortisol.

- Other sites: bladder, organ of Zuckerkandl near the bifurcation of the aorta, posterior mediastinum
    d. *N*-methyltransferase converts NOR to EPI.
        (1) Adrenal medulla and the organ of Zuckerkandl contain the enzyme.
            - Pheochromocytoma produces NOR and EPI.

(2) Other sites lack the enzyme.
- Tumors in other sites produce only NOR.

e. Associations

(1) Neurofibromatosis

(2) MEN IIa and IIb

(3) von Hippel–Lindau disease (often bilateral tumors)

2. Clinical findings

a. Diastolic hypertension
- Sustained with occasional paroxysmal bursts

b. Palpitations
- These are *not* present in essential hypertension.

c. Anxiety
- This is *not* present in essential hypertension.

d. Drenching sweats
- This is *not* present in essential hypertension.

e. Headache, chest pain from subendocardial ischemia

3. Laboratory findings

a. Increased 24-hour urine for VMA and metanephrine

b. Hyperglycemia
- Increased glycogenolysis and gluconeogenesis

c. Neutrophilic leukocytosis
- Inhibition of neutrophil adhesion molecules

F. **Adrenal medulla hyperfunction; neuroblastoma**

1. Epidemiology

a. Malignant tumor

b. Most often occurs in children < 5 years old

c. Primarily located in the adrenal medulla
- Occasionally located in the posterior mediastinum

2. Clinical findings

a. Palpable abdominal mass

b. Diastolic hypertension

3. Laboratory findings
- Increased urine VMA, metanephrines, and HVA

G. **Adrenocortical hypofunction (primary hypocortisolism)**

1. Acute adrenocortical insufficiency

a. Etiology

(1) Abrupt withdrawal of corticosteroids

(2) Waterhouse-Friderichsen syndrome

(3) Anticoagulation therapy

b. Waterhouse-Friderichsen syndrome

(1) Usually associated with septicemia from *Neisseria meningitidis*

(2) Patients develop endotoxic shock.
- Release of tissue thromboplastin causes disseminated intravascular coagulation (DIC)

(3) Bilateral adrenal hemorrhage
- Fibrin thrombi in vessels cause hemorrhagic infarction

2. Chronic adrenal insufficiency (Addison's disease)

Pheochromocytoma: palpitations, anxiety, drenching sweats

Neuroblastoma: abdominal mass + hypertension

Abrupt withdrawal corticosteroids: most common cause acute adrenocortical insufficiency

Miliary TB: most common cause Addison's in developing countries

a. Etiology
   (1) Autoimmune destruction
       • Most common cause
   (2) Miliary tuberculosis/histoplasmosis
   (3) Adrenogenital syndrome
   (4) Metastasis
       • Most often from a primary lung cancer
b. Clinical findings
   (1) Weakness and hypotension
       • Due to sodium loss from mineralocorticoid and glucocorticoid deficiency
   (2) Diffuse hyperpigmentation (Fig. 10-7)
       • Increased plasma ACTH stimulates melanocytes
c. Laboratory findings
   (1) Short and prolonged ACTH stimulation test
       • No increase in cortisol or 17-OH

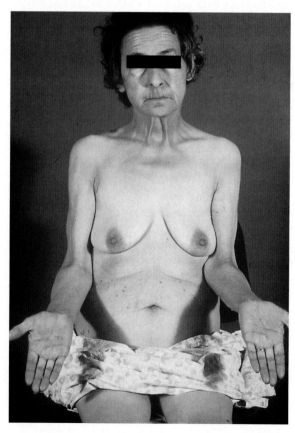

10-7: Addison's disease. Note the increased pigmentation in sun-exposed areas (face, neck, forearms) and in the palmar creases. (From Savin J, Hunter JA, Hepburn NC: Diagnosis in Color: Skin Signs in Clinical Medicine. London, Mosby-Wolfe, 1997, Fig. 6.15.)

(2) Metyrapone test (see Table 10-2)
- Increased ACTH but no increase in 11-deoxycortisol

(3) Increased plasma ACTH

(4) Electrolyte findings (see Chapter 2)
- Hyponatremia, hyperkalemia, and metabolic acidosis

d. Fasting hypoglycemia
- Due to decrease in cortisol (cortisol is gluconeogenic)

e. Eosinophilia, lymphocytosis, and neutropenia
- Due to decrease in cortisol (see Chapter 6)

3. Adrenogenital syndrome

a. Epidemiology
- Group of autosomal recessive disorders with variable electrolyte and clinical findings

b. Pathogenesis

(1) Enzyme deficiency causes hypocortisolism.

(2) Corresponding increase in ACTH
- Produces adrenocortical hyperplasia and diffuse skin pigmentation

(3) In females, an increase in 17-KS, testosterone, and DHT causes:
- Ambiguous genitalia primarily due to DHT

(4) In males, an increase in 17-KS, testosterone, and DHT causes:
- Precocious puberty due to increase in androgens

(5) Some have an increase in mineralocorticoids:
- Cause sodium retention leading to hypertension

(6) Some have a decrease in mineralocorticoids:
- Causes sodium loss (hyponatremia), hyperkalemia, and hypotension

(7) Substrates proximal to the enzyme block increase.

(8) Substrates distal to the enzyme block decrease.

c. 21-Hydroxylase deficiency

(1) Most common enzyme deficiency (95% of cases)

(2) Ambiguous genitalia in females
- Increase in 17-KS, testosterone, and DHT

(3) Precocious puberty in males
- Increase in 17-KS, testosterone, and DHT

(4) Hypotension
- Sodium loss due to decrease in mineralocorticoids

(5) Decrease in 17-OH

(6) Increase in 17-hydroxyprogesterone
- Excellent screening test

d. 11-Hydroxylase deficiency

(1) Ambiguous genitalia in females
- Increase in 17-KS, testosterone, and DHT

(2) Precocious puberty in males
- Increase in 17-KS, testosterone, and DHT

(3) Hypertension
- Increase in mineralocorticoids (11-deoxycorticosterone)

> Most common cause of Addison's disease in children: adrenogenital syndrome

> 21-Hydroxylase deficiency: most common adrenogenital syndrome

**TABLE 10-5
Summary of
Adrenogenital
Syndromes**

Laboratory	21-OHase	11-OHase	17-OHase
17-Ketosteroids	↑	↑	↓
17-hydroxyprogesterone	↑	↑	↓
17-hydroxycorticoids	↓	↑	↓
Mineralocorticoids	↓	↑	↑

      (4) Increase in 17-OH (11-deoxycortisol)
      (5) Increase in 17-hydroxyprogesterone
    e. 17-Hydroxylase deficiency
      (1) Hypogonadism in females
        (a) Decrease in 17-KS, testosterone, and DHT; decreased estrogen (see X.K)
        (b) Recall that estrogen comes from aromatization of androgens.
      (2) Male pseudohermaphroditism
        • Male external genitalia development requires DHT (see below)
      (3) Hypertension
        • Due to sodium retention from increase in mineralocorticoids
      (4) Decrease in 17-OH and 17-hydroxyprogesterone
    f. Summary of adrenogenital syndromes (Table 10-5)

VII. **Islet Cell Tumors**
    • See Table 10-6.

VIII. **Multiple Endocrine Neoplasia (MEN) Syndromes**
    • See Table 10-7.

IX. **Male Endocrine Disorders**
    A. **Klinefelter's syndrome**
      1. Pathogenesis
        a. XXY karyotype
        b. Nondisjunction
          • Unequal separation of sex chromosome in first phase of meiosis
        c. Fibrosis of seminiferous tubules
          (1) Azoospermia (no sperm)
          (2) Loss of Sertoli cells with decrease in inhibin
            • Increased FSH due to loss of negative feedback
        d. Hyperplasia of Leydig cells
          (1) Increased FSH causes increased synthesis of aromatase.
          (2) Aromatization of testosterone to estrogen
          (3) Decreased testosterone causes increase in LH.
          (4) Increase in LH causes Leydig cell hyperplasia.
      2. Clinical and laboratory findings
        a. Female secondary sex characteristics (Fig. 10-8)
          (1) Due to increased estrogen
          (2) Persistent gynecomastia

Klinefelter's syndrome:
↓ testosterone and
inhibin; ↑ LH and FSH,
respectively

TABLE 10-6
Summary of Islet Cell Tumors

Tumor	Discussion
Glucagonoma	Malignant tumor of α-islet cells Clinical: hyperglycemia, rash (necrolytic migratory erythema) Hyperglycemia: due to increase in gluconeogenesis
Insulinoma	Benign tumor of β-islet cells; most common islet cell tumor; approximately 80% have MEN I syndrome Clinical: fasting hypoglycemia causing mental status abnormalities Laboratory: fasting hypoglycemia; increase in serum insulin and C-peptide; C-peptide is an endogenous marker of insulin produced in β-islet cells Surreptitious injection of insulin: fasting hypoglycemia, increased insulin, decreased C-peptide
Somatostatinoma	Malignant tumor of δ-islet cells; somatostatin is an inhibitory hormone Inhibition of gastrin causes achlorhydria (absent gastric acidity) Inhibition of cholecystokinin causes cholelithiasis and steatorrhea Inhibition of gastric inhibitory peptide causes diabetes mellitus Inhibition of secretin causes steatorrhea
VIPoma (pancreatic cholera)	Malignant tumor with excessive secretion of vasoactive intestinal peptide (VIP) Clinical: secretory diarrhea, achlorhydria Hypokalemia, normal anion gap metabolic acidosis (loss of bicarbonate in stool)
Zollinger-Ellison	Malignant islet cell tumor that secretes gastrin producing hyperacidity; MEN I association (20–30% of cases) Clinical: peptic ulceration, diarrhea, maldigestion of food Serum gastrin > 1000 pg/mL

MEN, multiple endocrine neoplasia.

TABLE 10-7
Multiple Endocrine Neoplasia (MEN) Syndromes

Syndrome	Discussion
MEN I	Pituitary adenoma: usually nonfunctioning Parathyroid adenoma: primary hyperparathyroidism Pancreatic tumor: insulinoma or Zollinger-Ellison syndrome
MEN IIa	Medullary carcinoma of thyroid: malignancy of C-cells; calcitonin tumor marker Parathyroid adenoma Pheochromocytoma
MEN IIb	Medullary carcinoma Pheochromocytoma Mucosal neuromas (lips/tongue)

   (3) Soft skin
   (4) Female hair distribution
  b. Delayed sexual maturation (hypogonadism)
   • Testicular atrophy (decreased testicular volume)
  c. Disproportionately long legs, learning disabilities
 3. Laboratory findings
  a. One Barr body
   • One of the two X chromosomes is randomly inactivated.

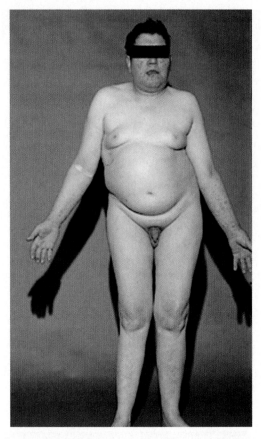

10-8: *Klinefelter's syndrome is characterized by female secondary sex characteristics, including gynecomastia (breast development) and a female distribution of pubic hair. The legs are disproportionately long. (From Bouloux P-M: Self-Assessment Picture Tests: Medicine, Vol. 1. St. Louis, Mosby, 1996, p 82.)*

     b. Decreased testosterone
       • Aromatized to estrogen
     c. Increased serum LH
       • Due to decreased testosterone
     d. Increased serum FSH
       • Due to decreased inhibin

B. **Testicular feminization**
    1. Overview of male sex organ development
      a. Presence of the Y chromosome
        • Causes germinal tissue to differentiate into testes
      b. Sertoli cells in seminiferous tubules
        (1) Synthesize müllerian inhibitory factor (MIF)
        (2) Causes müllerian tissue to undergo apoptosis
      c. Leydig cells
        (1) Synthesize testosterone

Y chromosome: determines differentiation of germinal tissue

Fetal testosterone: develops male accessory structures

        (2) Converts wolffian duct structures to epididymis, seminal vesicles, vas deferens

    d. 5α-Reductase

        (1) Converts testosterone to dihydrotestosterone (DHT)

        (2) DHT develops the prostate gland.

        (3) DHT develops the external male genitalia.

         • Genitalia is phenotypically female before DHT is produced.

> Fetal DHT: develops external genitalia, prostate gland

  2. Epidemiology

    a. X-linked recessive disorder

      • Androgen receptors are deficient or defective

    b. Male pseudohermaphrodite (Fig. 10-9)

      • Phenotypically female but genotype is a male (XY)

  3. Pathophysiology

    a. Fetal DHT and testosterone are unable to function without a receptor.

    b. Testicles are present in the inguinal canal or abdominal cavity.

    c. Müllerian structures are absent because MIF is synthesized by Sertoli cells.

        (1) Absence of fallopian tubes, uterus, cervix, upper vagina

        (2) Lower vagina is present and ends as a blind pouch.

         • Develops from the urogenital sinus

> Testicular feminization: deficiency of androgen receptors

    d. Male accessory structures are absent.

        (1) No testosterone effect on the wolffian duct structures

        (2) Absence of epididymis, seminal vesicles, vas deferens

    e. External genitalia remain female in appearance.

        (1) No DHT effect

        (2) Vagina ends as a blind pouch.

    f. Hormone levels

        (1) Normal male levels of testosterone and DHT

        (2) Estrogen activity is unopposed, because estrogen receptors are present.

  4. Majority of patients are reared female

C. Male hypogonadism

  1. Classification

    a. Primary hypogonadism

        (1) Due to Leydig cell dysfunction

        (2) Luteinizing hormone (LH) is increased.

         • Loss of negative feedback imposed by testosterone

        (3) Hypergonadotropic (increased LH) hypogonadism

    b. Secondary hypogonadism

        (1) Due to hypothalamic/pituitary dysfunction (see II.B, III.B)

        (2) LH is decreased.

        (3) Hypogonadotropic (decreased LH) hypogonadism

  2. Primary hypogonadism: Leydig cell dysfunction

    a. Etiology

        (1) Chronic alcoholic liver disease

         • Alcohol inhibits binding of LH to Leydig cells (? mechanism)

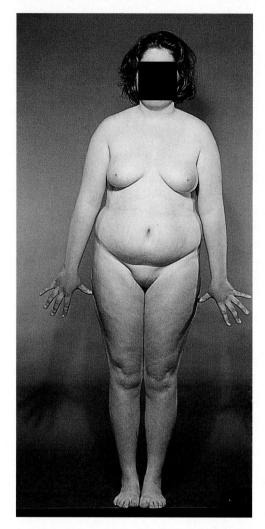

10-9: *Testicular feminization. The patient is genotypically male, but phenotypically female. The vagina ended as a blind pouch. (From Forbes C, Jackson W: Color Atlas and Text of Clinical Medicine, 2nd ed. St. Louis, Mosby, 2003, Fig. 7.55.)*

Leydig cell dysfunction: alcohol, chronic renal failure

    (2) Chronic renal failure
       • Toxins have a direct toxic effect on Leydig cell.
    (3) Irradiation, orchitis, trauma
  b. Laboratory findings in Leydig cell dysfunction
    (1) Decreased testosterone
       • Due to destruction of Leydig cells
    (2) Increased LH
       • Due to decreased testosterone
    (3) Decreased sperm count
       • Due to testosterone deficiency

Dysfunction	Testosterone	Sperm count	LH	FSH
Primary				
Leydig dysfunction	↓	↓	↑	Normal
Seminiferous dysfunction	Normal	↓	Normal	↑
Leydig cell + seminiferous tubule dysfunction	↓	↓	↑	↑
Secondary				
Hypopituitarism	↓	↓	↓	↓

TABLE 10-8
Summary of Causes of Male Hypogonadism

FSH, follicle-stimulating hormone; LH, luteinizing hormone; N, normal.

       (4) Normal FSH
- Inhibin is present in Sertoli cells
3. Primary hypogonadism: Leydig cell and seminiferous tubule dysfunction
   a. Etiology
- Same as Leydig cell dysfunction
   b. Laboratory findings
      (1) Decreased testosterone
- Due to destruction of Leydig cells
      (2) Increased LH
- Due to decreased testosterone
      (3) Decreased sperm count
- Due to testosterone deficiency and seminiferous tubule dysfunction
      (4) Increased FSH
- Due to decrease in inhibin
4. Etiology of secondary hypogonadism
   a. Constitutional delay in puberty
- A testicular volume >4 mL indicates puberty has begun.
   b. Kallmann's syndrome
      (1) Autosomal dominant disorder
      (2) Maldevelopment of the olfactory bulbs and GnRH-producing cells
      (3) Delayed puberty
      (4) Anosmia, color blindness
      (5) Laboratory findings
- Decreased FSH, LH, testosterone, and sperm count
   c. Hypopituitarism (see III.B)
5. Summary of causes of male hypogonadism (Table 10-8)
D. **Male infertility**
1. Etiology
   a. Decreased sperm count
   b. End-organ dysfunction
2. Decreased sperm count
   a. Primary testicular dysfunction

(1) Leydig cell dysfunction (see IX.C)
(2) Seminiferous tubule dysfunction
    (a) Causes include varicocele, Klinefelter's syndrome, orchitis
    (b) Normal testosterone and LH
       • Leydig cells are intact
    (c) Decreased sperm count
       • Loss of seminiferous tubules and decreased testosterone
    (d) Increased FSH
       • Inhibin is decreased
  b. Secondary hypogonadism
    • Pituitary or hypothalamic dysfunction (see II.B, III.B)
3. End-organ dysfunction
  a. Etiology
    (1) Obstruction of vas deferens
    (2) Disorders involving accessory sex organs or ejaculation
  b. Normal testosterone, FSH, LH, prolactin
  c. Sperm count variable
4. Semen analysis
  a. Gold standard test for infertility
  b. Components of semen
    (1) Spermatozoa derive from the seminiferous tubules.
    (2) Coagulant derives from the seminal vesicles.
    (3) Enzymes to liquefy semen derive from the prostate gland.
  c. Components evaluated in a standard semen analysis
    (1) Volume
       • Volume does *not* correlate with the number of sperm.
    (2) Sperm count
       • Normal count is 20 million to 150 million sperm per milliliter
    (3) Sperm morphology
       • Morphology is very abnormal in reconnections of a vasectomy.
    (4) Sperm motility

X. **Female Endocrine Disorders**
  A. **Sources and types of estrogen**
    1. Estradiol (Fig. 10-10)
      a. Primary estrogen in nonpregnant women
      b. Derived from aromatization of testosterone in granulosa cells
        • FSH increases synthesis of aromatase in granulosa cells
    2. Estrone
      a. Weak estrogen produced during menopause
      b. Primarily derived from adipose cell aromatization of androstenedione
        (1) Androstenedione is synthesized in the adrenal cortex.
        (2) Ovaries undergo atrophy in the menopause.
    3. Estriol
      a. End product of estradiol metabolism
      b. Primary estrogen of pregnancy
        • Derives from fetal adrenal, placenta, and maternal liver (see X.G)

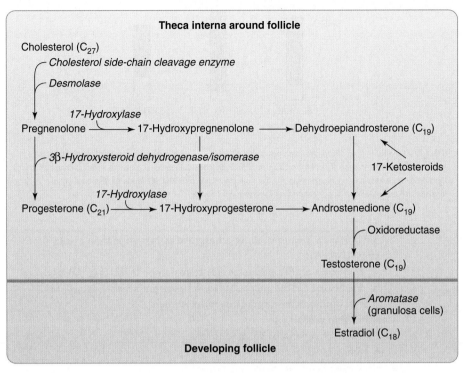

Theca interna around follicle

Cholesterol (C_{27})

— Cholesterol side-chain cleavage enzyme

— Desmolase

17-Hydroxylase

Pregnenolone ⟶ 17-Hydroxypregnenolone ⟶ Dehydroepiandrosterone (C_{19})

— 3β-Hydroxysteroid dehydrogenase/isomerase

17-Ketosteroids

17-Hydroxylase

Progesterone (C_{21}) ⟶ 17-Hydroxyprogesterone ⟶ Androstenedione (C_{19})

— Oxidoreductase

Testosterone (C_{19})

— Aromatase (granulosa cells)

Estradiol (C_{18})

Developing follicle

10-10: *Synthesis of sex hormones in the ovaries. Luteinizing hormone is responsible for stimulation of hormone synthesis in the theca interna surrounding the developing follicle. Follicle-stimulating hormone increases the synthesis of aromatase in granulosa cells. Aromatase converts testosterone to estradiol. (From Goljan EF: Rapid Review Pathology, 2nd ed. St. Louis, Mosby, 2007, Fig. 21-5.)*

B. **Sources and types of androgens**
  1. Androstenedione
     • Equal derivation from ovaries and adrenal cortex
  2. DHEA
     a. Primarily synthesized in the adrenal cortex (80% of the total)
     b. Remainder is synthesized in the ovaries
     c. DHEA-sulfate
        • Almost exclusively synthesized in the adrenal cortex
  3. Testosterone
     a. Derived from conversion of androstenedione to testosterone
     b. Primarily synthesized in the ovaries.
        • Small amount is synthesized in the adrenal cortex
C. **Sex hormone-binding globulin (SHBG)**
  1. Binding protein for testosterone and estrogen
     a. SHBG is primarily synthesized in the liver.
        • Also true for males
     b. Estrogen increases synthesis of SHBG in the liver.
     c. Androgens, obesity, hypothyroidism all decrease synthesis of SHBG.

DHEA-sulfate: almost exclusively synthesized in the adrenal cortex

10-11: *Alterations in sex hormone–binding globulin (SHBG). **A** shows the normal relationship of SHBG levels and free testosterone (FT). An increase in SHBG (**B**) causes increased binding of testosterone to SHBG leading to a corresponding decrease in FT levels. A decrease in SHBG (**C**) leads to less binding of testosterone to SHBG and a corresponding increase in FT levels.*

    2. SHBG has a greater binding affinity for testosterone than estrogen (Fig. 10-11A).
        a. Increased SHBG decreases free testosterone levels (Fig. 10-11B).
        b. Decreased SHBG increases free testosterone levels (Fig. 10-11C).
          • Common cause of hirsutism in women

D. **Cervical Pap smear**
    1. Presence of superficial squamous cells
        • Indicates adequate estrogen
    2. Presence of intermediate squamous cells
        • Indicates adequate progesterone
    3. Presence of parabasal cells
        • Indicate a lack of estrogen and progesterone.
    4. Normal nonpregnant adult women
        • 70% superficial squamous cells, 30% intermediate squamous cells
    5. Pregnant women
        • 100% intermediate squamous cells from progesterone effect
    6. Elderly women with lack of estrogen and progesterone
        • Atrophic smear with parabasal cells and inflammation
    7. Women with continuous exposure to estrogen without progesterone
        • 100% superficial squamous cells

E. **Summary of the normal menstrual cycle**
    1. Proliferative phase
        a. Estrogen-mediated proliferation of glands.
        b. Most variable phase of the cycle
        c. Estrogen surge occurs 24 to 36 hours prior to ovulation.
          (1) Stimulates luteinizing hormone (LH)
            • Positive feedback
          (2) Inhibits follicle-stimulating hormone (FSH)
            • Negative feedback; serum LH > FSH
        d. LH surge initiates ovulation.
    2. Ovulation
        a. Occurs between days 14 and 16
        b. Ovulation indicators

Proliferative phase: estrogen-mediated

(1) Increase in body temperature
- Effect of progesterone

(2) Subnuclear vacuoles in endometrial cells

Subnuclear vacuoles: sign of ovulation

(3) Mittelschmerz
- Peritoneal irritation from blood from the ruptured follicle

3. Secretory phase
   a. Progesterone-mediated
   b. Least variable phase of the cycle

> In fertility workups, endometrial biopsies are commonly performed on day 21 to see if ovulation has occurred. Presence of secretory endometrium on day 21 confirms that ovulation has occurred.

Secretory phase: progesterone-mediated

4. Menses
   - Initiated by drop-off in serum levels of estrogen and progesterone

5. Functions of FSH
   a. Prepares the follicle of the month
   b. Increases aromatase synthesis in the granulosa cells (see Fig. 10-10)
   c. Increases the synthesis of LH receptors

6. Functions of LH (see Fig. 10-10)
   a. LH in the proliferative phase
      (1) Increases the synthesis of 17-ketosteroids (KS) in the theca interna
         - 17-KS are DHEA and androstenedione.
      (2) DHEA is converted to androstenedione.
         - Androstenedione is converted to testosterone.
      (3) Testosterone enters granulosa cells and is aromatized to estradiol.
   b. LH surge is induced by a sudden increase in estrogen.
      - Induces ovulation when LH is higher than FSH
   c. LH in the secretory phase
      - Theca interna primarily synthesizes 17-hydroxyprogesterone.

F. **Human chorionic gonadotropin (hCG) in pregnancy**
   1. Function of hCG
      a. Synthesized in the syncytiotrophoblast lining the chorionic villus

hCG: maintains corpus luteum of pregnancy

      b. Acts as an LH analogue by maintaining the corpus luteum of pregnancy
      c. Corpus luteum synthesizes progesterone for ~8 to 10 weeks.
      d. Corpus luteum involutes after ~8 to 10 weeks.
         - Placenta synthesizes progesterone for the remainder of the pregnancy.
   2. Pregnancy tests
      a. Tests detect β-subunit of hCG
         (1) More specific for pregnancy
         (2) Peaks 10 weeks from last menstrual period
         (3) Doubles every 1.4 to 2.1 days
      b. Urine tests are used for initial screening.
         (1) Less sensitive than serum tests

Urine pregnancy test: screening test

(2) Positive at β-hCG levels of 25 IU/mL or higher
  • False negative values are below 25 IU/mL.
(3) Usually positive 24 to 26 days after the last menses

c. Serum tests

Serum pregnancy test: more sensitive than urine tests

  (1) More sensitive than urine tests
  (2) Can detect β-hCG at levels below 25 IU/mL
d. Uses of serum tests
  (1) Equivocal urine test results
  (2) Detect very early pregnancy
    • Example—24 to 48 hours after implantation
  (3) Used to rule out ectopic pregnancy
    • Serial levels of β-hCG are frequently used and often correlated with ultrasound.
  (4) Diagnosis and follow-up of molar pregnancies
    • Examples—hydatidiform mole (benign tumor of chorionic villus), choriocarcinoma (malignant tumor of trophoblastic tissue)
  (5) Diagnosis of gonadal (i.e., testes, ovaries) trophoblastic tumors
    • Trophoblast consists of syncytiotrophoblast (synthesizes hCG) and cytotrophoblast.

G. **Urine estriol in pregnancy**
  1. Derived from the fetal adrenal, placenta, and maternal liver
    a. Fetal zone of the adrenal cortex
      (1) Converts pregnenolone synthesized in the placenta to DHEA-sulfate
      (2) Fetal zone is absent in anencephaly (absent brain).

Estriol: derived from fetal adrenal, placenta, maternal liver

    b. Fetal liver
      • DHEA-sulfate is 16-hydroxylated to 16-OH-DHEA-sulfate.
    c. Maternal placenta
      (1) Placental sulfatase cleaves off the sulfate from 16-OH-DHEA-sulfate.
      (2) 16-OH-DHEA is converted by aromatase to free unbound estriol.
    d. Maternal liver
      (1) Free estriol is conjugated to estriol.
      (2) Estriol is excreted in maternal urine and bile.
  2. Decreased levels of estriol
    • Sign of fetal-maternal-placental dysfunction

Down syndrome triad:
↓ urine estriol, AFP
↑ β-hCG

  3. Down syndrome triad
    a. Decreased urine estriol
    b. Decreased AFP
    c. Increased β-hCG
    d. All three present
      • Sensitivity ~70%, specificity ~95%

H. **Menopause**
  1. Mean age 52 years old
  2. Ovaries undergo atrophy

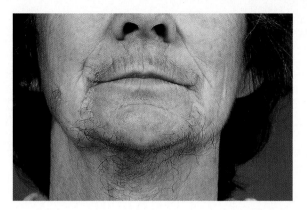

10-12: *Hirsutism showing excess hair above the lip and on the chin. (From Forbes C, Jackson W: Color Atlas and Text of Clinical Medicine, 2nd ed. St. Louis, Mosby, 2003, Fig. 2.99.)*

- Ovaries should *not* be palpable in menopause.
3. Increase in FSH and LH
   a. Due to drop in estrogen and progesterone, respectively
   b. Serum FSH is the best screen.
4. Clinical findings
   a. Secondary amenorrhea
   b. Hot flushes, night sweats

I. **Hirsutism and virilization**
1. Epidemiology and pathogenesis
   a. Excess androgen-dependent terminal hairs in female patients
      (1) Male-pattern distribution
         - Example—excess facial hair (Fig. 10-12)
      (2) Virilization is hirsutism plus male secondary sex characteristics
         - Clitoromegaly (enlarged clitoris; gold standard), acne, increased muscle mass
   b. Classification
      (1) Idiopathic
      (2) Familial
      (3) Drugs
         - Testosterone, danazol, phenothiazines, anabolic steroids, acetazolamide
      (4) Androgen excess from ovarian disorders
         - Polycystic ovarian syndrome, ovarian tumors
      (5) Androgen excess from adrenal disorders
         - Cushing's syndrome, adrenogenital syndrome
2. Laboratory tests
   a. Ovarian causes of hyperandrogenicity
      - Total or free testosterone increased
   b. Adrenal causes of hyperandrogenicity
      - DHEA-sulfate is primarily increased.
3. Polycystic ovarian syndrome (POS)

Menopause: ↑ FSH best marker

Hirsutism and virilization: androgen-dependent

a. Pathogenesis
   (1) Increased pituitary synthesis of LH and decreased synthesis of FSH
   (2) Increased LH increases androgen synthesis.
      • Hirsutism occurs more often than virilization.
   (3) Androgens are aromatized to estrogen in the adipose.
   (4) Increased estrogen has a positive feedback on LH.
      • Serum LH increases.
   (5) Increased estrogen has a negative feedback on FSH.
      • Serum FSH is decreased.
   (6) Suppression of FSH causes follicle degeneration.
      • Fluid accumulation produces subcortical cysts that enlarge the ovaries.

POS: ↑ LH, ↓ FSH; LH:FSH ratio >2

b. Clinical findings
   (1) Menstrual irregularities
      • Oligomenorrhea is the most common complaint.
   (2) Hirsutism, infertility, obesity (50% of cases)
c. Laboratory findings
   (1) Serum LH:FSH ratio > 2
   (2) Increased serum testosterone and androstenedione
   (3) Increased estrogen

J. **Dysfunctional uterine bleeding (DUB)**
1. Epidemiology and pathogenesis
   a. Excessive bleeding *unrelated* to an anatomic cause
   b. Caused by a hormonal imbalance

Anovulatory DUB: most common type of DUB

2. Anovulatory DUB
   a. Occurs at the extremes of reproductive life
      (1) Menarche to age 20
      (2) Perimenopausal period
   b. Excessive estrogen stimulation relative to progesterone
      (1) Absent secretory phase of the cycle
      (2) Produces endometrial hyperplasia and bleeding
3. Inadequate luteal phase
   a. Ovulatory type of DUB
   b. Inadequate maturation of the corpus luteum
      (1) Inadequate synthesis of progesterone
         • Delay in development of the secretory phase
      (2) Decreased serum 17-hydroxyprogesterone on day 21
4. Irregular shedding of the endometrium
   a. Ovulatory type of DUB
   b. Persistent luteal phase
      • Continued secretion of progesterone
   c. Mixture of proliferative and secretory glands in the menstrual effluent

K. **Amenorrhea**
1. Epidemiology
   a. Primary amenorrhea
      (1) Absence of menses by 16 years of age

(2) Most cases are due to constitutional delay.
  - Family history of delayed onset of menses.

  b. Secondary amenorrhea
   (1) Absence of menses for 3 months
   (2) Most cases are due to pregnancy

2. Pathogenesis
  a. Hypothalamic and/or pituitary disorder
   (1) Decreased synthesis of FSH and LH
     - Hypogonadotropic ($\downarrow$ FSH and LH) hypogonadism
   (2) Decreased synthesis of estrogen and progesterone
   (3) *No* withdrawal bleeding after receiving progesterone
     - Indicates that the endometrial mucosa is *not* estrogen-stimulated
   (4) Examples
     - Hypopituitarism, prolactinoma, anorexia nervosa

> Anorexia nervosa is a condition in which there is self-induced starvation leading to protein energy malnutrition. Patients have a distorted body image and see themselves as fat even though they have excessive weight loss. Excessive loss of weight and body fat leads to decreased synthesis and release of gonadotropin-releasing hormone, which, in turn, causes decreased serum FSH and LH and secondary amenorrhea due to lack of estrogen stimulation of the endometrial mucosa. The stress hormones (e.g., cortisol, growth hormone) are increased in these patients. The most common cause of death in anorexia nervosa is a ventricular arrhythmia.

  b. Ovarian disorder
   (1) Decreased synthesis of estrogen and progesterone
   (2) Increase in serum FSH and LH, respectively
     - Hypergonadotropic ($\uparrow$ FSH and LH) hypogonadism
   (3) *No* withdrawal bleeding after receiving progesterone
     - Indicates that the endometrial mucosa is *not* estrogen-stimulated
   (4) Examples
     - Turner syndrome (see X.L), surgical removal of ovaries
  c. End-organ defect
   (1) Prevents the normal egress of blood
     - More likely a cause of primary amenorrhea
   (2) Normal levels of FSH, LH, estrogen, and progesterone
   (3) *No* withdrawal bleeding after receiving progesterone
   (4) Examples
     - Imperforate hymen, Asherman syndrome (removal of stratum basalis owing to repeated curettage)

3. Summary of amenorrhea (Table 10-9)

Primary amenorrhea: most cases due to constitutional delay

Secondary amenorrhea: most cases due to pregnancy

Primary amenorrhea + poor female secondary sex characteristics: probable Turner syndrome

TABLE 10-9
Differential Diagnosis of Amenorrhea

Disorder	FSH and LH	Estrogen	Examples
Hypothalamic/pituitary disorder	↓	↓	Hypopituitarism Anorexia nervosa, prolactinoma
Ovarian disorder	↑	↓	Turner syndrome
End-organ defect	Normal	Normal	Imperforate hymen, Asherman syndrome
Constitutional delay	Normal	Normal	Family history of delayed onset of menses

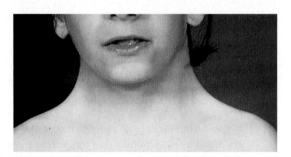

10-13: *Turner syndrome is characterized by a webbed neck. Other findings include short stature, primary amenorrhea, and delayed secondary sex characteristics (e.g., underdeveloped breasts). (From Bouloux P-M: Self-Assessment Picture Tests: Medicine, Vol. 1. St. Louis, Mosby, 1996, p 45.)*

L. **Turner syndrome**
 1. Sex chromosome disorder
 2. Pathogenesis
   a. Nondisjunction
     • 45,X karyotype (~60% of cases)
   b. Mosaicism
     • 45,X/46,XX karyotype (~40% of cases)
 3. Clinical and laboratory findings
   a. Short stature
     (1) Cardinal finding
     (2) Normal GH and IGF-1
   b. Lymphedema in hands and feet in infancy
     • Webbed neck is caused by dilated lymphatic channels (cystic hygroma) (Fig. 10-13).
   c. Streak gonads
     • Ovaries devoid of oocytes by 2 years of age
   d. Primary amenorrhea with delayed sexual maturation
     (1) Decreased serum estradiol
     (2) Increased FSH and LH
   e. No Barr bodies

Turner syndrome: 45,X karyotype

Most common genetic cause of primary amenorrhea: Turner syndrome

Questions

Refer to the following chart for questions 1 through 5:

	Serum T$_4$	Serum free T$_4$	Serum TSH	^{131}I Uptake
A.	↓	↓	↑	↔
B.	↓	N	N	↔
C.	↑	↑	↓	↓
D.	↑	↑	↓	↑
E.	↑	N	N	↔

N, normal; TSH, thyroid-stimulating hormone; ↔, not indicated.

Each lettered set of options relates to laboratory thyroid test results. For questions 1 through 5, select the *one* lettered option that is most closely associated with it. Each lettered option may be selected once, more than once, or not at all.

1. A 35-year-old obese woman has a history of palpitations that keep her up at night. She states that she has lost weight over the last few months while attending a weight loss clinic. Physical examination shows a nonpalpable thyroid gland, sinus tachycardia, and brisk deep tendon reflexes. There is no exophthalmos or pretibial myxedema.

2. A 20-year-old woman complains of intermittent fluttering in her chest. Physical examination reveals a normal thyroid, no lid stare or exophthalmos, a regular heart rate of 108 beats/minute, normal deep tendon reflexes, and blood pressure of 100/80 mm Hg. A midsystolic click and murmur is heard at the apex. She is currently taking oral contraceptive pills.

3. A 28-year-old woman has complaints of chronic constipation and progressive weight gain over the last 6 months in spite of being on a pure vegan diet. She is currently on no prescription or over-the-counter medications. Physical examination exhibits a young woman with periorbital puffiness; dry, yellow-colored skin; delayed deep tendon reflexes; and proximal muscle weakness in her lower extremities.

4. A 24-year-old college wrestler complains of fatigue. Physical examination reveals a muscular individual with cystic acne. The thyroid gland and deep tendon reflexes are normal.

5. A 30-year-old woman complains of palpitations that keep her awake at night. She states that she has a good appetite, but she has lost more than 4.5 kg (10 lb) over the past 3 months. Physical examination reveals proptosis of the eyes, diffuse enlargement of the thyroid gland, sinus tachycardia, and brisk tendon reflexes.

6. A 4-year-old boy who is below the normal percentile for height and weight for his age is brought to the family physician for evaluation. Both parents are small statured. The physical examination on the boy is normal. A magnetic resonance imaging study of the brain is normal. Serum gonadotropins are normal. The serum alkaline phosphatase is 130 U/L. What is the most likely diagnosis?
A. Growth hormone deficiency
B. Hypopituitarism
C. Hypothalamic disorder
D. Normal child

Refer to Figure 10-14 for questions 7 and 8.

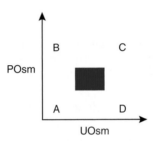

10-14: *Refer to questions 7 and 8.*

Each set of options relate plasma osmolality (POsm) to urine osmolality (UOsm). For questions 7 and 8, select the *one* lettered option that is most closely associated with it. Each lettered option may be selected once, more than once, or not at all. The square represents the normal values for POsm and UOsm.

7. A 25-year-old woman with a previous history of head trauma now has polyuria and increased thirst. A water deprivation test is abnormal.

8. A 55-year-old smoker has a centrally located mass on a chest radiograph, mental status abnormalities, and a serum sodium concentration of 110 mEq/L

9. A 52-year-old woman complains of fatigue, weakness, and lightheadedness when she stands up quickly. Physical examination reveals a patchy brown pigmentation of the buccal mucosa and increased pigmentation in the creases of the palms. The physician suspects a disorder involving the adrenal glands. Which of the following laboratory findings is most likely present?
A. Decreased plasma ACTH and 11-deoxycortisol after metyrapone stimulation
B. Increased plasma ACTH and decreased serum cortisol
C. Increased plasma ACTH and 11-deoxycortisol after metyrapone stimulation
D. Increased serum sodium and decreased serum potassium
E. Increased urine 17-hydroxycorticoids with prolonged ACTH stimulation

10. A 25-year-old woman who has not menstruated for the past 8 months complains of a milky discharge from her nipples that has been present for the past 6 months. Physical examination is unremarkable except for the milky discharge from the breasts. A urine pregnancy test is negative. Serum thyroid-stimulating hormone (TSH) is normal. Which of the following is the most likely diagnosis?
A. Cushing's syndrome
B. Graves' disease
C. Hypopituitarism
D. Primary hypothyroidism
E. Prolactinoma

11. A 32-year-old woman complains of menstrual irregularities and increased weight gain. Physical examination reveals a moon facies, hirsutism, and truncal obesity with purple stria. The extremities are thin. Multiple blood pressure readings show diastolic hypertension. A magnetic resonance imaging study shows a mass lesion in the anterior pituitary gland. Which of the following laboratory findings is most likely present?
A. Decreased plasma adrenocorticotropic hormone (ACTH)
B. Decreased serum cortisol with high-dose dexamethasone
C. Decreased 24-hour urine for 17-hydroxycorticoids
D. Decreased 24-hour urine for 17-ketosteroids
E. Increased 24-hour urine for metanephrine

12. For the past 5 years, a 48-year-old man has had episodic "attacks" of headache, palpitations, anxiety, and profuse sweating, the latter often drenching his bed sheets. His pulse is 160/minute and the average of three blood pressure readings is 180/120 mm Hg. A CT of the adrenal glands reveals a mass lesion in the right adrenal. Which of the following laboratory tests would be most useful in finding the cause of the hypertension?
A. Complete urinalysis
B. Serum electrolytes
C. Urine for free cortisol, 24 hours
D. Urine for 17-ketosteroids, 24 hours
E. Urine for metanephrines, 24 hours

13. A lethargic 2-month-old infant is noted to have ambiguous external genitalia. Laboratory studies show a decrease in serum cortisol and an increase in plasma ACTH. A random urine sodium is markedly increased and serum potassium is increased. A chromosome study shows an XX genotype. The patient most likely has a deficiency of which of the following enzymes involved in adrenal steroid synthesis?
A. 11-Hydroxylase
B. 17-Hydroxylase
C. 18-Hydroxylase
D. 21-Hydroxylase

14. A 20-year-old man complains of persistent breast enlargement. Findings on physical examination include eunuchoid proportions (arm span greater than height), soft skin, a female hair distribution, bilateral tender subareolar masses, and diminished volume of both testicles. When asked if he has erections at night, he states that he does not have any. Which of the following laboratory findings is most likely present?
A. Decreased concentration of follicle-stimulating hormone (FSH)
B. Decreased concentration of luteinizing hormone (LH)
C. Increased concentration of serum estradiol
D. Normal concentration of serum testosterone

15. A 17-year-old girl has primary amenorrhea. Examination reveals decreased stature, webbing of the neck, and underdevelopment of the breasts. Which of the following laboratory findings is most likely present?
A. Decreased concentration of luteinizing hormone (LH)
B. Decreased concentration of serum growth hormone
C. Increased concentration of follicle-stimulating hormone (FSH)
D. Increased concentration of serum estradiol

16. An obese 29-year-old woman has an 8-year history of infertility and problems with hirsutism. Both ovaries are enlarged on bimanual pelvic examination. An ultrasound study of the ovaries reveals subcapsular cysts. Which of the following laboratory findings is most likely present?
A. Decreased serum estrone
B. Increased dehydroepiandrosterone (DHEA) sulfate
C. Increased follicle-stimulating hormone (FSH)
D. Increased luteinizing hormone (LH)

17. A 16-year-old female with normal secondary female sex characteristics has primary amenorrhea. Physical examination shows discrete masses in both inguinal canals. Speculum examination of the vagina shows it ending in a blind pouch. Which of the following laboratory findings is most likely present?
A. Chromosome study with XO genotype
B. Chromosome study with XY genotype
C. Decreased serum testosterone
D. Normal androgen receptors

18. A 40-year-old man complains of headaches and dyspnea. Physical examination shows bilateral inspiratory crackles in the lungs, enlarged hands and feet, a prominent jaw with spacing between the teeth, and frontal bossing. A chest radiograph shows generalized enlargement of the heart and lung infiltrates consistent with congestive heart failure. Which of the following is the most sensitive screening test for this disorder?
A. Serum cortisol
B. Serum glucose
C. Serum insulin-like growth factor-I
D. Serum thyroid-stimulating hormone (TSH)

Answers

1. **C** is correct. The patient is taking excess hormone (increased serum T_4 and free T_4), leading to thyrotoxicosis. This suppresses the TSH causing the thyroid gland to undergo atrophy (nonpalpable) leading to a decrease in ^{131}I uptake. Also note the absence of signs specific for Graves' disease such as exophthalmos and pretibial myxedema.

2. **E** is correct. The patient is taking oral contraceptive pills. The estrogen in the pill is increasing liver synthesis of thyroid-binding globulin. This increases the total serum T_4 without affecting the serum TSH or free T_4 level. Mitral valve prolapse (midsystolic click and murmur) is producing the intermittent palpitations.

3. **A** is correct. The clinical findings in the patient are classic for primary hypothyroidism, most likely due to Hashimoto's thyroiditis. In primary hypothyroidism, the serum T_4 and free T_4 are decreased and serum TSH is increased.

4. **B** is correct. The patient is most likely taking anabolic steroids, which causes a decrease in liver synthesis of thyroid-binding globulin. This decreases serum T_4 without affecting free T_4 or TSH.

5. **D** is correct. The patient has classic Graves' disease (exophthalmos) and signs of thyrotoxicosis. In this disease, there is an IgG antibody directed against the TSH receptor causing continued stimulation of the gland. Serum T_4 and free T_4 are increased and serum TSH is suppressed. The ^{131}I uptake is increased, which distinguishes Graves' disease from thyrotoxicosis due to taking excess hormone or early phases of thyroiditis.

6. **D** (normal child) is correct. The child's parents are both small statured and there is no evidence of hypothalamic or pituitary disease. Serum alkaline phosphatase, though increased for an adult, is normal when age adjusted (70–140 U/L). Recall that normal growing children have increased osteoblastic activity in their growing bones and have increased levels of alkaline phosphatase and serum phosphorus to ensure adequate bone mineralization. This also underscores the fact that children's values are frequently not age-adjusted and can be misinterpreted as increased.

A (growth hormone deficiency) is incorrect. This hormone deficiency is usually associated with hypopituitarism, which is not present in this patient. Serum gonadotropins are the first pituitary hormones to decrease in hypopituitarism and these are normal in this patient.

B (hypopituitarism) is incorrect. The most common cause of hypopituitarism in children is a craniopharyngioma, which is excluded by the normal MRI study. Furthermore, the serum gonadotropin levels are normal.

C (hypothalamic disorder) is incorrect. A hypothalamic disorder would produce a decrease in serum gonadotropins. They are normal in this patient.

7. **B** (increased POsm, decreased UOsm) is correct. The patient has central diabetes insipidus due to transection of the pituitary stalk from her head trauma. Owing to a lack of antidiuretic hormone (ADH), the patient is always diluting her urine and never concentrating urine. Therefore, in a water deprivation test, the POsm will increase, due to excess loss of free water in the urine, and the UOsm will decrease, due to excess free water in the urine (dilution).

8. **D** (decreased POsm, increased UOsm) is correct. The patient has ectopic secretion of ADH by a small cell carcinoma of the lung. This is called the syndrome of inappropriate secretion of ADH (SIADH). With constant stimulation by ADH, the kidneys are constantly reabsorbing free water out of the urine (concentration) leading to a dilutional hyponatremia (decreased POsm) and increased UOsm.

9. **B** (increased plasma ACTH and decreased serum cortisol) is correct. Hyperpigmentation of the buccal mucosa and palmar creases, plus a history of fatigue, weakness, and signs of hypovolemia (lightheadedness when standing up suddenly) suggests a diagnosis of Addison's disease. Most cases of Addison's disease are due to autoimmune destruction of the adrenal cortex. This produces deficiencies of mineralocorticoids (e.g., aldosterone), glucocorticoids (e.g., cortisol), and sex hormones (e.g., androstenedione, testosterone). Hypocortisolism causes an increase in plasma ACTH due to a negative feedback relationship. ACTH has melanocyte-stimulating properties that increase the synthesis of melanin on the skin and mucosal surfaces. Hypovolemia is related to the loss of sodium in the urine due to aldosterone deficiency.

A (decreased plasma ACTH and 11-deoxycortisol after metyrapone stimulation) is incorrect. Metyrapone is a drug that blocks 11-hydroxylase in the adrenal cortex. This enzyme is normally responsible for conversion of the glucocorticoid 11-deoxycortisol to cortisol. Therefore, a normal response to metyrapone is a decrease in cortisol with a subsequent increase in ACTH and 11-deoxycortisol proximal to the enzyme block. If both plasma ACTH and 11-deoxycortisol are decreased, then hypopituitarism is the cause of hypocortisolism. Because of a decrease in ACTH there would be no signs of hyperpigmentation. In Addison's disease, the test causes an increased (not decreased) plasma ACTH and a decreased 11-deoxycortisol, because the adrenal cortex is destroyed.

C (increased plasma ACTH and 11-deoxycortisol after metyrapone stimulation) is incorrect. Metyrapone is a drug that blocks 11-hydroxylase in the adrenal cortex. This enzyme is normally responsible for conversion of the glucocorticoid 11-deoxycortisol to cortisol. Therefore, a normal response to metyrapone is a decrease in cortisol with a subsequent increase in ACTH and 11-deoxycortisol proximal to the enzyme block. In Addison's disease, the test results in an increased plasma ACTH and a decreased (not increased) 11-deoxycortisol, because the adrenal cortex is destroyed.

D (increased serum sodium and decreased serum potassium) is incorrect. Aldosterone normally maintains Na^+-K^+ channels in the late distal and collecting tubules that increase sodium reabsorption from urine in exchange for potassium, which is lost in the urine. In Addison's disease, hypoaldosteronism causes Na^+ loss in the urine (which causes hyponatremia not hypernatremia) and retention of K^+ (hyperkalemia, not hypokalemia).

E (increased urine 17-hydroxycorticoids with prolonged ACTH stimulation) is incorrect. The adrenal cortex is destroyed; therefore, urine 17-hydroxycorticoids (cortisol and 11-deoxycortisol) remain decreased after prolonged ACTH stimulation if the patient has Addison's disease. Patients with hypopituitarism have increased 17-hydroxycorticoids in urine after prolonged ACTH stimulation.

10. **E** (prolactinoma) is correct. The patient has a prolactinoma. Excess prolactin suppresses the release of gonadotropin-releasing hormone from the hypothalamus. This causes a decrease in follicle-stimulating hormone (FSH) and luteinizing hormone (LH) by the anterior pituitary gland leading to secondary amenorrhea. Prolactin also stimulates milk production in the breasts, causing galactorrhea.

A (Cushing's syndrome) is incorrect. Cushing's syndrome is characterized by signs of hypercortisolism (e.g., moon facies, truncal obesity with purple stria), which are not present in this patient. Furthermore, amenorrhea and galactorrhea are not features of Cushing's syndrome.

B (Graves' disease) is incorrect. Graves' disease is characterized by exophthalmos and thyromegaly, which are not present in this patient. Excess thyroid hormone causes menstrual irregularities but not galactorrhea.

C (hypopituitarism) is incorrect. Hypopituitarism is associated with amenorrhea (decreased FSH and LH). However, other expected findings of anterior pituitary hypofunction (e.g., secondary hypothyroidism) are not present in this patient.

D (primary hypothyroidism) is incorrect. Primary hypothyroidism may cause amenorrhea and galactorrhea, because a decrease in serum thyroxine increases both serum TSH and thyrotropin-releasing hormone. Thyrotropin-releasing hormone is a potent stimulator of prolactin release. However, the serum TSH is normal in this patient, which excludes primary hypothyroidism.

11. **B** (decreased serum cortisol with high-dose dexamethasone) is correct. The patient most likely has pituitary Cushing's syndrome, because the MRI shows a mass lesion in the anterior pituitary gland. The pituitary adenoma is secreting excess ACTH leading to hypercortisolism. Dexamethasone, a cortisol analogue, is used as a suppression test to differentiate pituitary Cushing's syndrome from adrenal Cushing's syndrome (cortisol-secreting adenoma) or ectopic Cushing's syndrome (e.g., ACTH-secreting small cell carcinoma of the lung). A normal response to dexamethasone is suppression of ACTH (negative feedback) and a decrease in cortisol production in the adrenal cortex. A low dose of dexamethasone is used as a screening test for hypercortisolism. It does not suppress cortisol production in pituitary, adrenal, or ectopic Cushing's syndrome. However, a high dose of dexamethasone suppresses ACTH production in pituitary Cushing's syndrome and results in a drop in cortisol levels. Cortisol remains increased in adrenal and ectopic Cushing's syndromes.

A (decreased plasma ACTH) is incorrect. In pituitary Cushing's syndrome, the ACTH is increased (not decreased).

C (decreased 24-hour urine for 17-hydroxycorticoids) is incorrect. In pituitary Cushing's syndrome, the 24-hour urine for 17-hydroxycorticoids is increased (not decreased). 17-Hydroxycorticoids (11-deoxycortisol and cortisol) are glucocorticoids.

D (decreased 24-hour urine for 17-ketosteroids) is incorrect. In pituitary Cushing's syndrome, the 24-hour urine for 17-ketosteroids is increased (not decreased). 17-Ketosteroids (dehydroepiandrosterone and androstenedione) are weak androgens.

E (increased 24-hour urine for metanephrine) is incorrect. Metanephrine is an end product of epinephrine metabolism in the adrenal medulla. It is primarily increased in tumors that originate in the adrenal medulla (e.g., pheochromocytoma).

12. **E** (urine for metanephrines, 24 hours) is correct. This patient has hypertension due to a pheochromocytoma, which is a benign tumor originating in the adrenal medulla. He demonstrates the classic triad of headache, palpitations, and excessive perspiration. Hypertension is characterized as sustained, sustained with paroxysms (most common), or paroxysmal only. A 24-hour urine test for metanephrines (most sensitive test) and vanillylmandelic acid are most often used as screening tests.

A (complete urinalysis) is incorrect. Although a urinalysis is useful in the workup of hypertension related to renal disease, it does not provide adequate information in screening for a pheochromocytoma.

B (serum electrolytes) is incorrect. Serum electrolytes are most useful in diagnosing primary aldosteronism, a tumor arising in the adrenal cortex.

Excess aldosterone causes hypertension along with hypernatremia, hypokalemia, and metabolic alkalosis. Hypokalemia produces muscle weakness, a very characteristic finding in primary aldosteronism that is not present in a pheochromocytoma. Furthermore, the classic triad listed above for pheochromocytoma is not present in primary aldosteronism.

C (urine for free cortisol, 24 hours) is incorrect. Increased urine free cortisol is a characteristic finding in Cushing's syndrome. Hypertension is present in Cushing's syndrome; however, it is not episodic and associated with headache, palpitations, and drenching sweat. Adrenal Cushing's syndrome is most often due to a benign adenoma in the adrenal cortex.

D (urine for 17-ketosteroids, 24 hours) is incorrect. Increased urine 17-ketosteroids (dehydroepiandrosterone and androstenedione) is a characteristic finding in Cushing's syndrome. It is not increased in a pheochromocytoma.

13. **D** (21-hydroxylase) is correct. The patient has adrenogenital syndrome, which is a group of autosomal recessive disorders characterized by enzyme deficiencies (in this patient, 21-hydroxylase deficiency) that cause a decrease in cortisol and an increase in ACTH. There is an increase in steroid compounds proximal to the enzyme block, including the 17-ketosteroids (dehydroepiandrosterone and androstenedione), testosterone, and dihydrotestosterone. There is a decrease in compounds distal to the enzyme block, including the mineralocorticoids (e.g., corticosterone) and the 17-hydroxycorticoids (11-deoxycortisol and cortisol). In the presence of excess dihydrotestosterone, female-appearing external genitalia in a fetus undergo male differentiation. The clitoris is often elongated (clitoromegaly) and the labia are often fused and appear as scrotal sacs. A decrease in serum cortisol causes an increase in ACTH, which has melanocyte-stimulating properties that produces increased skin pigmentation. A decrease in mineralocorticoids causes loss of sodium in the urine that may lead to hypovolemic shock. Serum potassium is increased, because potassium excretion in the kidneys is augmented by mineralocorticoids. A chromosome study is necessary to determine the sex of the patient. Genotypically, the patient is a female, and phenotypically, she has ambiguous genitalia; therefore, she is classified as a female pseudohermaphrodite.

A (11-hydroxylase) is incorrect. 11-Hydroxylase deficiency causes an increase in 11-deoxycortisol; 17-ketosteroids (dehydroepiandrosterone and androstenedione); and 11-deoxycorticosterone, a weak mineralocorticoid. The increase in deoxycorticosterone produces salt retention (not loss in the urine) and hypertension.

B (17-hydroxylase) is incorrect. 17-Hydroxylase deficiency causes an increase in the synthesis of mineralocorticoids (salt retention [not loss in the urine] and hypertension) and a decrease in 17-ketosteroids and 17-hydroxycorticoids.

C (18-hydroxylase) is incorrect. 18-Hydroxylase deficiency is uncommon and causes an isolated deficiency of aldosterone, resulting in hyponatremia, hyperkalemia, and acidosis. Disorders involving glucocorticoids and 17-ketosteroids do not occur.

14. C (increased concentration of serum estradiol) is correct. The patient has Klinefelter's syndrome. Characteristic findings in Klinefelter's syndrome include an XXY phenotype with 47 chromosomes, signs of hyperestrinism (gynecomastia, female distribution of pubic hair), eunuchoid proportions, and impotence (lack of erections). Diminished testicular volume is due to testicular atrophy. The testicles show fibrosis of the seminiferous tubules and hyperplasia of the Leydig cells. Loss of the seminiferous tubules leads to absence of spermatogenesis (azoospermia) and absence of Sertoli cells, which normally contain the hormone inhibin. Inhibin has a negative feedback relationship with follicle-stimulating hormone (FSH); therefore, a decrease in inhibin causes an increase in FSH. FSH, in turn, increases the synthesis of aromatase in the hyperplastic Leydig cells leading to conversion of all the testosterone to estradiol, which produces the signs of hyperestrinism that are present in the patient. Serum testosterone levels are decreased, which leads to a decrease in libido (sexual desire) and impotence (failure to sustain an erection).

A (decreased concentration of follicle-stimulating hormone) is incorrect. In Klinefelter's syndrome, decreased levels of inhibin cause a corresponding increase in FSH.

B (decreased concentration of luteinizing hormone) is incorrect. In Klinefelter's syndrome, there is a decreased testosterone and a corresponding increase in serum LH.

D (normal concentration of serum testosterone) is incorrect. In Klinefelter's syndrome, there is decreased serum testosterone, because it is aromatized to estradiol.

15. C (increased concentration of follicle-stimulating hormone) is correct. The patient has Turner syndrome. Characteristic signs of Turner syndrome are primary amenorrhea, short stature, underdeveloped breasts, and a webbed neck. Most patients have 45 chromosomes with an XO phenotype. This is due to nondisjunction of the sex chromosomes in the first stage of meiosis. No Barr bodies (randomly inactivated X chromosomes) are present. The ovaries of patients with Turner syndrome lack oocytes, which leads to decreased synthesis of estradiol and a corresponding increase in FSH.

A (decreased concentration of luteinizing hormone) is incorrect. In Turner syndrome, the ovaries lack oocytes. Because no progesterone is synthesized, serum LH levels increase.

B (decreased concentration of serum growth hormone) is incorrect. In Turner syndrome, growth hormone is normal.

D (increased concentration of serum estradiol) is incorrect. In Turner syndrome, the ovaries lack oocytes. This results in decreased synthesis of estradiol.

16. **D** (increased luteinizing hormone) is correct. The patient has polycystic ovary syndrome (PCOS). The ultrasound showed subcapsular cysts. In PCOS, the serum LH is increased. This stimulates the ovaries to produce increased amounts of 17-ketosteroids (DHEA and androstenedione) and testosterone. These androgen compounds cause hirsutism (abnormal hairiness in normal hair-bearing areas). In obese patients, an increase in adipose allows greater conversion of androgens to estrogens (aromatization). Therefore, androstenedione is converted to estrone and testosterone to estradiol by aromatase. Increased estrogen has a negative feedback on the release of FSH and a positive feedback on LH; therefore, LH remains increased and FSH is suppressed. Decreased FSH causes degeneration of the follicles, resulting in the formation of subcapsular cysts. In PCOS, the LH : FSH ratio is >2 : 1.

A (decreased serum estrone) is incorrect. Estrone is increased due to aromatization of androstenedione into estrone, a weak estrogen.

B (increased DHEA sulfate) is incorrect. DHEA sulfate is a 17-ketosteroid that is primarily synthesized in the adrenal cortex (95%). It is not increased in PCOS. DHEA-sulfate is one of the androgens responsible for producing hirsutism when there is adrenal cortical hyperfunction (e.g., Cushing's syndrome).

C (increased follicle-stimulating hormone) is incorrect. Serum FSH is decreased in PCOS due to a negative feedback relationship with estrogen.

17. **B** (chromosome study with XY genotype) is correct. The patient has testicular feminization syndrome, which is an X-linked recessive disorder with absence of the androgen receptors. The testes are present and either remain in the abdominal cavity or present as masses in the inguinal canal (patient in this case). Concentrations of testosterone and dihydrotestosterone (DHT) are normal, but the lack of androgen receptors prevents the development of male secondary sex characteristics and external genitalia. Testosterone effects normal fetal male development of the epididymis, seminal vesicles, and vas deferens from the mesonephric duct. DHT converts female-appearing external genitalia into a penis and scrotal sac and develops the prostate gland. The Sertoli cells in the seminiferous tubules, produce müllerian inhibitory factor, which causes müllerian structures (fallopian tubes, uterus, cervix, upper one third of vagina) to undergo apoptosis. In testicular feminization, due to a lack of testosterone effect, there is no epididymis, seminal vesicles, and vas deferens. Owing to a lack of DHT effect, there is no prostate gland; the vagina ends as a blind pouch (lower two thirds of the vagina develops from the urogenital sinus), and, the external genitalia remains female. Breast development and female secondary sex characteristics are normal, because estrogen receptors are present.

A (chromosome study with XO genotype) is incorrect. An XO genotype occurs in Turner syndrome. The ovaries lack germinal follicles; therefore, estrogen is not produced, resulting in primary amenorrhea and underdeveloped female sex characteristics.

C (decreased serum testosterone) is incorrect. In testicular feminization, testosterone levels are normal (negative feedback with luteinizing hormone).

D (normal androgen receptors) is incorrect. In testicular feminization, the androgen receptors are either deficient or defective.

18. **C** (serum insulin-like growth factor-I) is correct. The patient has signs of acromegaly and has a cardiomyopathy with congestive heart failure. Pituitary adenomas secreting excess growth hormone are often quite large and extend out of the sella turcica, causing headache, visual field defects, and hydrocephalus. Gigantism occurs if the tumor is present before the epiphyses have fused, whereas acromegaly develops if the epiphyses have closed. Excess growth hormone causes hyperglycemia (growth hormone is gluconeogenic) and increased amino acid uptake in muscle and other tissues. Excess growth hormone also stimulates the liver to synthesize and release increased amounts of insulin-like growth factor-I. This hormone increases linear and lateral bone growth and also causes visceromegaly. Although growth hormone is used as a screening test in cases of suspected acromegaly, insulin-like growth factor-I is a more sensitive and reliable test.

A (serum cortisol) is incorrect. Serum cortisol is a screening test for adrenocortical hypofunction or hyperfunction disorders, neither of which produces the changes noted in this patient.

B (serum glucose) is incorrect. Serum glucose is a screening test for diabetes mellitus, types 1 and 2. The patient most likely has diabetes mellitus due to excess growth hormone (gluconeogenic hormone). A glucose tolerance test is used to confirm acromegaly. Excess glucose should suppress growth hormone; however, in acromegaly, growth hormone and insulin growth factor-1 remain increased.

D (serum thyroid-stimulating hormone) is incorrect. TSH is used to screen for thyroid hypofunction and hyperfunction. TSH is decreased in hyperthyroidism and hypopituitarism and increased in primary hypothyroidism. It is normal in acromegaly.

Body Fluid Analysis

I. **Cerebrospinal Fluid (CSF)**
  A. **Overview of CSF**
     1. CSF derives from the choroid plexus in the ventricles.
     2. CSF enters the subarachnoid space.
        • Cushions the brain and spinal cord
     3. CSF is reabsorbed by arachnoid granulations.
        • Drained into dural venous sinuses
  B. **CSF analysis**
     1. Usually obtained by a lumbar puncture
     2. Three tubes for CSF analysis are usually collected.
        a. First tube
           • Microbiologic studies
        b. Second tube
           (1) Chemistry
              • Glucose, total protein
           (2) Cytologic test
              • If primary cancer or metastasis is suspected
           (3) Serologic tests
              (a) Syphilis serology (e.g., Venereal Disease Research Laboratory, VDRL)
              (b) Rapid plasma reagin (RPR) test *cannot* be used on CSF.
        c. Third tube
           • WBC count and differential
     3. Gross appearance
        a. Normal CSF
           • Clear and colorless
        b. Turbidity; causes:
           (1) Increased protein
           (2) Increase in cellular elements
           (3) Presence of microbial pathogens
           (4) Combinations of the above
        c. Bloody CSF taps; causes:
           (1) Most often iatrogenic
           (2) Pathologic hemorrhage into subarachnoid space
              • Examples—ruptured berry aneurysm, intracerebral bleed near surface of the brain or ventricles

Hydrocephalus: obstruction to outflow of CSF from ventricles or subarachnoid space

(3) CSF color changes in pathologic bleeds

    (a) Pink, yellow, or orange-tinged CSF after centrifugation

    (b) Pink color is due to oxyhemoglobin (oxyHb) from ruptured RBCs.

      • Color first occurs 2 to 4 hours after bleed; peaks in 24 to 36 hours; subsides in 4 to 8 days.

Xanthochromia: sign of pathologic bleed

    (c) Yellow to orange color (xanthochromia) is due to oxyHb breakdown to bilirubin.

      • First appears 12 hours after bleed; peaks in 2 to 4 days; subsides in 2 to 4 weeks.

4. CSF protein

    • Normal, <40 mg/dL

  a. CSF prealbumin and albumin

    (1) Normal levels derive from plasma.

    (2) Increased levels of prealbumin and albumin

      • Due to increased capillary permeability (e.g., inflammation)

  b. CSF gamma (γ) globulins

    (1) Normal levels derive from synthesis of IgG by plasma cells within the central nervous system (CNS).

      • Represents <12% of the total protein in CSF electrophoresis.

Increased CSF protein: acute inflammation, demyelinating disease

    (2) Increased IgG levels; causes:

    (a) Increased synthesis of IgG from plasma cells in CNS

      • Occurs in demyelinating disorders (e.g., multiple sclerosis, MS)

    (b) Increased capillary vessel permeability

      • Example—acute meningitis

    (3) CSF IgG index distinguishes acute inflammation from demyelinating diseases

    (a) CSF IgG index = CSF IgG × serum albumin/CSF albumin × serum IgG

    (b) Increased values indicate demyelinating disease; decreased values indicate acute inflammation.

    (4) Routine CSF electrophoresis

      • Quantitates the amount of γ-globulins when CSF protein is increased

    (5) High-resolution CSF electrophoresis

    (a) Most useful in detecting demyelinating disease

      • Examples—MS, neurosyphilis, Guillain-Barré syndrome

Oligoclonal bands: CSF electrophoresis sign of demyelination

    (b) Detects oligoclonal bands in the γ-globulin region (Fig. 11-1)

      • Discrete, discontinuous bands originating from single clones of immunocompetent B cells

  c. Myelin basic protein (MBP) in MS

    (1) Protein present in myelin

    (2) Antibodies attack MBP in myelin.

    (3) Increased CSF MBP occurs with active demyelinating disease.

      • CSF MBP is decreased when MS is in remission.

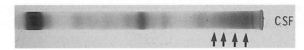

11-1: Cerebrospinal high-resolution electrophoresis showing oligoclonal bands in a patient with multiple sclerosis. The arrows show discrete, discontinuous bands in the γ-globulin region. (From Perkin GD: Mosby's Color Atlas and Text of Neurology. St. Louis, Mosby, 2002, Fig. 10.14.)

5. CSF glucose
   a. Slightly less concentration than in serum
      (1) Normal, 50 to 75 mg/dL
      (2) Should be ~66% of a serum sample obtained 30 to 90 minutes *before* the lumbar puncture
         • Example—serum glucose 100 mg/dL, CSF glucose 66 mg/dL
   b. Decreased CSF glucose (hypoglycorrhachia)
      (1) Defined as a glucose <40 mg/dL
      (2) Increased uptake of glucose by cellular elements
         • Examples—neutrophils (acute bacterial meningitis), malignant cells
      (3) Defective glucose carrier system
         • Frequently occurs in bacterial/fungal meningitis
   c. CSF levels usually normal:
      (1) Viral meningitis, neurosyphilis, demyelinating disease, cerebral abscess
      (2) Exceptions (when viral meningitis is associated with decreased CSF glucose):
         • Mumps, herpes simplex, lymphocytic choriomeningitis
6. CSF WBC count
   a. Normal, 0 to 5 mononuclear cells/mm³
      • Neutrophils are *not* normally present in the CSF.
   b. Etiology of increased CSF WBC count
      (1) Usually meningitis due to microbial pathogens
      (2) Bacterial meningitis
         (a) Predominance of neutrophils
         (b) Neonatal meningitis
            • Group B streptococcus (most common), *Escherichia coli, Listeria monocytogenes*
         (c) Meningitis in children 1 month to 18 years old
            • *Neisseria meningitidis* (most common), *Streptococcus pneumoniae*
         (d) Meningitis in those over 18 years old
            • *Streptococcus pneumoniae*
         (e) Tuberculous meningitis
            • Thick pellicle (exudate containing protein) should have acid-fast stain and be cultured
      (3) Viral meningitis
         (a) Initial neutrophil response in first 24 hours

CSF glucose: ↓ bacterial, fungal, metastatic disease to meninges

Bacterial meningitis: ↑ neutrophils

**TABLE 11-1
Cerebrospinal
Fluid (CSF)
Findings in Viral,
Bacterial, and
Fungal Meningitis**

CSF	Normal	Bacterial	Viral	Fungal
Total WBC count	0–5 cells/mm^3	>1000 cells/mm^3	<1000 cells/mm^3	<500 cells/mm^3
Differential count	Mononuclear cells; no neutrophils	>90% neutrophils	Lymphocytes	Lymphocytes/ monocytes
CSF glucose	50–75 mg/dL	<40 mg/dL	Usually normal 50–100 mg/dL	<40 mg/dL
CSF protein	<40 mg/dL	>150 mg/dL		>150 mg/dL

Viral meningitis:
↑ lymphocytes

        (b) Changes to lymphocyte response in 2 to 3 days
        (c) Common viral pathogens
            • Coxsackievirus (most common), mumps, herpes simplex virus, *Varicella*, HIV
    (4) Fungal meningitis
        (a) Predominance of mononuclear cells
            • Lymphocytes, monocytes
        (b) *Cryptococcus neoformans*
            • Most common pathogen in immunocompromised host
        (c) *Candida, Coccidioides, Mucor, Aspergillus*
    (5) Parasitic meningitis
        (a) Mixed inflammatory infiltrate
            • Pathogens include *Entamoeba histolytica, Naegleria*
        (b) Eosinophils suggest a helminth infection.
            • Cysticercosis, trichinosis
  7. Detection of pathogens in CSF
    a. Gram stain
        • Most useful for bacteria (75–80% sensitivity)
    b. Culture
    c. India ink for *Cryptococcus neoformans*
        • Sensitivity is 50%.
    d. Antigen detection
      (1) Latex agglutination and coagglutination
        (a) CSF or urine can be used.
        (b) Sensitivity depends on the pathogen.
        (c) Specificity is 96% to 100%.
      (2) Enzyme immunoassay
        • High sensitivity and specificity (96–100% in both)
      (3) Polymerase chain reaction
        • Detects DNA; high sensitivity (94%) and specificity (96%)
  8. Summary of CSF findings due to bacteria, virus, fungi (Table 11-1)
  9. Multiple sclerosis (MS)
    a. Epidemiology
      (1) Most common demyelinating disease
      (2) Female predominance (~2:1)
        • Typically a woman 20 to 40 years of age

    b. Pathogenesis
        (1) CD8 T-cell destruction of myelin sheaths
        (2) Antibodies directed against MBP
    c. Clinical findings
        (1) Episodic course punctuated by acute relapses and remissions
        (2) Sensory and motor dysfunction
            • Paresthesias, muscle weakness
    d. Laboratory findings
        (1) Increased CSF WBC count
            • Primarily T lymphocytes
        (2) Increased CSF protein
            (a) Primarily an increase in γ-globulins (IgG in particular)
            (b) Increased CSF IgG ratio or index
        (3) Increased CSF myelin basic protein
            • Indicates active disease
        (4) Normal CSF glucose
        (5) High-resolution electrophoresis shows oligoclonal bands

> Multiple sclerosis: autoimmune destruction of myelin sheath

II. **Pleural Fluid (PF) Analysis**
  A. **Movement of pleural fluid**
    1. Fluid moves from parietal pleura to pleural space to lungs
    2. Movement depends upon the balance of Starling's pressures (see Chapter 2)
        a. Parietal capillary hydrostatic pressure greater than visceral capillary hydrostatic pressure
        b. Parietal capillary oncotic pressure equals visceral capillary hydrostatic pressure
  B. **Etiology and pathogenesis of pleural effusions**
    1. Increased hydrostatic pressure in visceral pleura
        • Example—congestive heart failure
    2. Decreased oncotic pressure
        • Example—nephrotic syndrome
    3. Obstruction of lymphatic drainage from the visceral pleura
        • Example—lung cancer
    4. Increased vessel permeability of visceral pleural capillaries
        • Examples—pulmonary infarction, pneumonia
    5. Metastasis to the pleura
        • Example—metastatic breast cancer
  C. **Types of pleural effusions**
    1. Transudates
        a. Ultrafiltrate of plasma involving disturbances in Starling's pressures
        b. Examples
            (1) Increased hydrostatic pressure in congestive heart failure
            (2) Decreased oncotic pressure in nephrotic syndrome
    2. Exudates
        a. Protein-rich and cell-rich fluid
            • Due to an increased vessel permeability in acute inflammation
        b. Examples—pneumonia, infarction, metastasis

**TABLE 11-2
Pleural Fluid (PF)
Transudates
versus Exudates**

PF Component	Transudate	Exudate
PF protein/serum protein	<0.5	>0.5
PF LDH/serum LDH	<0.6	>0.6
PF LDH	<200 U/L	>200 U/L

LDH, lactate dehydrogenase; ULN, upper limit of normal.

3. Chylous fluid
   a. Indicates interruption of the thoracic duct
   b. Etiology
      (1) Malignancy (most common)
         • Blocks lymphatic drainage
      (2) Trauma
         • Iatrogenic tear during surgery or pathologic
   c. Turbid, milky appearance
      (1) Due to chylomicrons (diet-derived triglyceride; see Chapter 9)
      (2) Chylomicrons form a supranate in a test tube after refrigeration
   d. PF triglyceride >110 mg/dL is diagnostic.
4. Pseudochylous fluid
   a. Turbid, milky appearance
   b. Caused by inflammation with increased amount of necrotic debris
      • PF cholesterol increased
   c. Most commonly caused by rheumatoid lung disease

Congestive heart failure: most common overall cause of a pleural effusion

5. Laboratory distinction of transudates versus exudates (Table 11-2)
   a. PF and serum concentrations of LDH and protein are most useful.
      • Ratios of PF protein and LDH to serum protein and LDH increase test sensitivity and specficity
   b. Test sensitivity is 99% and specificity is 98% if at least one of the three criteria for an exudate is present.

Tuberculosis and malignancy: most common causes of a pleural exudate

6. Causes of bloody PF
   a. Trauma (iatrogenic or otherwise)
   b. Malignancy
   c. Pulmonary infarction
7. PF pH
   a. pH > 7.40 is usually a transudate.
   b. pH < 7.40 is usually an exudate.
8. Causes of a neutrophil-predominant exudate
   a. Empyema (pus in the cavity) from pneumonia
   b. Pulmonary infarction

Lymphocyte-predominant PF: tuberculosis most common cause

9. Causes of a lymphocyte-predominant exudate
   a. Tuberculosis (most common)
   b. Lymphatic blockage by tumor
   c. Viral pneumonia
   d. Metastatic leukemia or lymphoma
10. Causes of an eosinophil-predominant exudate
    a. Hemothorax (bleeding into pleural cavity)

    b. Pneumothorax

    c. Resolving bacterial pneumonia

    d. Coccidioidomycosis

    e. Mesothelioma

       (1) Malignancy of pleura associated with asbestos exposure

       (2) Malignant mesothelial cells are also present

11. PF glucose

    a. Parallels blood glucose

    b. Causes of decreased PF glucose (i.e., <60 mg/dL)

       (1) Bacterial pneumonia

       (2) Rheumatoid arthritis

          (a) Selective glucose block

          (b) *Not* present in other collagen disorders involving lungs

> Rheumatoid lung disease: characteristic decrease in PF glucose

12. PF cytology

    a. Indication

       • Distinguish effusion of tuberculosis versus malignancy

    b. Malignant effusion

       (1) Cytology and pleural biopsy have a similar sensitivity (65%)

       (2) Repeat pleural taps increase sensitivity of cytologic test

    c. Tuberculous effusion

       • Culture plus pleural biopsy has highest sensitivity.

13. Causes of increased PF amylase

    a. Acute pancreatitis (10% of cases)

       • Left-sided effusion

    b. Rupture of the esophagus (Boerhaave's syndrome)

> Complicated effusion triad: whenever pH < 7.0, glucose < 40 mg/dL, LDH > 1000 mg/dL

III. **Gastric Analysis**

  A. **General remarks**

    1. Uncommon test due to medical treatment of peptic ulcer disease

    2. Performed in the fasting state and after pentagastrin stimulation

  B. **Fasting basal acid output (BAO)**

    1. Based on a 1-hour collection of gastric juice via nasogastric tube

    2. Normal BAO is <5 mEq/hour.

  C. **Maximal acid output (MAO)**

    1. Performed after pentagastrin stimulation

    2. Normally MAO is 5 to 20 mEq/hour.

    3. Normal BAO/MAO ratio is 0.20.

  D. **Test interpretation**

    1. Gastric ulcers

       • Usually have a normal BAO and MAO

    2. Duodenal ulcer

       a. BAO is 5 to 15 mEq/hour.

       b. MAO is 20 to 60 mEq/hour.

       c. BAO/MAO ratio is 0.40 to 0.60.

    3. Zollinger-Ellison syndrome (see Chapter 10)

       a. BAO is >20 mEq/hour.

↑ MAO: duodenal ulcer,
Zollinger-Ellison
syndrome

b. MAO is >60 mEq/hour.
c. BAO/MAO ratio is >0.60.
4. Achlorhydria
   a. Gastric pH never falls below 6 after pentagastrin stimulation
   b. Causes
      • Pernicious anemia, gastric cancer, severe iron deficiency

IV. **Stool Analysis**
   A. **Stool for occult blood**
      1. Useful screening test
         • Identifies upper and lower gastrointestinal bleeding
      2. Guaiac-based chemical tests
         • Examples—Hemoccult, Seracult, Coloscreen

Stool guaiac test: most
often used in United
States; rapidly being
replaced by
immunochemistry testing
(antibodies against
human blood)

   a. Do *not* differentiate Hb from myoglobin
      (1) Tests are based on the peroxidase activity of heme in Hb.
         • Myoglobin also has peroxidase activity.
      (2) Peroxidase catalyzes the oxidation of a reagent (guaiac) by peroxide.
         • Reaction produces a color change.
   b. Varying levels of sensitivity and specificity
      (1) False positives
         (a) Myoglobin in meat
         (b) Plant peroxidases (e.g., radishes)
      (2) False negatives
         • Excess ascorbic acid (>250 mg)
   B. **Blood in the stool**
      1. Melena
         a. Passage of dark, tarry stools
            (1) Gastric acid converts Hb to hematin (black pigment)
            (2) Sign of upper gastrointestinal bleed
               (a) Approximately 90% of all bleeds are upper gastrointestinal.
               (b) Bleeding is proximal to the ligament of Treitz
                  • Where duodenum joins jejunum

Most common cause of
melena: peptic ulcer
disease

         b. Etiology
            (1) Peptic ulcer disease
               (a) Duodenal and gastric ulcers
               (b) Also the most common cause of hematemesis
                  • Vomiting of blood
            (2) Esophageal varices
            (3) Hemorrhagic gastritis

Most common cause of
hematemesis: peptic ulcer
disease

      2. Hematochezia
         a. Passage of bright red blood in the stool
            (1) Colonic bleeding below the ileocecal valve (90%)
            (2) Distal small bowel bleeding (10%)

Most common cause of
hematochezia: sigmoid
diverticulosis

         b. Etiology
            (1) Sigmoid diverticulosis (most common)
            (2) Angiodysplasia
               • Rupture of dilated small vessels in cecum, right colon

**TABLE 11-3
Invasive,
Secretory, and
Osmotic Diarrhea**

Type	Characteristics	Causes	Screening Tests
Invasive	Pathogens invade enterocytes Low volume Dysentery: diarrhea with blood and leukocytes	*Shigella* spp., *Campylobacter jejuni,* *Entamoeba histolytica*	Fecal smear for leukocytes: positive Stool culture and stool for O and P
Secretory	Loss of isotonic fluid High volume Mechanisms: Chemicals in laxatives Enterotoxins: stimulate Cl^- channels regulated by cAMP and cGMP Serotonin: increases bowel motility No inflammation in bowel mucosa	Phenanthracene laxatives Enterotoxin production: *Vibrio cholerae* Enterotoxigenic *E. coli* Serotonin: carcinoid syndrome	Fecal smear for leukocytes: negative Increased 5-HIAA: carcinoid syndrome Stool osmotic gap <50 mOsm/kg
Osmotic	High-volume diarrhea Osmotically active substance in bowel lumen: hypotonic salt solution is drawn into the bowel lumen No inflammation in bowel mucosa	Disaccharidase deficiency: e.g., lactase Ingestion of poorly absorbable solutes: e.g.,magnesium sulfate in laxatives	Fecal smear for leukocytes: negative Stool osmotic gap >100 mOsm/kg

cAMP, cyclic adenosine monophosphate; cGMP, cyclic guanosine monophosphate; HIAA, hydroxyindoleacetic acid; O and P, ova and parasites.

3. Blood coating stool
   a. Internal hemorrhoids (most common)
   b. Left-sided bowel cancer
   c. Anal fissure

Most common cause of blood coating stool: internal hemorrhoids

> Newborns may have blood in the stool due to swallowing of maternal blood during delivery or to bleeding from a lesion in the gastrointestinal tract (e.g., Meckel's diverticulum). The Apt test is performed on the stool and distinguishes maternal Hb from fetal Hb on the basis of the resistance of fetal Hb to acid and alkaline denaturation. However, the test has a low sensitivity.

C. **Diarrheal diseases (excluding malabsorption)**
   1. Diarrhea
      a. Defined as >250 g of stool per day
      b. Acute: <3 weeks
      c. Chronic: >4 weeks
      d. Invasive, osmotic, secretory types (Table 11-3)
   2. Important screening tests
      a. Fecal smear for leukocytes
         (1) Indicates invasive diarrhea and acute inflammation
         (2) Sensitivity ~75%

Types of diarrhea: osmotic, secretory, invasive

(3) Noninvasive causes of positive smear for leukocytes
    (a) Pseudomembranous colitis
        • Due to *Clostridium difficile*

Pseudomembranous colitis: cytotoxin assay of stool test of choice

> *Clostridium difficile* is normally present in up to 3% of normal people. Carrier rate increases in hospitalized patients (21%) due to contact with spores in the hospital environment. Antibiotic exposure (e.g., quinolones, clindamycin, ampicillin) causes overgrowth of the organisms with toxin production leading to pseudomembranous colitis. Toxins release proinflammatory mediators and cytokines that attract neutrophils and stimulate excess fluid secretion (watery diarrhea). Pseudomembranes are composed of cellular debris, leukocytes, fibrin, and mucin. Nonspecific laboratory findings include neutrophilic leukocytosis with left shift, fecal leukocytes, and decreased serum albumin. Cytotoxin assay of stool has greater specificity (75–100%) than culture of stool (75–80%) for securing the diagnosis. Treatment is metronidazole.

    (b) Ulcerative colitis
  b. Stool osmotic gap
    (1) 300 mOsm/kg (value used to represent normal POsm) − 2 × (random stool Na^+ + random stool K^+)
    (2) Gap of <50 mOsm/kg from POsm is a secretory diarrhea.
        • Indicates that diarrheal fluid approximates POsm

Secretory diarrhea: loss of isotonic fluid

Osmotic diarrhea: loss of hypotonic fluid

    (3) Gap >100 mOsm/kg from POsm is an osmotic diarrhea.
        • Indicates a hypotonic loss of stool due to presence of osmotically active substances
  c. Stool pH
    (1) Normal stool pH is 7.0 to 8.0.
    (2) Stool pH <6.0 suggests lactase deficiency (see below).

> Lactase deficiency is a common genetic defect in Native Americans, Asian-Americans, and black Americans. Lactase is a disaccharidase in the brush border of the small intestine that hydrolyzes lactose to glucose and galactose. In lactase deficiency, colon anaerobes degrade undigested lactose into lactic acid (decreases stool pH) and H_2 gas, leading to abdominal distention with explosive diarrhea. Diagnostic tests include measurement of stool pH and the H_2 breath test after administration of oral lactose (best test). Treatment is to avoid dairy products or to orally take lactase before eating dairy products.

3. Confirmatory test for invasive diarrheas
   • Stool culture (gold standard)

D. **Malabsorption**
   1. Definition
      a. Increased fecal excretion of fat plus
      b. Concurrent deficiencies of fat-soluble vitamins, minerals, carbohydrates, and proteins
   2. Pathogenesis
      - Pancreatic insufficiency, bile salt/acid deficiency, small bowel disease
   3. Pancreatic insufficiency
      a. Most often caused by chronic pancreatitis
         - Most commonly due to alcohol in adults and cystic fibrosis in children
      b. Pathogenesis
         (1) Maldigestion of fats
            (a) Due to diminished lipase activity
            (b) Undigested neutral fats and fat droplets are in stool.
         (2) Maldigestion of proteins
            (a) Due to diminished trypsin
            (b) Undigested meat fibers are in stool.
         (3) Carbohydrate digestion is *not* affected.
            (a) Amylase is present in salivary glands.
            (b) Disaccharidases are present in the brush border of intestinal epithelium.
   4. Bile salt deficiency
      a. Required to micellarize monoglycerides and fatty acids
      b. Etiology and pathogenesis
         (1) Inadequate production of bile salts/acids from cholesterol (e.g., cirrhosis)
         (2) Intrahepatic/extrahepatic blockage of bile
            - Examples—primary biliary cirrhosis, stone in common bile duct
         (3) Bacterial overgrowth in small bowel with destruction of bile salts
            - Example—small bowel diverticula
         (4) Excess binding of bile salts
            - Example—cholestyramine
         (5) Terminal ileal disease
            (a) Prevents recycling of bile salts/acids
            (b) Examples—Crohn's disease, resection of ileum
   5. Small bowel disease
      a. Villi are required to reabsorb micelles into enterocytes.
         - Villi increase the absorptive surface of the small intestine.
      b. Etiology and pathogenesis
         (1) Inability to reabsorb micelles
            (a) Due to loss of villous surface
            (b) Examples—celiac disease, Whipple's disease
         (2) Lymphatic obstruction
            - Examples—Whipple's disease, abetalipoproteinemia (see Chapter 9)

Causes of malabsorption: pancreatic insufficiency, bile salt/acid deficiency, small bowel disease

Pancreatic insufficiency: malabsorption of fat and proteins

Bile salts/acids: required to micellarize monoglycerides and fatty acids

General screening tests
for malabsorption: stool
for fat, serum beta
carotene

D-Xylose: decreased
reabsorption indicates
small bowel disease

Acute pancreatitis:
increased clearance of
amylase in urine

Serum lipase: more
specific and lasts longer
than amylase in acute
pancreatitis

Serum immunoreactive
trypsin: excellent
newborn screen for cystic
fibrosis

6. General screening tests for fat malabsorption
   a. Quantitative stool for fat
      (1) 72-hour collection of stool
      (2) Best screening test
      (3) Positive test, >7 g of fat/24 hours
   b. Qualitative stool for fat
      (1) Stains are used to identify fat in stool
      (2) Lacks sensitivity
   c. Decreased serum beta carotene
      • Precursor for fat-soluble retinoic acid (vitamin A)
   d. D-Xylose screening test
      (1) Xylose does *not* require pancreatic enzymes for absorption.
      (2) Lack of reabsorption of orally administered xylose
         • Indicates small bowel disease
7. Tests to evaluate pancreatic function
   a. Serum amylase
      (1) *Not* specific for pancreatitis
      (2) Also present in salivary glands
         • Increased in mumps
      (3) Amylase in acute pancreatitis
         (a) Sensitivity 85%, specificity 70%
         (b) Initial increase over 2 to 12 hours; peaks in 12 to 30 hours; returns to normal in 2 to 4 days
            • Increased renal clearance
         (c) Present in urine for 1 to 14 days
         (d) Persistent increase in serum amylase >7 days
            • Suggests pancreatic pseudocyst (collection of amylase-rich fluid around pancreas)
         (e) Urine amylase
            • Initial increase over 4 to 8 hours; peaks in 18 to 36 hours; returns to normal in 7 to 10 days
      (4) Amylase in chronic pancreatitis
         (a) Less reliable than in acute disease
         (b) Values either normal, borderline, or slightly increased
   b. Serum lipase
      (1) More specific for pancreatitis
         • Is *not* excreted in urine
      (2) Lipase in acute pancreatitis
         (a) Sensitivity 80%, specificity 75%
         (b) Initial increase over 3 to 6 hours; peaks in 12 to 30 hours; returns to normal in 7 to 14 days
      (3) Lipase in chronic pancreatitis
         • *Not* clinically useful
   c. Serum immunoreactive trypsin
      (1) Trypsin is specific for the pancreas.
      (2) Excellent newborn screen for cystic fibrosis
      (3) Serum immunoreactive trypsin in acute pancreatitis

        (a) Sensitivity 95 to 100%

        (b) Increases 5 to 10 times normal

        (c) Remains increased for 4 to 5 days

    (4) Serum immunoreactive trypsin in chronic pancreatitis

      • Decreased concentration

  d. Tests for pancreatic insufficiency

    (1) CT scan of pancreas shows dystrophic calcification.

      • Sign of chronic pancreatitis

    (2) Functional tests

        (a) Secretin stimulation test (requires instrumentation)

          • Tests ability of pancreas to secrete fluids and electrolytes

        (b) Bentiromide test

          • Tests ability of pancreatic chymotrypsin to cleave orally administered bentiromide to para-aminobenzoic acid (measured in urine)

  e. Tests for bile salt/acid deficiency

    (1) Total bile acids can be measured.

      • Decreased in liver disease (e.g., cirrhosis)

    (2) Bile breath test (oral radioactive test)

      • Decreased amount of radioactive cholylglycine in breath indicates bacterial overgrowth or terminal ileal disease.

8. Clinical findings in malabsorption

  a. Steatorrhea

    • Excessive, large, sticky, stools that float

  b. Fat-soluble vitamin deficiencies

    • Fat-soluble vitamins are A, D, E, K

  c. Water-soluble vitamin deficiencies

    • Particularly folate and vitamin B_{12}

  d. Combined anemias

    • Example—folate and iron deficiency

  e. Ascites and pitting edema

    • Due to hypoproteinemia

9. Selected disorders (Table 11-4)

> Ransom's criteria are prognostic indicators for morbidity and fatality in acute pancreatitis on admission and within 48 hours. They are subdivided into acute pancreatitis due to gallstones or not due to gallstones. Key factors evaluated on admission are age, WBC count, serum glucose, serum LDH, and serum aspartate aminotransferase (AST). In general, increasing values for all of these parameters is associated with increased mortality rate. Key factors evaluated within 48 hours include the hematocrit, serum blood urea nitrogen (BUN), serum calcium, serum phosphorus, serum albumin, base deficit, and fluid deficit. In general, these parameters correlate with serious complications associated with acute pancreatitis including hemorrhage in and around the pancreas, the degree of enzymatic fat necrosis, and the degree of volume depletion from fluid accumulation around the pancreas.

**TABLE 11-4
Selected Small
Bowel and
Pancreatic
Disorders**

Disorder	Epidemiology/Pathogenesis	Discussion
Celiac disease	Autoimmune disease: antibodies against gliadin fraction in gluten Usually begins in infancy Female dominant Primarily involves duodenum and jejunum; flattened villi	Steatorrhea, abdominal bloating Associations: dermatitis herpetiformis (autoimmune vesicular skin disease), type 1 diabetes, IgA deficiency Restrict or eliminate gluten from diet Antigliadin IgG and IgA antibodies: best screening test; sensitivity 96%, specificity 97% Antiendomysial IgG and IgA antibodies: sensitivity/specificity almost 100% Antireticulin IgG and IgA antibodies: variable sensitivity and specificity
Acute pancreatitis	Epidemiology Alcohol abuse and gallstones in pancreatic duct: major causes Other: infections (e.g., CMV, mumps), trauma, hypercalcemia Pathogenesis: activation of pancreatic proenzymes (inactive enzymes) leads to autodigestion of the pancreas	Fever, nausea and vomiting Severe, boring midepigastric pain with radiation into the back Shock: hemorrhage and loss of enzyme-rich fluid around the pancreas Hypocalcemia: caused by enzymatic fat necrosis; calcium binds to fatty acids leading to a decrease in ionized calcium. Left-sided pleural effusion: exudate rich in amylase
Chronic pancreatitis	Epidemiology Majority of cases are idiopathic Known causes: alcohol abuse most common cause in adults, cystic fibrosis in children; malnutrition Pathogenesis Repeated attacks of acute pancreatitis produce duct obstruction Calcified concretions occur along with dilation of the ducts	Severe pain radiating into the back Malabsorption: decreased lipase Type 1 diabetes mellitus: destruction of β-islet cells

CMV, cytomegalovirus.

Cirrhosis: most common cause of ascites

V. **Peritoneal Effusion (Ascites)**
   A. **Etiology and pathogenesis of effusions**
      1. Increased hydrostatic pressure
         • Example—cirrhosis, portal vein thrombosis
      2. Decreased oncotic pressure
         • Examples—cirrhosis, nephrotic syndrome
      3. Increased hepatic lymph formation
         a. Due to intrasinusoidal fibrosis
         b. Example—cirrhosis
      4. Increased vessel permeability of peritoneum
         • Example—acute peritonitis

5. Metastasis to the peritoneum
   • Example—seeding from surface-derived ovarian cancer
6. Secondary aldosteronism
   a. Decreased liver uptake and metabolism of aldosterone (e.g., cirrhosis)
   b. Decreased cardiac output with activation of renin-angiotensin-aldosterone system (e.g., congestive heart failure)
   c. Causes retention of sodium and water
7. Leakage of fluid into peritoneal cavity
   • Bile peritonitis (ruptured gallbladder), acute pancreatitis, chylous effusions
8. Meigs' syndrome
   • Benign fibroma of ovary, ascites, right-sided pleural effusion
B. **Types of peritoneal effusions**
1. Transudates
   a. Ultrafiltrate of plasma involving disturbances in Starling's pressures
   b. Example—increased hydrostatic pressure and decreased oncotic pressure in cirrhosis
2. Exudates
   a. Protein-rich and cell-rich fluid
      • Due to an increased vessel permeability in acute inflammation
   b. Examples—peritonitis from ruptured bowel, spontaneous peritonitis, malignancy
3. Chylous fluid
   • Obstruction of lymphatics; malignancy (most common)
C. **Clinical findings**
1. Bulging of the flanks
2. Shifting dullness to percussion
   • Fluid moves from one side to the other with patient repositioning
3. Ultrasound
   • Useful in confirming the presence of ascites.
D. **Peritoneal fluid analysis**
1. Gradient between serum albumin and ascitic fluid albumin
   a. Differentiates ascites of liver origin (transudate) from ascites of peritoneal origin (exudate)
   b. Difference > 1.1 g/dL
      • Ascites is of liver origin.
   c. Difference < 1.1 g/dL
      (1) Ascites is of peritoneal origin (e.g., peritonitis).
      (2) Increased vessel permeability with loss of protein into ascitic fluid
2. Peritoneal fluid protein
   a. Concentration < 2.5 g/dL
      • Consistent with a transudate
   b. Concentration > 2.5 g/dL
      • Consistent with an exudate
3. Peritoneal fluid WBC count
   a. WBC count < 300 cells/mm^3 + neutrophils < 25% of the total count
      • Consistent with a transudate

b. WBC count >300 cells/mm^3 + neutrophils >25% of the total count
  - Consistent with an exudate
4. Bloody peritoneal fluid
   a. Iatrogenic post-peritoneal tap
   b. Trauma
      - Ruptured spleen or liver
   c. Ruptured ectopic pregnancy
   d. Ruptured hepatic adenoma
      - Associated with long-term oral contraceptive pill usage
   e. Ruptured cavernous hemangioma of liver
   f. Hepatocellular carcinoma
E. **Spontaneous bacterial peritonitis**
   1. Occurs in ~15% of patients with ascites due to cirrhosis or nephrotic syndrome
   2. *Escherichia coli* most common cause in adults
   3. *Streptococcus pneumoniae* most common cause in children.
   4. Clinical findings
      - Fever, rebound tenderness
   5. Laboratory findings in peritoneal fluid
      - WBC count > 300 cells/mm^3 with > 25% of cells representing neutrophils

VI. **Synovial fluid (SF) Analysis**
   A. **Overview**
      1. SF is secreted by synovial cells
         - Viscosity of SF is due to hyaluronic acid.
      2. Functions
         a. Lubricant for joints
         b. Nourishment for articular cartilage
   B. **Routine studies**
      1. Gross appearance
         a. Clear, pale yellow
            (1) Normal
            (2) Noninflammatory joint disease
               (a) Group I joint disorders
               (b) Examples—osteoarthritis, neuropathic joint
         b. Turbidity (noninfectious)
            (1) Group II inflammatory joint disease
            (2) Examples—rheumatoid arthritis, gout, seronegative spondyloarthropathies
         c. Purulent
            (1) Group III joint disease
            (2) Example—septic arthritis
            (3) Common pathogens:
               - *Neisseria gonorrhoeae, Staphylococcus aureus, Streptococcus pyogenes, Salmonella* species

Spontaneous peritonitis: ascites due to cirrhosis or nephrotic syndrome

Synovial fluid: joint lubricant

   d. Bloody
      (1) Group IV joint disease
      (2) Examples—trauma, severe coagulation factor deficiency, scurvy
2. WBC count and differential
   a. Normal WBC count < 200/mm^3
      • Neutrophils < 25% of the total count
   b. Increased WBC count
      (1) Examples—inflammatory joint disease, septic arthritis
      (2) Reiter's cells
         (a) Monocytes with phagocytosed neutrophils
         (b) Present in Reiter's syndrome
            • HLA-B27 positive arthritis plus urethritis due to *Chlamydia trachomatis*
      (3) Ragocytes
         (a) Neutrophils containing cytoplasmic granules
            • Granules represent phagocytosed rheumatoid factor
         (b) Present in rheumatoid arthritis
3. Crystal analysis (see item C in this section)
4. Culture and Gram stain
   • If WBC count is increased
5. Other less common tests
   a. Rheumatoid factor
      • Immunocomplex with IgM antibody against Fc portion of IgG
   b. Complement
   c. SF viscosity (mucin clot test)
      (1) Acetic acid is added to SF to form a clot.
      (2) Firm clot indicates adequate viscosity.
      (3) Clot breaks apart in inflammatory joint disease.
   d. Glucose
      (1) Normal SF glucose < 10 mg/dL difference from serum
      (2) SF glucose difference > 25 mg/dL
         • Inflammatory type of joint disease

C. **Crystal analysis**
1. Crystals are identified by viewing SF under polarized light.
   • Background is black and crystals are white.
2. Crystal identification
   a. Monosodium urate (MSU)
      (1) Needle-shaped (monoclinic) crystal
      (2) Free in SF and phagocytosed by neutrophils
      (3) Sign of gouty arthritis
   b. Calcium pyrophosphate dihydrate crystals (CPPD)
      (1) Monoclinic-like (needle or rod-shaped) or triclinic (rhomboid) crystals
      (2) Signs of pseudogout
      (3) Triclinic crystal is specific for CPPD
   c. Distinguishing monoclinic MSU from monoclinic-like CPPD crystals

↑ Synovial fluid WBC count: inflammatory joint disease, septic arthritis

Important types of crystals: monoclinic, triclinic

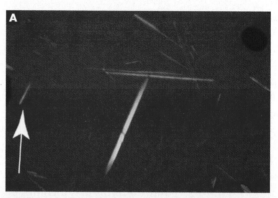

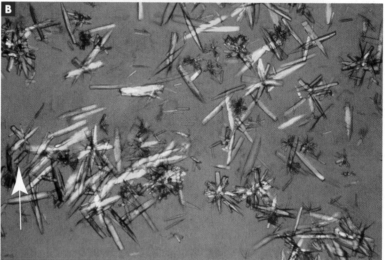

11-2: *Synovial fluid with special polarization in a patient with gout. A special first-order red filter inserted into the microscope causes the background in both synovial fluid specimens (**A** and **B**) to be red. The needle-shaped, monoclinic crystals are yellow and blue. In gout (**A**), the crystal that is aligned parallel to the axis of the red filter (white arrow represents the axis) is yellow. This orientation defines negative birefringence and the presence of a monosodium urate crystal. The crystals in part **B** are blue when aligned parallel to the axis of the red filter (white arrow). This defines positive birefringence and the presence of calcium pyrophosphate dihydrate (CPPD) crystals. (**A** from Henry JB: Clinical Diagnosis and Management by Laboratory Methods, 20th ed. Philadelphia, WB Saunders, 2001, plate 19–7. **B** from McKee PH, Colonje JE, Granter SR: Pathology of the Skin, 3rd ed. St. Louis, Mosby, 2005, Fig. 12.131.)*

(1) Microscope requires a first-order red filter (red compensator).
    (a) Background is red and the crystals have yellow and blue colors.
    (b) Blue crystals are aligned in a different direction than the yellow crystals.
(2) Crystals are aligned parallel to the axis of the red compensator.
    (a) Crystal is yellow when parallel to the axis (Fig. 11-2A).
       • Defines negative birefringence and the presence of MSU crystals

MSU crystals: negative birefringence

(b) Crystal is blue when parallel to the axis (Fig. 11-2B).
- Defines positive birefringence and the presence of CPPD crystals

D. **Gouty arthritis**
- See Chapter 9

E. **Pseudogout (chondrocalcinosis)**
1. Degenerative joint disease
    a. Usually involves the knee
    b. CPPD crystals produce linear deposits in articular cartilage.
        - Visible on a bone radiograph
2. Crystals phagocytosed by neutrophils show positive birefringence.

Questions

1. A febrile 56-year-old male alcoholic has pain in his right big toe that wakes him up at night. The right toe is swollen, hot, and exquisitely sensitive to touch. Laboratory studies show a neutrophilic leukocytosis and left shift. A synovial tap is performed. Which of the following best applies to this case?
   A. HLA-B27 positive spondyloarthropathy
   B. Negative birefringent crystal
   C. Overproduction of uric acid
   D. Septic joint disease
   E. Triclinic crystal disease

2. A 48-year-old man with a lengthy history of alcohol abuse has epigastric pain that radiates into the back. Over 3 days he develops shock and respiratory problems consistent with acute respiratory distress syndrome. A left-sided pleural effusion is present on a chest radiograph. Which of the following laboratory test results is most likely to be present?
   A. Decreased serum immunoreactive trypsin
   B. Decreased serum glucose
   C. Decreased total WBC count
   D. Increased serum calcium
   E. Increased serum lipase

3. A 48-year-old man with a lengthy history of alcohol abuse has chronic epigastric pain with radiation into the back and chronic diarrhea associated with bloating and fatty stools. Physical examination shows malnutrition, abdominal distention, and tender hepatomegaly. A plain radiograph of the abdomen shows multiple irregular densities in the left upper quadrant. Which of the following is the most likely diagnosis?
   A. Celiac disease
   B. Chronic pancreatitis
   C. Pancreatic carcinoma
   D. Peptic ulcer disease

4. A 25-year-old man has a 10-year history of chronic diarrhea with greasy stools. An endoscopic biopsy of the jejunum reveals flattening of the villi and hyperplastic glands with a pronounced chronic inflammatory infiltrate. Which of the following additional tests would be useful in confirming the diagnosis?
   A. Antigliadin antibodies
   B. Antinuclear antibodies

C. Fecal smear for leukocytes

D. Stool for ova and parasites

E. Stool osmotic gap

5. A 25-year-old Asian man develops explosive, watery diarrhea and abdominal distention after eating dairy products. A fecal smear for leukocytes is negative. Which of the following is the most likely cause of the diarrhea?

A. Autoimmune destruction of intestinal villi

B. Enterocolitis due to microbial pathogens

C. Intraluminal osmotically active solutes

D. Toxin activation of adenylate cyclase

E. Toxin activation of guanylate cyclase

6. A 45-year-old woman with postnecrotic cirrhosis secondary to hepatitis C has ascites and dependent pitting edema in the lower legs. Fluid accumulation in the peritoneal cavity and legs occurs by which of the following mechanisms?

A. Decreased plasma oncotic pressure

B. Increased plasma hydrostatic pressure

C. Increased vessel permeability due to histamine

D. Lymphatic obstruction with lymphedema

E. Movement of water into the intracellular compartment

7. A 2-year-old black-American child with sickle cell anemia has a high fever. Physical examination shows nuchal rigidity, scleral icterus, and splenomegaly. Complete blood cell count shows a normocytic anemia and a WBC count of 35,000 cells/mm^3 with left shift. Lumbar puncture shows increased protein, decreased glucose, and numerous neutrophils with phagocytosed bacteria. Which of the following types of bacteria is most likely to be found on Gram stain of cerebrospinal fluid (CSF)?

A. Gram-negative diplococci

B. Gram-negative rods

C. Gram-positive cocci

D. Gram-positive diplococci

E. Gram-positive rods

8. A 32-year-old woman has retro-orbital pain and blurry vision in the left eye. Physical examination shows flame hemorrhages around the disk vessels and a swollen optic disk. After treatment with systemic corticosteroids, vision is restored to normal. A few months later, the patient has slurry speech, an ataxic gait, and weakness and paresthesias in the arms and legs that eventually remit without sequelae. Which of the following findings is most likely present in the cerebrospinal fluid (CSF)?

A. Decreased glucose

B. Increased neutrophils

C. Normal protein

D. Oligoclonal bands

E. Positive Gram stain

9. A hospitalized 72-year-old woman who is being treated for pneumonia develops diarrhea. Proctoscopy reveals a yellow-gray exudate overlying the rectal mucosa. Which of the following is the best screening test for this disease?

A. Blood culture
B. Colon biopsy
C. Culture of stool
D. Cytotoxin assay of stool
E. Gram stain of stool

Answers

1. **B** (negative birefringent crystal) is correct. The patient has acute gouty arthritis. Monosodium urate (MSU) crystals are present in synovial fluid (SF) in the inflamed joint where they are both free and phagocytosed by neutrophils. MSU crystals are needle-shaped (monoclinic) and demonstrate negative birefringence when using a microscope with a first-order red filter (red compensator). This filter causes the background to become red and the crystals to have yellow and blue colors. When the MSU crystals are aligned parallel to the axis of the red compensator they have a yellow color, which defines them as negatively birefringent. If the crystals have a blue color, this defines them as positively birefringent crystals calcium pyrophosphate crystals.

A (HLA-B27 positive spondyloarthropathy) is incorrect. Gout has no relationship with any HLA markers. HLA-B27 is associated with ankylosing spondylitis and other seronegative (rheumatoid factor negative) joint disorders.

C (overproduction of uric acid) is incorrect. Gout is most often associated with underexcretion of uric acid by the kidneys (90% of cases).

D (septic joint disease) is incorrect. Septic joint disease does not usually affect the joints in the foot. Furthermore, the history of alcohol abuse in the patient favors gout. In alcohol abuse, there is an increase in both lactic acid and β-hydroxybutyric acid, which compete for excretion with uric acid in the proximal tubule causing an increase in uric acid and gouty arthritis.

E (triclinic crystal disease) is incorrect. Triclinic crystals are rhomboid-shaped and are present in pseudogout where there is deposition of calcium pyrophosphate in the articular cartilage and synovial fluid of a joint. Calcium pyrophosphate crystals can also have a monoclinic-like appearance as well, which is why it is important to use a first-order red filter (red compensator) in a microscope to distinguish them from MSU crystals.

2. **E** (increased serum lipase) is correct. The patient has acute pancreatitis complicated by acute respiratory distress syndrome and a pleural effusion on the left. Serum lipase is a more specific test for acute pancreatitis than serum amylase, which may be normal in the serum after 2 to 4 days. Lipase initially increases in 3 to 6 hours; peaks in 12 to 30 hours, and returns to normal in 7 to 14 days. Regarding the left-sided pleural effusion, it is also a potential complication of acute pancreatitis. It is an exudate with increased protein with a pleural fluid (PF) protein/serum protein >0.5, PF LDH/serum lactate dehydrogenase (LDH) >0.6, and a PF LDH > 200 U/L. PF amylase is also increased.

A (decreased serum immunoreactive trypsin) is incorrect. Serum immunoreactive trypsin is increased (not decreased) in 95% to 100% of cases of acute pancreatitis. It is decreased in chronic pancreatitis.

B (decreased serum glucose) is incorrect. In severe acute pancreatitis, as in this case, serum glucose is frequently increased (not decreased) due to destruction of β-islet cells in the pancreas.

C (decreased total WBC count) is incorrect. In acute pancreatitis, the total WBC count is usually increased (neutrophilic leukocytosis) and a left-shift is present (increased number of band neutrophils).

D (increased serum calcium) is incorrect. In severe acute pancreatitis, as in this case, the serum calcium is frequently decreased due to enzymatic fat necrosis in the pancreas (calcium binds to fatty acids).

3. **B** (chronic pancreatitis) is correct. The irregular densities in the left upper quadrant of the radiograph are foci of dystrophic calcification (calcification of damaged tissue) in the parenchyma of the pancreas. This is presumptive evidence of chronic pancreatitis, which is most often associated with chronic alcohol abuse. In chronic pancreatitis, recurrent attacks of acute pancreatitis lead to repair by fibrosis and loss of both exocrine and endocrine function. Loss of the pancreatic enzymes results in malabsorption, which is the cause of the patient's chronic diarrhea and malnutrition. Serum amylase is usually increased and serum immunoreactive trypsin is decreased, due to destruction of the pancreatic parenchyma. The D-xylose is test is normal, because xylose does not require pancreatic enzymes for reabsorption.

A (celiac disease) is incorrect. Celiac disease is an autoimmune disease that destroys intestinal villi, leading to malabsorption of fat, proteins, and carbohydrates. It is not associated with alcohol abuse or the type of pain described in this patient.

C (pancreatic carcinoma) is incorrect. Most pancreatic carcinomas involve the head of the pancreas, with subsequent obstruction of the common bile duct. This leads to jaundice, which is not present in this patient.

D (peptic ulcer disease) is incorrect. Peptic ulcer disease due to duodenal ulcers that penetrate posteriorly may produce acute pancreatitis. However, this is an unlikely cause of chronic pancreatitis and would not explain the presence of malabsorption in this patient.

4. **A** (antigliadin antibodies) is correct. The patient has celiac disease, which is an autoimmune disease that has antibodies against the gliadin fraction in gluten in wheat products. The antibodies interact with gluten reabsorbed in the small bowel villi leading to destruction of the villi and hyperplastic glands with pronounced chronic inflammation. Other antibodies present in celiac disease include antiendomysial and antireticulin antibodies. Treatment of celiac disease is to restrict gluten containing products.

B (antinuclear antibodies) is incorrect. The antibodies in celiac disease are not directed against nuclear proteins.

C (fecal smear for leukocytes) is incorrect. A fecal smear for leukocytes is used for evaluating diarrhea that may be caused by invasive microbial pathogens (e.g., *Campylobacter jejuni, Shigella sonnei*).

D (stool for ova and parasites) is incorrect. Testing the stool for ova and parasites is recommended in the workup of a patient with chronic diarrhea. Giardiasis is the most common cause of chronic diarrhea associated with malabsorption; however, the findings on endoscopy are consistent with those seen in celiac disease.

E (stool osmotic gap) is incorrect. A stool sample to calculate the osmotic gap is used for high-volume diarrheal states when a secretory or osmotic type of diarrhea is suspected. Secretory diarrheas are characterized by isotonic diarrheal fluid (e.g., due to certain types of laxatives, enterotoxigenic bacteria), whereas osmotic diarrheas are characterized by hypotonic stool because of the presence of osmotically active solutes (e.g., lactase deficiency with an excess of lactose). The stool osmotic gap is calculated with the following formula: 300 mOsm/kg (value used to represent normal POsm) $- 2 \times$ (random stool Na^+ + random stool K^+). A gap <50 mOsm/kg from the POsm is a secretory diarrhea. A gap >100 mOsm/kg from the POsm is an osmotic diarrhea.

5. C (intraluminal osmotically active solutes) is correct. The patient has a deficiency of lactase, which is a disaccharidase (brush border enzyme) that hydrolyzes lactose in dairy products to glucose and galactose. Anaerobes in the colon degrade lactose to lactic acid and hydrogen gas. The gas causes distention of the bowel and explosive diarrhea. Undigested lactose is osmotically active and causes the movement of a hypotonic salt solution from the bowel mucosa into the bowel lumen. The diarrhea is noninflammatory; therefore, the fecal smear for leukocytes is negative. Diagnostic tests include measurement of stool pH (<6) and the H_2 breath test after administration of oral lactose (best test). Treatment is to avoid dairy products or to orally take lactase before eating dairy products.

A (autoimmune destruction of intestinal villi) is incorrect. Autoimmune destruction of intestinal villi is a characteristic finding in celiac disease. The villi are normal in lactase deficiency.

B (enterocolitis due to microbial pathogens) is incorrect. Invasive diarrhea (enterocolitis) caused by microbial pathogens (e.g., *Campylobacter jejuni*) produces a low-volume diarrhea with blood and neutrophils in the stool. The fecal smear for leukocytes is positive, not negative, as in lactase deficiency.

D (toxin activation of adenylate cyclase) is incorrect. Toxins that stimulate adenylate cyclase (produced by *Vibrio cholerae* and some strains of enterotoxigenic *E. coli*) cause a secretory diarrhea (loss of isotonic fluid) by stimulating ionic pumps in the small intestine. The diarrhea is noninflammatory, and the fecal smear for leukocytes is negative. Toxin-induced secretory diarrhea is excluded, because the diarrhea only follows ingestion of dairy products.

E (toxin activation of guanylate cyclase) is incorrect. Toxins that stimulate guanylate cyclase (toxin produced by some strains of enterotoxigenic *E. coli*) cause a secretory diarrhea (loss of isotonic fluid) by stimulating ionic pumps in the small intestine. The diarrhea is noninflammatory, and the fecal smear for leukocytes is negative. Toxin-induced secretory diarrhea is excluded, because the diarrhea only follows ingestion of dairy products.

6. **A** (decreased plasma oncotic pressure) is correct. Edema is the accumulation of fluid in body cavities (e.g., ascites) and in the interstitial space (e.g., peripheral edema). Edema caused by cirrhosis of the liver involves alterations in vascular hydrostatic pressure and in oncotic pressure. In general, an increase in hydrostatic pressure or a decrease in plasma oncotic pressure (hypo-albuminemia) will cause outflow of a protein-poor (<3 g/dL) and cell-poor fluid into body cavities and interstitial spaces. This defines a transudate. In cirrhosis, the portal vein encounters increased resistance to emptying blood into the liver sinusoids (intrasinusoidal hypertension) due to compression of the sinusoids by regenerative nodules and fibrosis. This causes increased hydrostatic pressure (portal hypertension) that contributes to ascites formation (not pitting edema in the legs). The synthetic function of the liver is compromised in cirrhosis; therefore, hypoalbuminemia occurs, which decreases the plasma oncotic pressure, further contributing to ascites and peripheral edema (dependent pitting edema). Because transudates have decreased protein and cells, they obey the law of gravity and percolate through the interstitial tissue and settle in the most dependent portions of the body (e.g., feet).

B (increased plasma hydrostatic pressure) is incorrect. Increased hydrostatic pressure is involved only in ascites formation. It is not involved in dependent pitting edema in the legs. An example of increased hydrostatic pressure causing pitting edema in the legs is right-sided heart failure.

C (increased vessel permeability due to histamine) is incorrect. Increased vessel permeability due to histamine, which is a marker of acute inflammation, causes a nonpitting type of peripheral edema. The edema fluid is a protein-rich exudate (>3 g/dL) that contains polymorphonuclear leukocytes. Exudates also accumulate in body cavities (e.g., pleural effusion in pneumonia, spontaneous bacterial peritonitis).

D (lymphatic obstruction with lymphedema) is incorrect. Obstruction of lymphatic channels causes leakage of lymphatic fluid into the interstitial space (e.g., filariasis), producing a nonpitting lymphedema. Lymphatic fluid accumulates in body cavities (e.g., chylous effusions in the pleural cavities caused by a tear in the thoracic duct). Chylous effusion contain triglyceride from chylomicrons.

E (movement of water into the intracellular compartment) is incorrect. Movement of water between the extracellular fluid compartment (ECF) and the intracellular fluid compartment (ICF) is called osmosis. Alterations in the serum Na^+ concentration in the ECF compartment is the primary cause of water movement between the compartments. In hyponatremia, water moves from the ECF into the ICF compartment, whereas in hypernatremia, water moves from the ICF into the ECF compartment.

7. **D** (gram-positive diplococci) is correct. The child has sickle cell anemia complicated by bacterial meningitis (nuchal rigidity, neutrophils in CSF with phagocytosed bacteria). In sickle cell anemia, the spleen is typically dysfunctional by 2 years of age, which causes the patient to be susceptible to sepsis and meningitis resulting from *Streptococcus pneumoniae*, a gram-positive diplococcus.

A (gram-negative diplococci) is incorrect. *Neisseria meningitidis*, a gram-negative diplococcus, is the most common cause of meningitis in patients 1 month to 18 years of age with a normal spleen. The spleen is dysfunctional in this patient.

B (gram-negative rods) is incorrect. Meningitis caused by gram-negative rods (e.g., *E. coli*) most commonly occurs in newborns.

C (gram-positive cocci) in incorrect. Meningitis caused by gram-positive cocci (e.g., *Streptococcus agalactiae*) most commonly occurs in newborns.

E (gram-positive rods) is incorrect. Meningitis caused by gram-positive rods (e.g., *Listeria monocytogenes*) most commonly occurs in newborns and immunocompromised hosts.

8. **D** (oligoclonal bands) is correct. The patient has multiple sclerosis, an autoimmune disease characterized by destruction of the myelin sheaths by antibodies directed against myelin basic protein. The episodic course of acute relapses with optic neuritis (blurry vision), scanning speech, cerebellar ataxia, and sensory and motor dysfunction, followed by remissions, are characteristic of this disease. CSF shows an increase in CSF protein due to an increase in CSF IgG. High-resolution electrophoresis of CSF shows discrete bands of immunoglobulins in the γ-globulin region called oligoclonal bands. They are indicative of a demyelinating process.

A (decreased glucose) is incorrect. The CSF glucose is normal in multiple sclerosis.

B (increased neutrophils) is incorrect. T lymphocytes (not neutrophils) are increased in the CSF in multiple sclerosis.

C (normal protein) is incorrect. The CSF protein is increased (not normal) in multiple sclerosis. CSF IgG ratios or indexes are increased in demyelinating disease.

E (positive Gram stain) is incorrect. The Gram stain is negative (not positive) for microbial pathogens in multiple sclerosis.

9. **D** (cytotoxin assay of stool) is correct. The patient has pseudomembranous colitis caused by *Clostridium difficile*, which is normally present in up to 3% of normal people. Carrier rate increases in hospitalized patients (21%) due to contact with spores in the hospital environment. Antibiotic exposure (e.g., clindamycin) causes overgrowth of the organisms with toxin production leading to pseudomembranous colitis. Toxins release proinflammatory mediators and cytokines that attract neutrophils and stimulate excess fluid secretion (watery diarrhea). Pseudomembranes are composed of cellular debris, leukocytes, fibrin, and mucin. Nonspecific laboratory findings include neutrophilic leukocytosis with left shift, fecal leukocytes, and decreased serum albumin. Cytotoxin assay of stool has greater specificity (75–100%) than culture of stool (75–80%) for securing the diagnosis. Treatment is metronidazole.

A (blood culture) is incorrect. *C. difficile* is noninvasive; therefore, it does not cause septicemia.

B (colon biopsy) is incorrect. A colon biopsy is an invasive and expensive test; therefore, it is not recommended as a screening test.

C (culture of stool) is incorrect. *C. difficile* may normally be present in the colon; therefore, a stool culture positive for *C. difficile* does not always confirm the diagnosis of pseudomembranous colitis (specificity is 80%).

E (Gram stain of stool) is incorrect. *C. difficile* may normally be present in the colon; therefore, Gram stain of stool showing Gram-positive rods does not prove that pseudomembranous colitis is present.

12

Clinical Immunopathology

I. **B and T Lymphocytes**

  A. **B lymphocytes**

    1. Involved in humoral immune response

      a. Differentiate into plasma cells that produce immunoglobulins (Igs) (antibodies)

      b. Antibodies help kill encapsulated bacteria

        • Example—*Streptococcus pneumoniae*

    2. IgM synthesis begins at birth.

      a. Adult concentration achieved by 1 year of age

      b. Increased IgM in cord blood may indicate congenital infection.

        • Examples—cytomegalovirus (CMV), toxoplasmosis

      c. IgG synthesis begins at 2 months.

        (1) Adult levels achieved by 6 to 10 years old

        (2) Cord blood IgG is maternally derived IgG.

        (3) Maternally derived IgG lasts 3 to 4 months.

    3. B cell tests

      a. Peripheral lymphocyte count

        • B cells account for 10% to 20% of the total count.

      b. CD marker studies for surface receptors

        • Example—CD21 receptor for Epstein-Barr virus (EBV)

      c. Measure total Ig concentration

        • Concentration in descending order: IgG, IgA, IgM, IgD, IgE

      d. Lymph node histologic examination

        • Identify germinal follicles and plasma cells

      e. Mitogen stimulation (e.g., pokeweed)

        (1) Functional B cell test

        (2) B cells should respond by dividing.

  B. **T lymphocytes**

    1. Involved in cell-mediated immunity (CMI)

      • Type IV hypersensitivity reactions

    2. CD4 (helper T cell, T_H) and CD8 (cytotoxic/suppressor) cells

    3. Testing

      a. Peripheral lymphocyte count

        • T cells account for 60% to 70% of total count

      b. Cutaneous anergy testing of CMI

        (1) Host T-cell response to injected antigens

          • Example—*Candida*

        (2) No response is called anergy.

Newborns: IgM and IgG synthesis begin after birth

T cells: cell-mediated immunity

c. Mitogen stimulation (e.g., phytohemagglutinin)
(1) Functional T-cell test
(2) T cells should respond to the mitogen by dividing.
d. Lymph node histologic examination
- Identify T cells in parafollicular areas
e. Cluster designation (CD) marker studies
(1) CD3
- Transmembrane component of antigen recognition complex on all T cells
(2) CD4 and CD8
(a) Antigen binding site molecules
(b) Ratio of CD4 to CD8 is 2.

C. **Summary of congenital immunodeficiency disorders** (Table 12-1)

> Graft-versus-host (GVH) reaction is a potential complication in bone marrow and liver transplants and in blood transfusions given to patients with a T-cell immunodeficiency (e.g., DiGeorge syndrome). Donor T cells recognize host tissue as foreign and activate immunocompetent CD4 and CD8 T cells. Clinical findings include bile duct necrosis (jaundice), gastrointestinal mucosa ulceration (bloody diarrhea), and dermatitis. Newborns and patients with T-cell defects that require a transfusion must receive blood without the donor lymphocytes.

D. **Acquired immunodeficiency syndrome (AIDS)**

AIDS: most common acquired immunodeficiency disease worldwide

1. Modes of transmission
a. Sexual transmission (>75% of cases)
(1) Homosexual transmission
(a) Anal intercourse between men
(b) Most common cause in the United States
(2) Heterosexual transmission
- Most common in developing countries
b. Intravenous drug abuse
c. Other modes of transmission
(1) Vertical transmission
- Transplacental route, blood contamination during delivery, breastfeeding

Pediatric AIDS: most due to vertical transmission

(2) Accidental needlestick
(a) Risk per accident is 0.3%.
(b) Most common mode of infection in health care workers
(3) Blood products
d. Body fluids containing HIV
- Examples—blood, semen, breast milk
2. Etiology
a. RNA retrovirus
b. HIV-1
- Most common cause in the United States
c. HIV-2
- Most common cause in developing countries

TABLE 12-1
Summary of Congenital Immunodeficiency Disorders

Disorder	Defect	Clinical Findings
B cell		
Bruton's disease	XR disorder Failure of pre-B cells to become mature B cells Mutant tyrosine kinase	Recurrent SP infections; increased incidence *Streptococcus pneumoniae* infections Maternal antibodies protective from birth to 6 months of age All Igs decreased; flat γ-globulin peak Absent germinal follicles and plasma cells
IgA deficiency	Most common hereditary immunodeficiency Failure of IgA B cells to mature into plasma cells	SP infections, allergies, autoimmune disease, giardiasis Potential for anaphylaxis if exposed to blood products with IgA Decreased to absent serum IgA and secretory IgA if IgA is totally absent
CVID	Age bracket 15–35 yr old No consistent inheritance pattern Defect in B cell maturation to plasma cells	SP infections, malabsorption (celiac sprue); increased risk for autoimmune disease, non-Hodgkin's lymphoma, giardiasis All Igs decreased Hyperplastic germinal follicles
T cell		
DiGeorge's syndrome	Most result from 22q11 deletion or intrauterine insult to the facial neural crest Failure of 3rd and 4th pharyngeal pouch development; thymus and parathyroids fail to develop	Hypoparathyroidism (tetany), absent thymic shadow, PJP, candidiasis, danger of GVH Decreased total peripheral blood lymphocyte count Anergy to cutaneous testing: defective CMI
B and T cell		
SCID	40% have adenosine deaminase deficiency (AR); adenine toxic to B/T cells 50–60% have XR mutated cytokine receptors	PJP, disseminated CMV, risk for GVH reaction All Igs decreased; defective CMI Profound T cell defect; antibody synthesis impaired
Wiskott-Aldrich syndrome	XR disorder Progressive deletion of T cells	Triad: eczema, thrombocytopenia, SP infections Increased risk for malignant lymphoma/leukemia Decreased IgM, normal IgG, increased IgA and IgE; defective CMI late in disease
Ataxia telangiectasia	AR disorder Mutation in DNA repair enzymes; increased susceptibility for chromosomal mutations	Cerebellar ataxia, telangiectasias in eyes and skin Increased risk for lymphomas/leukemias Decreased IgA, IgE, IgG; increased serum α-fetoprotein; cutaneous anergy

AR, autosomal recessive; CMI, cell-mediated immunity; CVID, common variable immunodeficiency; GVH, graft-versus-host; Ig, immunoglobulin; PJP, *Pneumocystis jiroveci* pneumonia; SP, sinopulmonary; XR, sex-linked recessive.

**TABLE 12-2
Laboratory Tests
Used in HIV and
AIDS**

Test	Use	Comments
ELISA	Screening test	Detects anti-gp120 antibodies Sensitivity ~100% Positive within 6–10 weeks
Western blot	Confirmatory test	Used if ELISA is positive or indeterminate Positive test: presence of p24 and gp41 antibodies and either gp120 or gp 160 antibodies ~100% specificity
p24 antigen	Indicator of active viral replication Present *before* anti-gp120 antibodies	Positive *prior* to seroconversion and when AIDS is diagnosed (two distinct peaks)
CD$_4$ T-cell count	Monitoring immune status	Useful in determining when to initiate HIV treatment and when to administer prophylaxis against opportunistic infections
HIV viral load	Detection of actively dividing virus Marker of disease progression	Most sensitive test for diagnosis of acute HIV *before* seroconversion

ELISA, enzyme-linked immunoabsorbent assay.

3. Pathogenesis
   a. HIV envelope protein (gp120)
      • Attaches to the CD4 molecule of T cells
   b. HIV infects CD4 T cells
      (1) Direct cytotoxicity
      (2) Reverses CD4/CD8 ratio
   c. Macrophages and dendritic cells
      • Reservoirs for the virus
   d. Reverse transcriptase
      (1) Converts viral RNA into proviral double-stranded DNA
      (2) DNA is integrated into the host DNA.
4. HIV and AIDS testing (Table 12-2)
5. Clinical phases
   a. Acute phase
      • Mononucleosis-like syndrome 3 to 6 weeks after infection
   b. Latent (chronic) phase
      (1) Asymptomatic period 2 to 10 years after infection
      (2) CD4 T-cell count > 500 cells/mm³.
      (3) Viral replication occurs in dendritic cells (reservoir cells).
         • Located in germinal follicles of lymph nodes
   c. Early symptomatic phase
      (1) CD4 T-cell count 200 to 500 cells/mm³
      (2) Generalized painful lymphadenopathy
      (3) Non–AIDS-defining infections

HIV: cytotoxic to CD4 T cells; loss of CMI

Anti-gp120: detected in ELISA test screen

Western blot: confirms HIV

Reservoir cell for HIV: follicular dendritic cells in lymph nodes

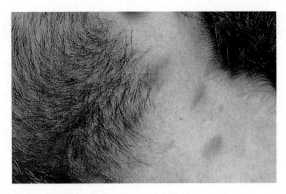

12-1: Kaposi's sarcoma in HIV. Skin lesions are raised, red, and nonpruritic. (From Forbes C, Jackson W: Color Atlas and Text of Clinical Medicine, 2nd ed. St. Louis, Mosby, 2003, Fig. 1-48.)

         (a) Hairy leukoplakia of tongue
- EBV glossitis

         (b) Oral candidiasis, shingles (varicella-zoster virus)

    (4) Fever, weight loss, diarrhea

  d. AIDS

    (1) Criteria
- HIV-positive with CD4 T-cell count $\leq$ 200 cells/mm^3 or with an AIDS-defining condition

    (2) Most common AIDS-defining infections
- *Pneumocystis jiroveci* pneumonia, systemic candidiasis

    (3) AIDS-defining malignancies

         (a) Kaposi's sarcoma (Fig. 12-1)
- Due to human herpesvirus type 8

         (b) Burkitt's lymphoma
- Due to EBV

         (c) Primary central nervous system (CNS) lymphoma
- Due to EBV

    (4) Summary of organ pathology (Table 12-3)

    (5) Causes of death
- Disseminated infections (CMV, *Mycobacterium avium* complex)

  e. Immunologic abnormalities

    (1) Lymphopenia
- Due to decreased CD4 T-cell count

    (2) Cutaneous anergy
- Defect in CMI

    (3) Hypergammaglobulinemia
- Due to polyclonal B-cell stimulation by EBV and CMV

    (4) CD4:CD8 ratio < 1

  f. CD4 count and risk for certain diseases
- Normal, 700 to 1500 cells/mm^3

    (1) 200 to 500 cells/mm^3
- Oral thrush, herpes zoster (shingles), hairy leukoplakia

Most common CNS fungal infection in AIDS: cryptococcosis

Most common malignancy in AIDS: Kaposi's sarcoma

TABLE 12-3
Organ Systems Affected by AIDS

Organ System	Condition	Comments
Central nervous system (CNS)	AIDS-dementia complex	Caused by HIV
	Primary CNS lymphoma	Caused by EBV
	Cryptococcosis	Most common CNS fungal infection
	Toxoplasmosis	Most common space-occupying lesions
	CMV retinitis	Most common cause of blindness
Gastrointestinal	Esophagitis	Caused by *Candida, herpes,* CMV
	Colitis	Caused by *Cryptosporidium,* CMV, MAC
Hepatobiliary	Biliary tract infection	Caused by CMV
Renal	Focal segmental glomerulosclerosis	Causes hypertension and nephrotic syndrome
Respiratory	Pneumonia	Caused by *Pneumocystis jiroveci* and *Streptococcus pneumoniae*
Skin	Kaposi's sarcoma	Caused by HHV-8
	Bacillary angiomatosis	Caused by *Bartonella henselae*

CMV, cytomegalovirus; CNS, central nervous system; EBV, Epstein-Barr virus; HHV-8, human herpesvirus type 8; MAC, Mycobacterium-avium complex.

(3) 100 to 200 cells/mm^3
  • *Pneumocystis jiroveci* pneumonia, dementia
(4) <100 cells/mm^3
  • Toxoplasmosis, cryptococcosis, cryptosporidiosis
(5) <50 cells/mm^3
  (a) CMV retinitis
  (b) *Mycobacterium avium* complex
  (c) Progressive multifocal leukoencephalopathy
  (d) Primary CNS lymphoma

II. **Major Histocompatibility Complex (MHC)**
  A. **Location**
    • Short arm of chromosome 6
  B. **Human leukocyte antigen (HLA) genes**
    1. Code for HLA proteins that are unique to each individual
    2. Inheritance
      a. One set of HLA genes is inherited from each parent.
      b. Both sets of genes produce gene products.
        • Codominant inheritance

> In a family, the chance of a sibling having a 0, 1, or 2 haplotype HLA match with another sibling is 25%, 50%, and 25%, respectively. Parents are a 1 haplotype match.

  C. **Class I MHC molecules**
    1. Coded by HLA-A, -B, and -C genes
    2. Present on the membranes of all nucleated cells
      • *Not* present on mature erythrocytes; present on platelets
    3. Recognized by CD8 T cells and natural killer cells

Class I MHC: present on nucleated cells

D. **Class II MHC molecules**
   1. Coded by HLA-DP, -DQ, and -DR genes
   2. Present on antigen-presenting cells (APCs)
      • B cells, macrophages, dendritic cells
   3. Recognized by CD4 T cells
E. **HLA association with disease**
   1. HLA-B27 with ankylosing spondylitis
   2. HLA-DR2 with multiple sclerosis
   3. HLA-DR3 and -DR4 with type 1 diabetes mellitus
F. **HLA testing**
   1. Clinical usefulness
      a. Matching recipients and donors for organ transplantation

      > Close matches of ABO blood groups and HLA-A, -B, and -D loci in both the donor and graft recipient increase the chance of graft survival.

      b. Identifying patients who are at risk for certain disorders
         • Example—HLA-B27 relationship with ankylosing spondylitis
   2. Transplantation tests
      a. Identify class I and II proteins on recipient and donor lymphocytes
         • React lymphocytes against a battery of anti-HLA antibodies
      b. Test for compatibility of recipient and donor class II antigens
         (1) Recipient and donor lymphocytes are mixed together in culture.
         (2) Compatible if lymphocytes do *not* undergo mitosis
         (3) Incompatible if lymphocytes undergo mitosis
      c. Lymphocyte crossmatch
         (1) Screen for the presence of anti-HLA antibodies in the recipient
         (2) Recipient serum is reacted against donor lymphocytes
         (3) Lysis of donor lymphocytes
            • Recipient has anti-HLA antibodies against donor lymphocytes
         (4) Absence of lysis of donor lymphocytes
            • Recipient does *not* have anti-HLA antibodies against donor lymphocytes.

III. **Hypersensitivity Reactions**
   A. **Type I (immediate) hypersensitivity**
      1. IgE antibody–mediated activation of mast cells
         • Produces an acute inflammatory reaction
      2. IgE antibody production (sensitization; first exposure)
         a. Allergens (e.g., pollen) are first processed by APCs.
         b. APCs interact with CD4 T_H2 cells.
            (1) Release of interleukins (ILs) stimulates B-cell maturation.
            (2) IL-4 causes plasma cells to switch from IgM to IgE synthesis.
      3. Mast cell activation (reexposure)
         a. Allergen-specific IgE antibodies are bound to mast cells.
         b. Specific allergens cross-link specific IgE antibodies on mast cell membranes.

APCs: B cells, macrophages, dendritic cells

HLA-B27: ankylosing spondylitis

Lymphocyte crossmatch: similar in concept to major crossmatch for blood transfusion

Type I hypersensitivity: IgE activation of mast cells

    c. Cross-linking triggers mast cell release of preformed mediators.
      (1) Early phase reaction
        • Release of histamine, chemotactic factors for eosinophils, proteases
      (2) Produces tissue swelling and bronchoconstriction
    d. Late-phase reaction
      (1) Mast cells synthesize and release prostaglandins and leukotrienes
      (2) Enhances and prolongs acute inflammatory reaction

> Desensitization therapy involves repeated injections of increasingly greater amounts of allergen, resulting in production of IgG antibodies that attach to allergens and prevent them from binding to mast cells.

  4. Tests used to evaluate type I hypersensitivity
    a. Scratch test (best overall sensitivity)
      • Positive response is a histamine-mediated wheal-and-flare reaction after introduction of an allergen into the skin
    b. Radioimmunosorbent test (RAST)
      • Detects specific IgE antibodies in serum that are against specific allergens
    c. Serum IgE levels
    d. CBC to identify eosinophils
      • Eosinophilia is *not* always present.
  5. Clinical examples of type I hypersensitivity (Table 12-4)

B. **Type II (cytotoxic) hypersensitivity**
  1. Antibody-dependent cytotoxic reactions
  2. Complement-dependent antibody reactions
    a. Lysis of target cells
      (1) Antibody (IgG/IgM) is directed against a specific antigen on the cell membrane
      (2) Leads to activation of the complement system
      (3) Membrane attack complex produces lysis of the target cell.
    b. Phagocytosis of target cells
      • Fixed macrophages (e.g., in spleen) phagocytose cells (e.g., RBCs) coated by IgG and complement (C3b).
  3. Complement-independent antibody reactions
    a. Antibody (IgG, IgE)-dependent cell-mediated cytotoxicity
      • Leukocytes with receptors for IgG or IgE lyse but do *not* phagocytose cells coated by antibodies.
    b. IgG autoantibodies directed against cell surface receptors
  4. Tests used to evaluate type II hypersensitivity
    a. Direct Coombs' test (see Chapter 5)
      • Detects IgG and C3b attached to RBCs
    b. Indirect Coombs' test (see Chapter 5)
      • Detects antibodies in serum (e.g., anti-D)
  5. Clinical examples of type II hypersensitivity (see Table 12-4)

Mast cells: early and late phase reactions

Anaphylactic shock: potentially fatal type I hypersensitivity reaction

Type II hypersensitivity: antibody-dependent cytotoxic reactions

TABLE 12-4
Hypersensitivity Reactions

Reaction	Pathogenesis	Examples
Type I	IgE-dependent activation of mast cells	Atopic disorders: hay fever, eczema, hives, asthma, reaction to bee sting Drug hypersensitivity: penicillin rash or anaphylaxis

Type II	Antibody-dependent reaction	Complement-dependent antibody reactions
		  Lysis of target cell: ABO mismatch, Goodpasture's syndrome, hyperacute transplantation rejection
		  Phagocytosis of target cell: warm (IgG) immune hemolytic anemia, ABO and Rh hemolytic disease of newborn
		Complement-independent antibody reactions
		  Antibody (IgG, IgE)-dependent cell-mediated cytotoxicity: natural killer cell destruction of neoplastic and virus-infected cells; helminth destruction by eosinophils
		  Antibodies directed against cell surface receptors: myasthenia gravis, Graves' disease

Type III	Deposition of antigen-antibody complexes	Systemic lupus erythematosus (DNA-anti-DNA) Rheumatoid arthritis (IgM-Fc receptor IgG) Poststreptococcal glomerulonephritis (bacterial antigen-antibody against antigen)
Type IV	Antibody-independent T cell–mediated reactions	Delayed type: contact dermatitis (e.g., poison ivy), tuberculous granuloma CD8 T-cell–mediated cytotoxic destruction of cells: tumor cells, virus-infected cells

C. **Type III (immunocomplex) hypersensitivity**
1. Circulating antigen-antibody complexes deposit in tissue
   - Example—DNA–anti-DNA immunocomplexes
   a. Immune complexes activate the complement system.
   b. Complement component C5a is produced.
   c. C5a attracts neutrophils, which, in turn, damage the tissue.
2. Tests used to evaluate type III hypersensitivity
   a. Measure immunocomplexes in blood
   b. Immunofluorescent staining of tissue biopsies
      - Example—glomeruli in glomerulonephritis
3. Clinical examples of type III hypersensitivity (see Table 12-4)
D. **Type IV hypersensitivity**
1. Antibody-independent T-cell–mediated reactions
   - Cell-mediated immunity
2. Delayed reaction hypersensitivity (e.g., granuloma)
   a. CD4 T cells interact with class II antigens on macrophages
   b. Release of cytokines from both cells
      (1) Macrophages release IL-12 and IL-1
         - IL-12 results in formation of memory CD4 T_H1 cells
      (2) CD4 T cells release IL-2 and γ-interferon (IF).
      (3) Cytokines produce an inflammatory reaction.
      (4) γ-IF activates macrophages.

Type III hypersensitivity: circulating antigen-antibody complexes activate complement system

Antibody-mediated hypersensitivity reactions: types I, II, and III

Type IV hypersensitivity: cellular immunity

(a) Kills pathogens processed by the macrophage

(b) Activated macrophages are called epithelioid cells.

3. Cell-mediated cytotoxicity

    a. CD8 cytotoxic T cells interact with altered MHC class I antigens.

      • Altered cells include tumor cells, virus-infected cells, or donor graft cells.

    b. Cytokines and chemical mediators are released by CD8 T cells.

      • Directly lyse cells or initiate apoptosis and death of cells

4. Test used to evaluate type IV hypersensitivity

    a. Patch test to confirm contact dermatitis

      • Example—suspected allergen (e.g., nickel) placed on an adhesive patch is applied to the skin to see if a skin reaction occurs.

    b. Cutaneous testing with antigens

      • Example—*Candida*

5. Clinical examples of type IV hypersensitivity (see Table 12-4)

IV. **Autoimmune Diseases**

  A. **Mechanisms of autoimmunity**

    1. Autoimmune dysfunction is associated with loss of self-tolerance

      • Leads to immune reactions directed against host tissue

    2. Types of mechanisms

      a. Emergence (usually from trauma) of a sequestered antigen

        • Examples—lens protein, spermatozoa, brain tissue

      b. Imbalance favoring CD4 T helper cells over CD8 T suppressor cells

      c. Alteration of self-antigens by drugs or by a pathogen

        (1) Drug example—methyldopa alters Rh antigens on RBCs.

        (2) Pathogen example—coxsackievirus alters β-islet cells.

      d. Cross-reactivity (mimicry) between self-antigens and foreign antigens

        • Example—group A streptococcus antigens are similar to antigens in the human heart in rheumatic fever.

      e. Abnormal immune response genes on chromosome 6 (Ir genes)

      f. Polyclonal activation of B lymphocytes

        • Polyclonal activators: EBV, CMV, endotoxins

  B. **Classification of autoimmunity**

    1. Organ-specific; examples:

      a. Addison's disease (see Chapter 10)

        • Immune destruction of the adrenal glands

      b. Pernicious anemia (see Chapter 5)

        • Immune destruction of parietal cells

      c. Hashimoto's thyroiditis (see Chapter 10)

    2. Systemic; examples:

      a. Systemic lupus erythematosus (SLE)

      b. Rheumatoid arthritis (RA)

      c. Systemic sclerosis

  C. **Laboratory assessment**

    1. Serum antinuclear antibody (ANA) test

      a. Most useful screen for systemic autoimmune diseases

  b. Antinuclear antibodies are directed against the following:
   (1) DNA
    • Double-stranded (ds) and single-stranded (ss) antibodies
   (2) Histones
   (3) Acidic proteins
    • Anti-Smith (Sm) and antiribonucleoprotein antibodies
   (4) Nucleolar antigens
  c. Serum ANA test is a fluorescent antibody test.
   (1) Provides a pattern of nuclear fluorescence (Table 12-5)
    • Identifies specific nuclear antigens listed earlier
   (2) Provides a titer of the antibody
 2. Specific antibody tests
  a. Utilized in documenting organ-specific diseases
  b. Example—antibodies against the proton pump in parietal cells in pernicious anemia
 3. Summary of autoantibodies (Table 12-6)
D. **Systemic lupus erythematosus (SLE)**
 1. Occurs predominantly in women of childbearing age
 2. Pathogenesis
  a. Polyclonal B-cell activation
  b. Sustained estrogen activity

TABLE 12-5 Immunofluorescent Nuclear Patterns in Autoimmune Disease

Pattern	Clinical Significance
Speckled	Most common pattern. Antibodies to non-DNA nuclear constituents (e.g., anti-Smith, anti-ribonucleoprotein, anti-SS-A, anti-SS-B) Disorders: Sjögren's syndrome, systemic sclerosis, MCTD, SLE
Homogenous (diffuse)	Second most common pattern. Antibodies to chromatin, histones, DNA (occasionally). Disorders: drug-induced lupus (>95% sensitivity), SLE, RA
Rim (membranous)	Antibodies to double-stranded DNA Disorder: SLE (usually implies renal disease)
Nucleolar	Antibodies to nucleolar proteins (RNA polymerase) Disorder: systemic sclerosis (high frequency)

MCTD, mixed connective tissue disease; RA, rheumatoid arthritis.

TABLE 12-6
Autoantibodies in Autoimmune Disease

Autoantibodies	Disease	Test Sensitivity
Anti-acetylcholine receptor	Myasthenia gravis	>85%
Anti–basement membrane	Goodpasture's syndrome	>90%
Anticentromere	CREST syndrome	90%
	Systemic sclerosis	25%
Anti-double-stranded DNA	SLE	50–90%
Antiendomysial	Celiac disease	100%
Antigliadin		97% (IgA)
Anti-insulin	Type 1 diabetes	50%
Anti–islet cell		75–80%
Anti-intrinsic factor	Pernicious anemia	60%
Antiparietal cell		90%
Antimicrosomal	Hashimoto's thyroiditis	97%
Antithyroglobulin		85%
Antimitochondrial	Primary biliary cirrhosis	90–100%
Antimyeloperoxidase	Microscopic polyangiitis	80% (p-ANCA)
Antinuclear (ANA)	SLE	99%
	Drug-induced lupus	90–95%
	Systemic sclerosis	70–90%
	Dermatomyositis/polymyositis	<30%
Anti-proteinase 3	Wegener's granulomatosis	>90% (c-ANCA)
Anti-ribonucleoprotein	MCTD	100%
Anti-RNA polymerase	Systemic sclerosis	20%
Anti-Smith (Sm)	SLE	20–30%
Anti-SS-A (Ro)	Sjögren's syndrome	70–95%
	SLE	30–50%
Anti-SS-B (La)	Sjögren's syndrome	60–90%
Anti-topoisomerase (Scl-70)	Systemic sclerosis	20–40%
Anti-TSH receptor	Graves' disease	85%

ANA, antinuclear antibody; c-ANCA, cytoplasmic antineutrophil cytoplasmic antibody; MCTD, mixed connective tissue disease; p-ANCA, perinuclear antineutrophilic cytoplasmic antibody; SLE, systemic lupus erythematosus; SS, Sjögren's syndrome; TSH, thyroid-stimulating hormone.

    c. Environmental triggers
      • Examples—sun, procainamide
   3. Clinical findings
    a. Hematologic
      • Autoimmune hemolytic anemia, thrombocytopenia, leukopenia
    b. Lymphatic
      (1) Generalized painful lymphadenopathy
      (2) Splenomegaly
    c. Musculoskeletal
      (1) Small-joint inflammation
        • Example—hands
      (2) Absence of joint deformity
    d. Skin
      (1) Immunocomplex deposition along basement membrane
        • Basis for the immunofluorescent test
      (2) Malar butterfly rash (Fig. 12-2)

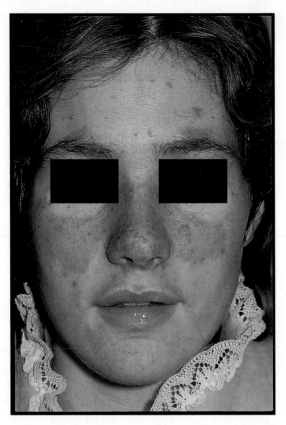

12-2: *Malar rash in systemic lupus erythematosus showing the butterfly-wing distribution. (From Forbes: Color Atlas and Text of Clinical Medicine, 2nd ed. St. Louis, Mosby, 1997, Fig. 3.77, p. 140.)*

  e. Renal
    (1) Diffuse proliferative glomerulonephritis
    (2) Associated with anti-ds DNA antibodies
  f. Cardiovascular
    • Fibrinous pericarditis with or without effusion
  g. Respiratory
    • Pleural effusion with friction rub
  h. Pregnancy-related
    (1) Complete heart block in newborns
       • Caused by IgG anti-SS-A (Ro) antibodies crossing the placenta
    (2) Recurrent spontaneous abortions
       • Caused by antiphospholipid antibodies (see Chapter 7)
4. Drug-induced lupus erythematosus
  a. Associated drugs
    • Procainamide, hydralazine
  b. Features that distinguish drug-induced lupus from SLE
    (1) Antihistone antibodies (>95% of cases)

Procainamide: most common drug associated with drug-induced lupus

Drug-induced lupus: antihistone antibodies

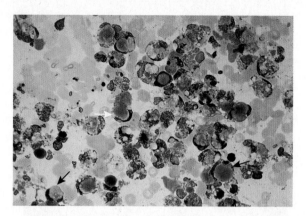

12-3: *Lupus erythematosus cell. The arrows point to neutrophils that have phagocytosed purple-staining, homogeneous nuclear material. (From McKee PH, Colonje JE, Granter SR: Pathology of the Skin, 3rd ed. St. Louis, Mosby, 2005, Fig. 16.34.)*

(2) Low incidence of renal and CNS involvement

(3) Disappearance of symptoms when the drug is discontinued

5. Laboratory findings in SLE

  a. Positive serum antinuclear antibody (ANA)

    (1) Sensitivity 99%, specificity 80%

    (2) Better screening test than confirmatory test (see Chapter 1)

  b. Anti-ds DNA antibodies

    (1) *Crithidia test* : sensitivity 50% to 90%, specificity 98% to 100%

    (2) Better confirmatory test than screening test

  c. Anti-Smith (Sm) antibodies

    (1) Sensitivity 20% to 30%, specificity 100%

    (2) Better confirmatory test than screening test (see Chapter 1)

  d. Antiphospholipid antibodies (see Chapter 7)

  e. Lupus erythematosus (LE) cell

    (1) Neutrophil-containing phagocytosed altered DNA (Fig. 12-3)

    (2) Sensitivity 76%, specificity 97%

  f. Decreased serum complement

    (1) Used up with activation of complement system

    (2) Sensitivity 40%, specificity 98%

  g. Immunocomplexes at the dermal-epidermal junction in skin biopsies

    • Band-like distribution of fluorescence along the dermal-epidermal junction

E. **Systemic sclerosis (scleroderma)**

1. Occurs predominantly in women of childbearing age

2. Pathogenesis

  a. Small-vessel endothelial cell damage produces blood vessel fibrosis and ischemic injury.

  b. T-cell release of cytokines results in excessive collagen synthesis.

3. Clinical findings

  a. Raynaud's phenomenon

Confirm SLE: anti-ds DNA and anti-Sm antibodies

Systemic sclerosis: excess collagen deposition

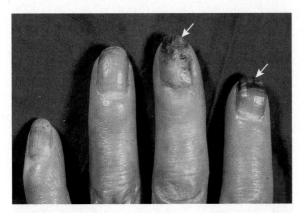

12-4: *Fingers in systemic sclerosis. The fingers are erythematous, shiny, and tapered. Blackened areas (arrows) are present at the tips of two of the fingers. These represent digital infarctions due to digital vessel fibrosis. (From McKee PH, Colonje JE, Granter SR: Pathology of the Skin, 3rd ed. St. Louis, Mosby, 2005, Fig. 16.81B.)*

      (1) Sequential color changes
          (a) Normal to white to blue to red
          (b) Caused by digital vessel vasculitis and fibrosis
      (2) Sclerodactyly (tapered fingers) and digital infarcts (Fig. 12-4)
   b. Skin
      (1) Skin atrophy and tissue swelling beginning in the fingers
        • Extends proximally
      (2) Parchment-like appearance
      (3) Tightened facial features
        • Radial furrowing around the lips (Fig. 12-5)
   c. Gastrointestinal tract
      (1) Dysphagia (difficult swallowing) for solids and liquids
          (a) No peristalsis in the lower two thirds of the esophagus.
          (b) Smooth muscle is replaced by collagen.
      (2) Lower esophageal sphincter relaxation with reflux
      (3) Malabsorption
        • Loss of villi
   d. Respiratory findings
      (1) Interstitial fibrosis of lungs
        • Restrictive lung disease (see Chapter 3)
      (2) Respiratory failure
        • Most common cause of death in systemic sclerosis
   e. Renal
     • Infarctions, malignant hypertension
  4. Laboratory findings in systemic sclerosis
   a. Serum ANA
     • Positive in 70% to 90% of cases
   b. Anti-topoisomerase antibody
     • Positive in 20% to 40% of cases

Raynaud's phenomenon: most common initial sign of systemic sclerosis

Systemic sclerosis: anti-topoisomerase antibodies

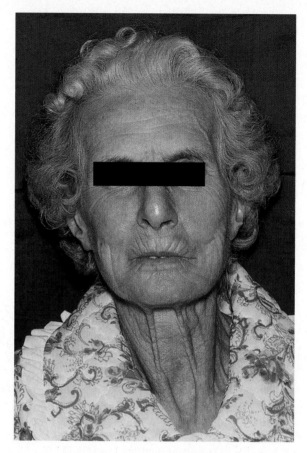

12-5: *Systemic sclerosis. The tightening of the skin produces radiating furrows around the mouth. This is caused by excess collagen. (From McKee PH, Colonje JE, Granter SR: Pathology of the Skin, 3rd ed. St. Louis, Mosby, 2005, Fig. 16.85.)*

  5. CREST syndrome
    a. Limited sclerosis
    b. Clinical findings
      (1) C: calcification in subcutaneous tissue
      (2) R: Raynaud's phenomenon
      (3) E: esophageal dysmotility
      (4) S: sclerodactyly
      (5) T: telangiectasis
        • Multiple punctate blood vessel dilations
    c. Laboratory findings
      • Anticentromere antibodies in 90% of cases
  F. **Dermatomyositis (DM) and polymyositis (PM)**
    • DM with skin involvement; PM without skin involvement
    1. Occurs predominantly in women 40 to 60 years of age
    2. Increased risk of malignant neoplasms (15–20% of cases)
      • Particularly lung cancer

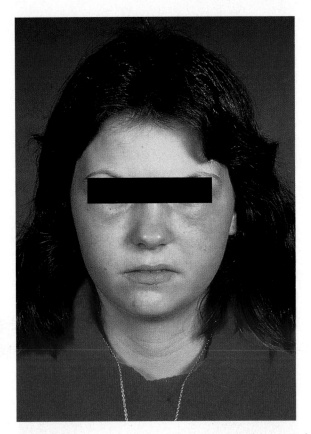

12-6: *Dermatomyositis. Note the red-mauve swelling and discoloration around the eyes with spreading into the cheeks. (From McKee PH, Colonje JE, Granter SR: Pathology of the Skin, 3rd ed. St. Louis, Mosby, 2005, Fig. 16.124.)*

3. Pathogenesis
   a. Antibody-mediated damage in DM
   b. T-cell–mediated damage in PM
4. Clinical findings
   a. Muscle pain and atrophy
   b. Heliotrope eyelids or "raccoon eyes"
      • Red-mauve eyelid discoloration (Fig. 12-6)
   c. Gottron's patches
      • Purple papules overlying joints in the hands (Fig. 12-7)
5. Laboratory findings
   a. Serum ANA is positive in <30% of cases.
   b. Increased serum creatine kinase
      (1) Due to inflammation of muscle
      (2) Muscle biopsy shows a lymphocytic infiltrate.
G. **Mixed connective tissue disease (MCTD)**
   1. Signs and symptoms similar to SLE, systemic sclerosis, and PM
   2. Renal disease is uncommon.

DM/PM: ↑ serum creatine kinase

MCTD: anti-ribonucleoprotein antibodies

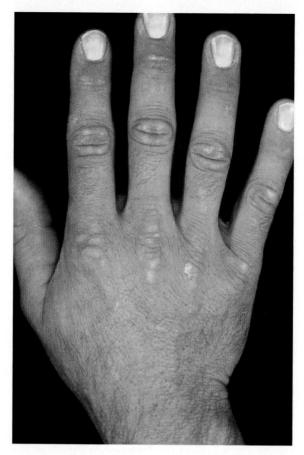

12-7: *Dermatomyositis. Note the light purple-colored papules overlying the skin of the knuckles and proximal interphalangeal and distal interphalangeal joints. (From McKee PH, Colonje JE, Granter SR: Pathology of the Skin, 3rd ed. St. Louis, Mosby, 2005, Fig. 16.127.)*

      3. Anti-ribonucleoprotein antibodies
- Positive in ~100% of cases

H. **Rheumatoid arthritis (RA)**
1. Epidemiology
   a. Predominantly occurs in women 30 to 50 years of age
   b. HLA-DR4 association
   c. Initial inciting agent may be EBV
2. Pathogenesis of joint disease; sequential changes occur:
   a. Synovial tissue produces rheumatoid factor (RF) complexes.
      (1) RF complexes are IgM autoantibodies against the Fc receptor of IgG.
         - Antibodies are sometime IgG or IgA.
      (2) Type III hypersensitivity reaction
   b. RF complexes activate complement.
      (1) Complement component C5a attracts neutrophils.

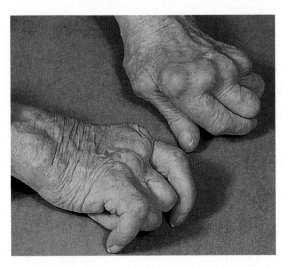

12-8: *Rheumatoid arthritis showing bilateral ulnar deviation of the hands and prominent swelling of the second and third metacarpophalangeal joints. (From Forbes C, Jackson W: Color Atlas and Text of Clinical Medicine, 2nd ed. St. Louis, Mosby, 2003, Fig. 3.3.)*

        (2) Neutrophils produce acute inflammation of synovial tissue.

        (3) Neutrophils phagocytose RF complexes.

          • Produces ragocytes (see Chapter 11)

    c. Chronically inflamed synovial tissue proliferates (forms a pannus).

        (1) Pannus releases cytokines that destroy articular cartilage.

        (2) End result is reactive fibrosis and joint fusion (ankylosis).

3. Clinical and laboratory findings

    a. Symmetric involvement of joints in the hands

        (1) Swelling and pain in metacarpophalangeal (MCP) and proximal interphalangeal (PIP) joints

        (2) Produces ulnar deviation, morning stiffness (Fig. 12-8)

        (3) Other joints are commonly involved

          • Knees, ankles, hips, cervical spine

    b. Lung disease

        • Chronic pleuritis with effusions (see Chapter 11), interstitial fibrosis

    c. Hematologic disease

        (1) Anemia of chronic disease (see Chapter 5)

        (2) Felty's syndrome

          • Autoimmune neutropenia and splenomegaly

    d. Serum ANA

        • Sensitivity 30%

    e. Serum RF complexes

        (1) Sensitivity 85%

        (2) False positives:

          • Normal people, infective endocarditis, tuberculosis

4. Sjogren's syndrome (SS)

    a. Female dominant autoimmune disease

> Rheumatoid factor: IgM autoantibody directed against Fc receptor of IgG

Sjögren's syndrome: autoimmune destruction of lacrimal glands, minor salivary glands

b. Pathogenesis
  • Autoimmune destruction of salivary glands and lacrimal glands
c. Clinical findings
  (1) Rheumatoid arthritis
  (2) Keratoconjunctivitis sicca
    • Dry eyes described as "sand in my eyes"
  (3) Xerostomia or dry mouth
    • Autoimmune destruction of salivary glands
d. Laboratory findings
  (1) Anti-SS-A antibodies (Ro)
    • Sensitivity 70% to 95%
  (2) Anti-SS-B antibodies (La)
    • Sensitivity 60% to 90%
  (3) Confirm with lip biopsy
    • Must demonstrate lymphoid destruction of minor salivary glands

V. **Complement System Disorders**
  A. **Overview**

Complement: augment natural host immune defense

  1. Synthesized in the liver
  2. Augment natural host immune defenses
  3. Circulate as inactive proteins
    a. System activated by
      • IgM, IgG, immunocomplexes, endotoxins
    b. Classical pathway
      (1) Complement components: C1, C4, C2
      (2) C1 esterase inhibitor
        (a) Inactivates the protease activity of C1 in the classical pathway
        (b) Deficient in hereditary angioedema
    c. Alternative pathway
      • Complement components: factor B, properdin, factor D
    d. Membrane attack complex (MAC)
      • Final common pathway for classical and alternative pathways
    e. Decay accelerating factor (DAF)
      (1) Present on cell membranes
      (2) Enhances degradation of C3 convertase and C5 convertase
      (3) Protects the cell against MAC destruction
      (4) Deficiency in paroxysmal nocturnal hemoglobinuria (see Chapter 5)

Complement: cleavage products are functional

  4. Functions of complement cleavage products
    a. C3a, C5a (anaphylatoxins)
      • Stimulate mast cell release of histamine
    b. C3b
      • Opsonization
    c. C5a
      (1) Activation of neutrophil adhesion molecules
      (2) Neutrophil chemotaxis

TABLE 12-7
Complement
Disorders

Disorder	Comments
Hereditary angioedema	AD disorder: deficiency of C1 esterase inhibitor Continued C1 activation: decreases C2 and C4; increases their cleavage products, which have anaphylatoxic activity; normal C3 Swelling of face and oropharynx
C2 deficiency	Most common complement deficiency Association with septicemia (usually *Streptococcus pneumoniae*) and lupus-like syndrome in children
C5–C9 deficiency	Increased susceptibility to disseminated *Neisseria gonorrhoeae* or *N. meningitidis* infections; MAC is necessary for phagocytosis of the pathogens
Paroxysmal nocturnal hemoglobinuria	Acquired stem cell disease Defect in molecule anchoring decay accelerating factor (DAF); DAF normally degrades C3 convertase and C5 convertase on hematopoietic cell membranes Complement-mediated intravascular lysis of RBCs (hemoglobinuria), platelets, and neutrophils; produces pancytopenia; increased risk for leukemia.

AD, autosomal dominant; MAC, membrane attack complex.

    d. C6 to C9 (membrane attack complex, MAC)
       • Cell lysis
  5. Testing of the complement system
    a. Total hemolytic complement assay (CH_{50})
       • Tests functional ability of both complement systems
    b. Tests indicating activation of classical system
      (1) Decreased C4, C3
      (2) Normal factor B
    c. Tests indicating activation of alternative system
      (1) Decreased factor B, C3
      (2) Normal C4
    d. Tests indicating activation of both systems
       • Decreased C4, factor B, C3
  7. Summary of complement disorders (Table 12-7)

Classical pathway activation: decreased C4, C3; normal factor B

Alternative pathway activation: decreased factor B, C3; normal C4

Questions

1. A 16-year-old girl with a recent history of a severe sore throat presents with fever, dyspnea, and polyarthritis. Cardiopulmonary examination demonstrates a grade III pansystolic murmur heard at the apex and bibasilar inspiratory crackles. Based only on this history and physical examination findings, which of the following laboratory test findings is most likely present?
   A. Increased antimitochondrial antibodies
   B. Increased antistreptolysin O titers
   C. Positive blood culture
   D. Positive serum antinuclear antibody test
   E. Positive serum double-stranded DNA antibody test

Refer to the following list when answering questions 2 through 12:

A. Anti-acetylcholine receptor antibody
B. Anti–basement membrane antibody
C. Anticentromere antibody
D. Anti-double-stranded DNA antibody
E. Antigliadin antibody
F. Antiparietal cell
G. Antimitochondrial antibody

H. Anti-ribonucleoprotein antibody
I. Anti-Smith (Sm) antibody
J. Anti-SS-A (Ro) antibody
K. Anti-topoisomerase
L. c-Antineutrophil cytoplasmic antibody
M. p-Antineutrophil cytoplasmic antibody

Options A through M describe different antibodies. For questions 2 through 13, select the *one* lettered option that is most closely associated with it. When answering these questions, each lettered option may be selected once, more than once, or not at all.

2. A 42-year-old man has repeated sinus infections, a saddle-nose deformity, nodular masses in the lungs, and glomerulonephritis with RBC casts. An antibody study is pending.

3. A 36-year-old woman complains of problems with swallowing both solids and liquids. She also complains of changes in her fingers. Physical examination reveals tapered fingers with digital infarctions and dilated vessels on her skin. A radiograph of her fingers reveals dystrophic calcification in subcutaneous tissue. There is no evidence of pulmonary or renal disease.

4. A 25-year-old man who recently finished a course of penicillin for a group A streptococcal pharyngitis develops palpable purpura over his trunk and extremities along with hematuria and RBC casts.

5. A 55-year-old woman complains of burning feet and a sore tongue. Examination reveals decreased vibratory sensation in both lower extremities and atrophy of the papillae of the tongue. A CBC shows pancytopenia with macrocytic indices and hypersegmented neutrophils in the peripheral blood.

6. A 55-year-old woman complains of generalized itching. Physical examination reveals xanthelasma on both eyelids and an enlarged, nontender liver. Serum alkaline phosphatase and γ-glutamyltransferase are markedly increased.

7. A 25-year-old woman presents with morning stiffness involving both hands, photophobia, and left-sided chest pain that increases with inspiration. Physical examination reveals dullness to percussion in the left lower lobe. A chest radiograph confirms the presence of a left-sided pleural effusion. The serum antinuclear antibody test is positive and a speckled pattern is present in high titer. (Select two antibodies.)

8. A 28-year-old man has a history of greasy stools since childhood. He now presents with a vesicular rash on his right elbow.

9. A 23-year-old woman complains of droopy eyes at the end of the day and generalized muscle weakness and fatigue. She also complains of difficulty in swallowing solids and liquids, which seem to "get stuck" in the upper part of her esophagus.

10. A 23-year-old man presents with dyspnea and hemoptysis. This is shortly followed by a sudden onset of acute renal failure with hematuria and RBC casts.

11. A 55-year-old woman with rheumatoid arthritis complains of dry eyes and a dry mouth.

12. A 56-year-old woman complains of problems swallowing solids and liquids, color changes and pain in her hands, and problems with breathing. Examination reveals pursing of the lips, sclerodactyly and swelling of the fingers, and dry inspiratory crackles at both lung bases.

13. A 22-year-old man complains of recurrent swelling of the face. On some occasions he also has difficulty breathing. Initial laboratory studies show normal concentrations of complement C3 and factor B and a decreased concentration of complement C4. Which of the following additional studies is most indicated?
  A. C1 esterase inhibitor assay
  B. Chromosome study
  C. Cutaneous skin testing to rule out anergy
  D. Quantitative immunoglobulin assay for IgG, IgA, and IgM
  E. Serum antinuclear antibody test

Refer to the following list in answering questions 14 to 20:

A. Ataxia telangiectasia
B. Bruton's agammaglobulinemia
C. Common variable immunodeficiency
D. DiGeorge's syndrome
E. Selective IgA immunodeficiency
F. Severe combined immunodeficiency
G. Wiskott-Aldrich syndrome

Options A through G describe different immunodeficiency disorders. For questions 14 through 20, select the *one* lettered option that is most closely associated with it. When answering these questions, each lettered option may be selected once, more than once, or not at all.

14. A 3-year-old boy has a disease characterized by the absence of plasma cells and germinal follicles in lymph nodes and failure of pre-B cells to differentiate into mature B cells.

15. A 25-year-old man has an immunodeficiency disorder associated with a failure of mature B cells to differentiate into plasma cells.

16. A 20-year-old woman has an immunodeficiency associated with recurrent sinopulmonary disease, allergies, malabsorption, and giardiasis due to lack of a secretory component.

17. A 5-year-old girl has an immunodeficiency associated with deficiency of adenosine deaminase leading to destruction of both B and T cells.

18. A newborn baby boy has an immunodeficiency associated with tetany and cyanotic congenital heart disease. A chest radiograph shows an absent thymic shadow.

19. A 6-year-old boy has an immunodeficiency syndrome associated with eczema, recurrent sinopulmonary infections, thrombocytopenia, and abnormalities involving immunoglobulins and cell-mediated immunity.

20. A 10-year-old girl has an immunodeficiency syndrome associated with vessel abnormalities, cerebellar disease, and increased serum α-fetoprotein levels.

21. A 20-year-old man with acquired immunodeficiency syndrome (AIDS) has recurrent candidiasis and a *Pneumocystis jiroveci* pneumonia. Which of the following laboratory test results is expected?
A. Hypergammaglobulinemia
B. Increase in CD4 helper T cell/CD8 suppressor T cell ratio
C. Intact cellular immunity
D. Normal phytohemagglutinin assay
E. Normal skin reaction to intradermal injection of *Candida*

22. Which of the following tests is used to confirm a positive or indefinite enzyme-linked immunoabsorbent assay (ELISA) test for HIV?
   A. CD4 T cell count
   B. HIV viral load
   C. p24 capture assay
   D. Western blot assay

Answers

1. **B** (increased antistreptolysin O titers) is correct. The patient has acute rheumatic fever (ARF) with polyarthritis, mitral regurgitation (pansystolic murmur), and left-sided heart failure (bibasilar crackles) due to a myocarditis. ARF is an autoimmune disease due to cross-reacting antibodies that attack both group A streptococci and human tissue, in this case, the heart and joints. This is a type II hypersensitivity reaction. In ARF, the initial group A streptococcal infection is usually in the pharynx. Within a few weeks of the infection, there is an increase in antistreptolysin O titers and anti-DNAase B titers, the former usually ordered to diagnose ARF.

   A (increased antimitochondrial antibodies) is incorrect. These antibodies occur in primary biliary cirrhosis, where there is autoimmune destruction of bile ducts in the portal triads.
   C (positive blood culture) is incorrect. A positive blood culture occurs in infective endocarditis. ARF is an immune destruction of valves due to cross-reacting antibodies.
   D (positive serum antinuclear antibody test) is incorrect. In ARF, antibodies are not directed against nuclear antigens.
   E (positive serum double-stranded DNA antibody test) is incorrect. In ARF, antibodies are not directed against nuclear antigens.

2. **L** (c-antineutrophil cytoplasmic antibody) is correct. Wegener's granulomatosis is characterized by necrotizing vasculitis (small vessels and small muscular arteries) and necrotizing granulomas involving the upper airways (i.e., sinuses, nasal cavity, trachea), lungs (pulmonary artery vasculitis and granulomas), and kidneys (glomerulonephritis with RBC casts, see Chapter 4). In over 90% of cases, c-antineutrophil cytoplasmic antibodies are present that contribute to the inflammatory reaction. The antibodies are directed against proteinase 3 in the cytoplasm of neutrophils.

3. **C** (anticentromere antibody) is correct. The patient has limited sclerosis or CREST syndrome: C, calcinosis and centromere antibodies; R, Raynaud's phenomenon (color changes produced by digital vasculitis/fibrosis); E, esophageal dysmotility (dysphagia for solids and liquids); S, sclerodactyly (tapered fingers); and T, telangiectasia (dilated vessels). The end stage of the vasculitis is fibrosis of the digital vessels and gangrene of the digits. Anticentromere antibodies are present in 90% of cases.

4. **M** (p-antineutrophil cytoplasmic antibody) is correct. The patient has microscopic polyangiitis (polyarteritis), which is a disorder that involves small vessels. Damage to small vessels produces acute inflammation and palpable purpura when the blood vessels rupture. It is associated with a nephritic type of glomerulonephritis (proteinuria and RBC casts) and antibodies directed against myeloperoxidase in the cytoplasm of neutrophils.

5. **F** (antiparietal cell) is correct. The patient has pernicious anemia an autoimmune disease with destruction of parietal cells leading to loss of intrinsic factor and the ability to reabsorb vitamin B_{12} in the terminal ileum. This produces a delay in nuclear maturation resulting in large, immature nuclei in erythroid, myeloid, and megakaryocytic cells producing a macrocytic anemia and pancytopenia.

6. **G** (antimitochondrial antibody) is correct. The patient has primary biliary cirrhosis in which there is autoimmune destruction of bile ducts within the portal triads leading to cirrhosis and intrahepatic cholestasis. Bile salts deposit in skin causing itching. Jaundice is a late finding. The obstructive liver enzymes alkaline phosphatase and γ-glutamyl transferase are markedly increased. Antimitochondrial antibodies are present in 90% to 100% of cases.

7. **I** (anti-Smith antibody) and **J** (anti-SS-A [Ro] antibody) are correct. The patient has systemic lupus erythematosus. The speckled immunofluorescence pattern is due to antibodies against non-DNA nuclear constituents. Anti-Sm has a sensitivity of only 20% to 30%; however, the specificity is 100%. Anti-SS-A (Ro) antibodies are present in 30% to 50% of cases. Anti-ds DNA antibodies (choice D) are also commonly increased in SLE; however, these produce a rim pattern and are associated with renal disease.

8. **E** (antigliadin antibody) is correct. The patient has celiac disease in which antibodies develop against the gliadin fraction in gluten in wheat products. There is autoimmune destruction of the small intestine villi leading to malabsorption of fat, protein, and carbohydrates. The vesicular lesion is dermatitis herpetiformis, which is an autoimmune disease of skin that has a very high association with celiac disease. Antigliadin antibodies (IgA) are present in 97% of cases. In addition, antiendomysial and reticulin antibodies are also increased.

9. **A** (anti-acetylcholine receptor antibody) is correct. The patient has myasthenia gravis. Autoantibodies are directed against the acetylcholine receptor, which is a type II hypersensitivity reaction. Muscle weakness is reversed by giving the patient acetylcholinesterase inhibitors, which is the basis of the Tensilon test.

10. **B** (anti–basement membrane antibody) is correct. The patient has Goodpasture's syndrome, in which antibodies are directed against collagen in the basement membrane of pulmonary capillaries and glomeruli, the former producing hemoptysis and the latter glomerulonephritis. It is a type II hypersensitivity reaction.

11. **J** (anti-SS-A [Ro] antibody) is correct. The patient has Sjögren's syndrome, in which there is autoimmune destruction of the lacrimal glands (dry eyes) and salivary glands (dry mouth). Anti SS-A and SS-B antibodies are present in 70% to 95% and 60% to 90% of cases, respectively.

12. **K** (anti-topoisomerase) is correct. The patient has systemic sclerosis, where there is a vasculitis of digital vessels and excess deposition of collagen in subcutaneous tissue. Interstitial fibrosis in the lungs (restrictive lung disease) and renal disease are common. Anti-topoisomerase antibodies are present in 20–40% of cases.

13. **A** (C1 esterase inhibitor assay) is correct. The patient most likely has hereditary angioedema caused by a deficiency of C1 esterase inhibitor. The resultant continued activation of C1 decreases the concentration of C2 and C4 in the classical pathway and increases the concentration of their cleavage products (C2a and C4a), both of which have anaphylatoxic activity. Anaphylatoxins directly stimulate the release of histamine from mast cells, leading to increased vascular permeability and swelling of the face and larynx. Factor B is present in the alternative complement pathway, which explains why it is normal. There is no activation of C3 in hereditary angioedema.

    B (chromosome study) is incorrect. Chromosome studies are usually ordered when a genetic disorder involving chromosome number (e.g., Down syndrome) or structure (e.g., translocation) is suspected. It would be normal in hereditary angioedema.

    C (cutaneous skin testing to rule out anergy) is incorrect. Cutaneous skin testing to rule out anergy is ordered when a defect in cellular immunity is suspected (e.g., T-cell deficiency in DiGeorge syndrome). Injection of *Candida* into the skin does not produce an inflammatory reaction when T cells are deficient. These studies would be normal in hereditary angioedema.

D (quantitative immunoglobulin assay for IgG, IgA, and IgM) is incorrect. Total immunoglobulins are ordered when B-cell immunodeficiency is suspected (e.g., Bruton's agammaglobulinemia). It would be normal in hereditary angioedema.

E (serum antinuclear antibody test) is incorrect. A serum antinuclear antibody test is ordered when autoimmune disease is suspected (e.g., systemic lupus erythematosus). It would be normal in hereditary angioedema.

14. **B** (Bruton's agammaglobulinemia) is correct. It is an X-linked recessive disorder in which a mutation in tyrosine kinase causes failure of pre-B cells to become mature B cells. Patients have recurrent sinopulmonary infections and an increased incidence of *Streptococcus pneumoniae* infections. All immunoglobulins (Igs) are decreased and there is a flat γ-globulin peak in a serum protein electrophoresis.

15. **C** (common variable immunodeficiency, CVID) is correct. CVID has no consistent inheritance pattern. It is the most common immunodeficiency in adults. It is characterized by recurrent sinopulmonary infections, malabsorption (celiac sprue), and an increased risk for autoimmune disease, non-Hodgkin's lymphoma, and giardiasis. All Igs are decreased.

16. **E** (selective IgA immunodeficiency) is correct. It is the most common hereditary immunodeficiency and is characterized by failure of IgA B cells to mature into plasma cells leading to decreased serum IgA and secretory IgA.

17. **F** (severe combined immunodeficiency) is correct. It is an autosomal recessive disease. In most cases, there is a deficiency of adenine deaminase leading to an accumulation of adenine in B and T cells resulting in death of the cells. All Igs are decreased and there is defective cell-mediated immunity (CMI).

18. **D** (DiGeorge's syndrome) is correct. In this immunodeficiency, there is failure of development of the third and fourth pharyngeal pouches. This leads to a pure T-cell immunodeficiency and hypoparathyroidism, the latter producing hypocalcemia and tetany. Cyanotic congenital heart disease due to a truncus arteriosus (common aorta and pulmonary artery) occurs in some cases.

19. **G** (Wiskott-Aldrich syndrome) is correct. It is an X-linked recessive disorder with progressive deletion of T cells. The classic triad is eczema, thrombocytopenia, and recurrent sinopulmonary infections. There is an increased risk for malignant lymphoma and leukemia. Immunoglobulins show a decreased IgM, normal IgG, and increased IgA and IgE. Defective CMI occurs late in the disease.

20. **A** (ataxia telangiectasia) is correct. It is an autosomal recessive disorder with a mutation in DNA repair enzymes leading to increased susceptibility for chromosomal mutations. In addition to the findings listed in the question patients have thymic hypoplasia and an increased risk for lymphomas/leukemias. Immunoglobulins show decreased IgA, IgE, and IgG, and there are defects in CMI. Serum α-fetoprotein is increased.

21. **A** (hypergammaglobulinemia) is correct. Acquired immune deficiency syndrome (AIDS) is the most common acquired immunodeficiency in the United States. It is caused by human immunodeficiency virus-1 (HIV-1), which is an RNA retrovirus containing reverse transcriptase. The virus infects and is cytolytic to CD4 T_H cells. Epstein-Barr virus (EBV) and cytomegalovirus infections are common in AIDS. They are potent polyclonal stimulators of B cells, which produce a polyclonal gammapathy (benign increase in γ-globulins); however, because patients are unable to mount an antibody response to a new antigen, they are still susceptible to bacterial infections.

B (increase in CD4 helper T cell/CD8 suppressor T cell ratio) is incorrect. The virus attacks and destroys CD4 helper T cells. This decreases the CD4 helper T-cell count (less than 200 cells/mm^3) and reverses the CD4 helper T cell/CD$_8$ suppressor T cell ratio from a normal of 2 to less than 1.
C (intact cellular immunity) is incorrect. The virus attacks and destroys CD4 helper T cells, thus impairing cell-mediated immunity (type IV hypersensitivity).
D (normal phytohemagglutinin assay) is incorrect. The virus attacks and destroys CD4 helper T cells, thus impairing cell-mediated immunity (type IV hypersensitivity). Therefore, in vitro stimulation of T-cell response to phytohemagglutinin, a potent T-cell mitogen, is impaired (not normal).
E (normal skin reaction to intradermal injections of *Candida*) is incorrect. Cellular immunity is impaired in AIDS. Therefore, intradermal injections of *Candida* does not elicit the expected T-cell immune response. This lack of immune response is called anergy. Defective cellular immunity is responsible for *Pneumocystis jiroveci* lung infection, which is the most common initial presentation in AIDS, and other opportunistic infections.

22. **D** (Western blot assay) is correct. This assay is the confirmatory test if the ELISA test is positive or indeterminate. The ELISA assay detects anti-gp120 antibodies. A positive Western blot assay requires the presence of p24 and gp41 antibodies and either gp120 or gp160 antibodies. The test has close to 100% specificity.

A (CD4 T cell count) is incorrect. This test is used to monitor the immune status of the patient. It is useful in determining when to initiate HIV treatment and when to administer prophylaxis against opportunistic infections.

B (HIV viral load) is incorrect. This test is used to detect actively dividing virus and is also used as a marker of disease progression. It is the most sensitive test for diagnosis of acute HIV before seroconversion.

C (p24 capture assay) is incorrect. The p24 antigen is an indicator of active viral replication. It is present before anti-gp120 antibodies are developed in the patient. It is positive at two different times in HIV infections: prior to seroconversion and when AIDS is diagnosed.

Common Laboratory Values

Test	Conventional Units	SI Units
Blood, Plasma, Serum		
Alanine aminotransferase (ALT, GPT at 30°C)	8–20 U/L	8–20 U/L
Amylase, serum	25–125 U/L	25–125 U/L
Aspartate aminotransferase (AST, GOT at 30°C)	8–20 U/L	8–20 U/L
Bilirubin, serum (adult): total; direct	0.1–1.0 mg/dL; 0.0–0.3 mg/dL	2–17 μmol/L; 0–5 μmol/L
Calcium, serum (Ca^{2+})	8.4–10.2 mg/dL	2.1–2.8 mmol/L
Cholesterol, serum	Rec: <200 mg/dL	<5.2 mmol/L
Cortisol, serum	8:00 AM: 6–23 μg/dL; 4:00 PM: 3–15 μg/dL	170–630 nmol/L; 80–410 nmol/L
	8:00 PM: ≤50% of 8:00 AM	Fraction of 8:00 AM: ≤0.50
Creatine kinase, serum	Male: 25–90 U/L	25–90 U/L
	Female: 10–70 U/L	10–70 U/L
Creatinine, serum	0.6–1.2 mg/dL	53–106 μmol/L
Electrolytes, serum		
Sodium (Na^+)	136–145 mEq/L	135–145 mmol/L
Chloride (Cl^-)	95–105 mEq/L	95–105 mmol/L
Potassium (K^+)	3.5–5.0 mEq/L	3.5–5.0 mmol/L
Bicarbonate (HCO_3^-)	22–28 mEq/L	22–28 mmol/L
Magnesium (Mg^{2+})	1.5–2.0 mEq/L	1.5–2.0 mmol/L
Estriol, total, serum (in pregnancy)		
24–28 wk; 32–36 wk	30–170 ng/mL; 60–280 ng/mL	104–590 nmol/L; 208–970 nmol/L
28–32 wk; 36–40 wk	40–220 ng/mL; 80–350 ng/mL	140–760 nmol/L; 280–1210 nmol/L
Ferritin, serum	Male: 15–200 ng/mL	15–200 μg/L
	Female: 12–150 ng/mL	12–150 μg/L
Follicle-stimulating hormone, serum/plasma (FSH)	Male: 4–25 mIU/mL	4–25 U/L
	Female:	
	Premenopause, 4–30 mIU/mL	4–30 U/L
	Midcycle peak, 10–90 mIU/mL	10–90 U/L
	Postmenopause, 40–250 mIU/mL	40–250 U/L
Gases, arterial blood (room air)		
pH	7.35–7.45	[H^+] 36–44 nmol/L
PCO_2	33–45 mm Hg	4.4–5.9 kPa
PO_2	75–105 mm Hg	10.0–14.0 kPa
Glucose, serum	Fasting: 70–110 mg/dL	3.8–6.1 mmol/L
	2 hr postprandial: <120 mg/dL	<6.6 mmol/L
Growth hormone–arginine stimulation	Fasting: <5 ng/mL	<5 μg/L
	Provocative stimuli: >7 ng/mL	>7 μg/L

continued

Test	Conventional Units	SI Units
Blood, Plasma, Serum—cont'd		
Immunoglobulins, serum		
IgA	76–390 mg/dL	0.76–3.90 g/L
IgE	0–380 IU/mL	0–380 kIU/L
IgG	650–1500 mg/dL	6.5–15 g/L
IgM	40–345 mg/dL	0.4–3.45 g/L
Iron	50–170 μg/dL	9–30 μmol/L
Lactate dehydrogenase, serum	45–90 U/L	45–90 U/L
Luteinizing hormone, serum/ plasma (LH)	Male: 6–23 mIU/mL	6–23 U/L
	Female:	
	Follicular phase, 5–30 mIU/mL	5–30 U/L
	Midcycle, 75–150 mIU/mL	75–150 U/L
	Postmenopause, 30–200 mIU/mL	30–200 U/L
Osmolality, serum	275–295 mOsm/kg	275–295 mOsm/kg
Parathyroid hormone, serum, N-terminal	230–630 pg/mL	230–630 ng/L
Phosphatase (alkaline), serum (p-NPP at 30°C)	20–70 U/L	20–70 U/L
Phosphorus (inorganic), serum	3.0–4.5 mg/dL	1.0–1.5 mmol/L
Prolactin, serum (hPRL)	<20 ng/mL	<20 μg/L
Proteins, serum		
Total (recumbent)	6.0–8.0 g/dL	60–80 g/L
Albumin	3.5–5.5 g/dL	35–55 g/L
Globulin	2.3–3.5 g/dL	23–35 g/L
Thyroid-stimulating hormone, serum or plasma (TSH)	0.5–5.0 μU/mL	0.5–5.0 mU/L
Thyroidal iodine (^{123}I) uptake	8–30% of administered dose/24 hr	0.08–0.30/24 hr
Thyroxine (T_4), serum	4.5–12 μg/dL	58–154 nmol/L
Triglycerides, serum	35–160 mg/dL	0.4–1.81 mmol/L
Triiodothyronine (T_3), serum (RIA)	115–190 ng/dL	1.8–2.9 nmol/L
Triiodothyronine (T_3) resin uptake	25–38%	0.25–0.38
Urea nitrogen, serum (BUN)	7–18 mg/dL	1.2–3.0 mmol urea/L
Uric acid, serum	3.0–8.2 mg/dL	0.18–0.48 mmol/L
Cerebrospinal Fluid		
Cell count	0–5 cells/mm^3	$0–5 \times 10^6$/L
Chloride	118–132 mEq/L	118–132 mmol/L
Gamma globulin	3–12% total proteins	0.03–0.12
Glucose	50–75 mg/dL	2.8–4.2 mmol/L
Pressure	70–180 mm H_2O	70–180 mm H_2O
Proteins, total	<40 mg/dL	<0.40 g/L
Hematology		
Bleeding time (template)	2–7 min	2–7 min
Erythrocyte count	Male: 4.3–5.9 million/mm^3	$4.3–5.9 \times 10^{12}$/L
	Female: 3.5–5.5 million/mm^3	$3.5–5.5 \times 10^{12}$/L
Erythrocyte sedimentation rate (Westergren)	Male: 0–15 mm/hr	0–15 mm/hr
	Female: 0–20 mm/hr	0–20 mm/hr
Hematocrit (Hct)	Male: 40–54%	0.40–0.54
	Female: 37–47%	0.37–0.47

Test	Conventional Units	SI Units
Hematology—cont'd		
Hemoglobin A$_{IC}$	≤6%	≤ 0.06%
Hemoglobin, blood (Hb)	Male: 13.5–17.5 g/dL	2.09–2.71 mmol/L
	Female: 12.0–16.0 g/dL	1.86–2.48 mmol/L
Hemoglobin, plasma	1–4 mg/dL	0.16–0.62 mmol/L
Leukocyte count and differential		
Leukocyte count	4500–11,000/mm^3	4.5–11.0 × 10^9/L
Segmented neutrophils	54–62%	0.54–0.62
Bands	3–5%	0.03–0.05
Eosinophils	1–3%	0.01–0.03
Basophils	0–0.75%	0–0.0075
Lymphocytes	25–33%	0.25–0.33
Monocytes	3–7%	0.03–0.07
Mean corpuscular hemoglobin (MCH)	25.4–34.6 pg/cell	0.39–0.54 fmol/cell
Mean corpuscular hemoglobin concentration (MCHC)	31–37% Hb/cell	4.81–5.74 mmol Hb/L
Mean corpuscular volume (MCV)	80–100 μm^3	80–100 fl
Partial thromboplastin time (activated) (aPTT)	25–40 sec	25–40 sec
Platelet count	150,000–400,000/mm^3	150–400 × 10^9/L
Prothrombin time (PT)	12–14 sec	12–14 sec
Reticulocyte count	0.5–1.5% of red cells	0.005–0.015
Thrombin time	<2 sec deviation from control	<2 sec deviation from control
Volume		
Plasma	Male: 25–43 mL/kg	0.025–0.043 L/kg
	Female: 28–45 mL/kg	0.028–0.045 L/kg
Red cell	Male: 20–36 mL/kg	0.020–0.036 L/kg
	Female: 19–31 mL/kg	0.019–0.031 L/kg
Sweat		
Chloride	0–35 mmol/L	0–35 mmol/L
Urine		
Calcium	100–300 mg/24 hr	2.5–7.5 mmol/24 hr
Creatinine clearance	Male: 97–137 mL/min	
	Female: 88–128 mL/min	
Estriol, total (in pregnancy)		
30 wk	6–18 mg/24 hr	21–62 μmol/24 hr
35 wk	9–28 mg/24 hr	31–97 μmol/24 hr
40 wk	13–42 mg/24 hr	45–146 μmol/24 hr
17-Hydroxycorticosteroids	Male: 3.0–9.0 mg/24 hr	8.2–25.0 μmol/24 hr
	Female: 2.0–8.0 mg/24 hr	5.5–22.0 μmol/24 hr
17-Ketosteroids, total	Male: 8–22 mg/24 hr	28–76 μmol/24 hr
	Female: 6–15 mg/24 hr	21–52 μmol/24 hr
Osmolality	50–1400 mOsm/kg	
Oxalate	8–40 μg/mL	90–445 μmol/L
Proteins, total	<150 mg/24 hr	<0.15 g/24 hr

Index

Note: Page numbers followed by f indicate figures; those followed by t indicate tables.